Aromatherapy For Holistic Therapists
by
Colin Paddon Ph.D., D.Ac., D.N.M.

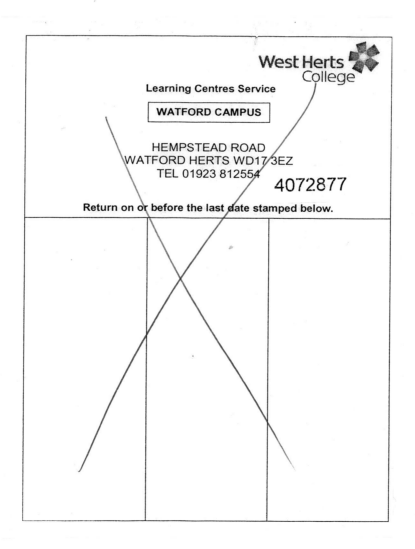

Aromatherapy For Holistic Therapists
by
Colin Paddon Ph.D., D.Ac., D.N.M.

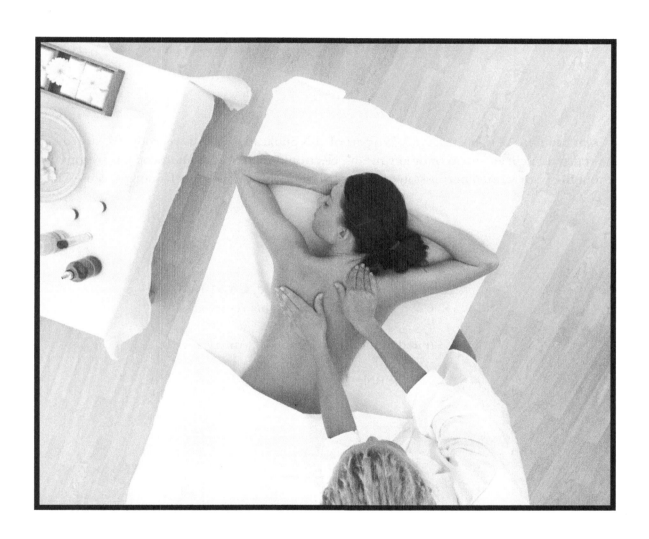

Airmid Holistic Books, Los Angeles

Airmid Holistic Books, Sunland, CA 91040
© Colin Paddon 2008. All rights reserved.
Published 2008.
Printed in the United States of America

ISBN 978-0-9820318-0-3

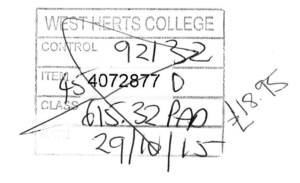

CONTENTS

AROMATHERAPY 101
FOR HOLISTIC PRACTITIONERS

To all practitioners in the healing field of Holistic health care and allopathic professionals, it often takes courage to embark in a new modality and dare to extend your knowledge in a new direction. During this program you will doubt yourself many times, become confused often and even entertain the thoughts of terminating your studies at some point in your program. Don't.

Certain actions will bring happiness and just around the corner is success and...
 if you care enough to heal you will care enough to study how to increase your ability to make a difference in this world one patient at a time.

Medical professionals throughout the world are using Holistic Medicine to enhance their practice, improve their income and become known as a true healer. Welcome to a new thought, called "intent".

Professor Anton Jayasuriya once said,

"if you cannot be a King, be a healer"

About the author - Colin T. Paddon Ph.D., D.Ac., F.I.A.M.A.

Colin is a world-renowned healer and teacher of Acupuncture, Aromatherapy, Reflexology, Cranial Sacral, Lymph drainage, Dark field microscopy, Biological terrain testing and Advanced Quantum medicine. Colin is also spiritually connected to the universe as a Christian and Spiritual Healer in Canada since 1991.

Acknowledgments
- Michelle Annes who guided my first steps in Canada and helped me become who I am today.
- Michael Coyle (deceased) who became my mentor and friend and guided me through Darkfield Microscopy and Biological Terrain.
- Dr Thomas Rau who took me to a new level in Biological Medicine.
- Dr. Anton Jayasuriya for teaching me about Acupuncture and Homeopathy.
- To Shirley and Len Price who took me gently through my learning years as an Aromatherapist
- Dr. Bill Nelson who led me into the Biofeedback world of Quantum Medicine.
- Dr. Mathias Nauts who guided my hands and led me in those early years when I was new to Canada and without whom I would not be the healer I am today.
- For my son Daniel who believed in me and still does.
- For all my students and friends who helped me on this journey we call life

Colin is affiliated with:
- Officially recognised by the World Health Organisation and accredited to the Open International University for Complementary Medicines.
- Indian Board of Alternative medicines in Calcutta, India.
- Open International University for Complementary Medicines.
- The American Naturopathic Medical Certification & Accreditation Board.
- The American Alternative Medical Association Commission on Accreditation The American Association of Drugless Practitioners Commission.
- The Canadian Council of Certified Acupuncturists
- The Canadian Examining Board of Health Care Practitioners
- The Hong Kong Association of Quantum Medicine
- NuLife Sciences, Petaluma, California. USA.
- The Canadian School of Natural Health Sciences
- Bioscience Research Institution.

Colin has designed courses and delivered teaching modules for:
- Mohawk College in Hamilton, Ontario, as part of a Health Sciences Degree
- Canadore College in North Bay, Ontario, as part of a Post Graduate Health Sciences Diploma Fanshawe College in London, Ontario, as a Diploma Course
- Algonquin College in Ottawa, Ontario, as a Diploma Course
- Homewood Health Psychiatric Hospital, as a Psycho-Aromatherapy Course

How to use this study course in three steps...

1. First, read the book from cover to cover.
2. Refer to the questions and attempt to answer them from memory. Then reread the chapter and paragraph on that subject to either validate the answer or to seek out the answer that you did not know.
3. Using the answer sheets, insert the correct answer and return these sheets to your instructor.

Certificate of completion

Should you require a certificate of Completion then scan your answer pages and email them to aroma-therapy101@airmidbooks.com along with your full name and return address. We will send you a request via PayPal for an administrative charge (email us first to request current charge) to cover costs, and will send you your score and cerificate on receipt of this fee.

LESSON ONE

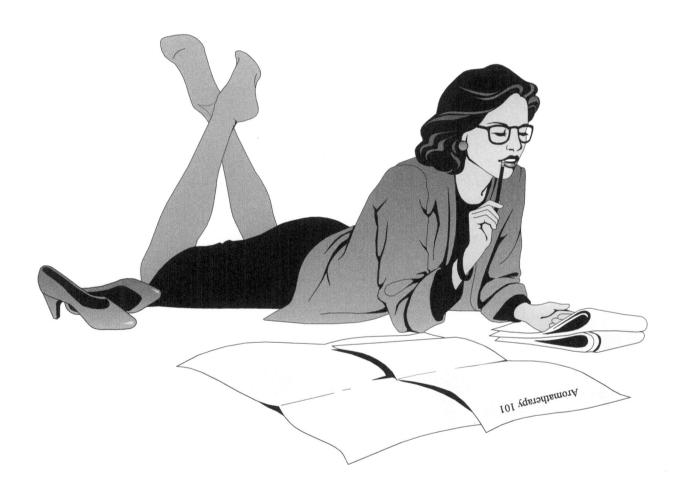

Lesson #1

Table of Contents

Introduction to the History of Aromatherapy

In **Lascaux** *(pronounced, "La-Soo")* in the Dordoigne area in France, there are references on the cave walls in the form of paintings that suggest the medicinal use of plants. These paintings are recorded by carbon-dating samples that belong to an era according to many authorities that date back as far as **18000 B.C.**.

In **3000 B.C.** in China the *Yellow Emperor, Huang Ti,* included herbal medicine in his book on disease called *"The Yellow Emperor's Classic of Internal Medicine."*

In **4500 B.C.** Egyptians used balsams, perfumed oils, scented barks, and resins, spices and aromatic vinegars. Perfumery at that time was firmly linked to religion. Each deity had their own special fragrance, and statues would be covered with scented oils. The Pharaohs had a perfume for war, one for meditation, one for love, and so on. They set great importance on perfume for both public and private use. On important state occasions, incense would be burned, and slaves danced with cones of perfume on their heads. These cones would melt and gradually disperse the scent into the air as they performed, the reason behind this practice was to enhance her attraction and so increase the slaves value.

Translations of hieroglyphics found in the temple of Edfu south of the Valley of Kings in Egypt, indicate that aromatic substances were formulated by the priests to make perfumes and medicines. Papyrus manuscripts during the reign of Khufu about 2800 BC, record the use of many medicinal herbs and aromatic essences. We know from these Egyptian papyrus documents about some of the plants they used medicinally, as well as the other methods of use. They made pills, powders, suppositories, medicinal cakes and purees, ointment and pastes for external use from a wide variety of plants and trees. They also utilized the plant ashes and smoke. Some of the plants used included *aniseed, cedar, onion, garlic, cumin, coriander, caster oil, grapes and watermelons.* The Egyptians were in fact , experts in cosmetology and famous for their herbal preparations and ointments. Possibly the most famous of these old preparations is known as *"Kyphi"*, which is a mixture of sixteen different ingredients. Kyphi is used as an incense, a perfume and even as a medicine because of its antiseptic properties; it is balsamic, soothing and an antidote to poison.

Their embalming knowledge was considerable. The priests of that time predicted that the embalmed bodies of the deceased Pharaohs would last 3,000 years. They embalmed their Pharaohs in essential oils to kill and inhibit bacteria, thus limiting decomposition. This has proved to be true; as bandages from mummies have been found to contain traces of *galbanum resin, cedar, myrrh and spices such as clove, cinnamon and nutmeg.*

Strangely, for a civilization that was so technologically advanced, there is no written evidence that the Egyptians knew how to distill essential oils. They prepared aromatic oils and incense by soaking plant materials in base oils or fats, but recent findings indicate that there are records that show that they did in fact import large quantities of essential oils such as *cedar and cypress.*

Note: *Although most books on aromatherapy claim that the Egyptians did not distill their own oils, Shirley Price's book "Aromatherapy Workbook" outlines the first crude beginnings of Egyptian distillation of cedarwood. Cedarwood fragments were placed into a clay pot beneath a layer of wool, this clay pot was then heated by fire. As the temperature rose, the essential oils contained within the fragments would begin to evaporate, and the wool cover would catch the evaporating cedarwood oil as it was released from the wood. When this procedure had run its course, the wool would be squeezed to release the water and essential aromatic oil trapped in the wool, because essential oil is lighter than water, the separation is simple.*

Natural aromatic herbs and essential oils constituted one of the earliest trade items of the ancient world. As mentioned in the Bible, the Jews began their exodus from Egypt to Israel around 1240 BC. They took with them not only the herbs but also the knowledge of how to use them. In the book of Exodus, the Lord gave Moses the formula for a special oil for anointing the priesthood. **Myrrh, cinnamon, calamus, cassia and olive oil** were among the ingredients. This **Holy Oil** was used to consecrate Aaron and his sons into the priesthood. This tradition continued for many generations. Frankincense and myrrh were two aromatic oils given as gifts to the baby Jesus at his birth; possibly because it was valuable not only as currency, but also because the aroma of this perfume was very popular in those days as well as its therapeutic properties.

Around the same time (3000 years ago) as the Egyptians were using essential oils, another traditional medicine called *"Ayur Veda"* from India was also **incorporating essential oils into their healing potions.** A principal feature of Ayurvedic medicine is aromatic massage using infused oils made from indigenous herbs and woods. The word Ayur, means *"life",* and Veda means *"Knowledge",* so the whole word Ayur-Veda means *"Knowledge of life".* Ayur-Veda combines holistic assessment and diagnosis with diet, exercise and herb/mineral medication.

The knowledge of the Egyptians was acquired and catalogued by the **Greeks** between **500** and **400 BC.** They continued making further discoveries of their own, such as the fact that the odour of certain flowers was stimulating and refreshing, while that of others was relaxing and soporific. **Greek soldiers carried into battle an ointment** made from *myrrh* for the treatment of wounds. One of the most famous Greek preparations, made from myrrh, cinnamon and cassia, was called *"Megaleion"* after its creator Megallus. It had the dual purpose of being a perfume and medication for healing wounds and reducing inflammation.

Hippocrates, (*pronounced; Hip-poc cra-tees*) born in Greece around 460 BC described the effects of 300 plants and their uses, and wrote a treatise on herbal medicine, placing more importance on the moral qualities needed to be a doctor, such as discernment and devotion.

To this day Hippocrates is still revered as the *" Father of Medicine ", and the "Hippocratic Oath"* continues to be taught to medical students today.

Many Greek doctors were employed by Rome as military surgeons. One of these Greek surgeons was **Galen.** Born in Pergamon in Asia Minor around 131-199 AD., Galen reworked many of the old Hippocratic ideas, and formalized his theories in medical texts used extensively by the Romans and medieval Arab physicians. He became the physician to **the Roman Emperor Marcus Aurelius** and served as a surgeon to a school of gladiators. **It was recorded that no gladiator died of his wounds during Galen's term of office**. Perhaps this is not surprising, since he was familiar with and used several *essential oils* from which he prepared his remedies. He wrote a great deal on the theory of plant medicine and divided plants into various medicinal categories, which are still known as *"Galenic"*. He also invented the original *"Cold Cream"*, which was the prototype of virtually all ointments in current use.

The healing knowledge used so extensively by the Egyptians and Greeks greatly influenced the Romans. One of these Roman doctors was the Greek **Dioscorides,** *(pronounced; di-o-scor-ides)*. Having made a detailed study of the application of plants and aromatics, he compiled an account of his works and wrote in **50 AD.** five-huge volumes called *"De Materia Medica"* also known as the *Herbarius*. This remained the standard text for 1,500 years, in which he gave a detailed account of the healing properties of many herbs. This was later translated into Persian, Hebrew, Anglo-Saxon and many other languages.

980-1037 AD. Ali-Ibn Sina, known to us as **Avicenna** (pronounced; Av-vi-seen-na) the Arab, wrote books on the properties of over 800 plants and their effects on the human body. However, his greatest achievement as far as the history of aromatherapy is concerned, is that he is credited with having discovered the method of distilling essential oils. Whether or not Avicenna himself invented or discovered the process of distillation is not certain, but Arabic manuscript from his lifetime contained drawings of stills whose basic principles of operation have not changed, even if the method of construction may be more sophisticated. By this time, the Arabs were famous for their perfumes and medications.

Knowledge of herbal medicine gained during the **Crusades** in the Middle East and Islands of the Mediterranean was disseminated throughout Western Europe by the Knights and their armies. Not only did they bring back the actual perfumes, but also many of the plants and the knowledge of how to distill them. Lacking the Aromatic (fragrant smell) gum yielding trees of the Mediterranean, the Europeans substituted *lavender, rosemary, and thyme*. Eventually many of the aromatic shrubs that were native to the Mediterranean, were cultivated much further north.

During the **Bubonic Plague** in the *17th century, frankincense and pine* were burned in the streets. Indoors, incense, perfumed gums and resins were worn around the neck. During the Black Death era, aromatics were the best antiseptics available. Exactly how effective these measures were, can only be surmised. History reported that those in closest contact with aromatics especially the perfumers, were virtually immune. Since all **aromatics are antiseptic** it is likely that some of those used were indeed effective protection against the plague.

Until the 19th century, medical practitioners carried a small *cassoulet filled with aromatics on top of their walking sticks.* This acted as a personal antiseptic, and would be held up to the nose when visiting any contagious patients.

In the Middle Ages, many herbal books were written in Latin. In his **16th century** writings **William Turner, The Father of Botany** was the first to describe herbs and their medicinal properties in English and thus helping to popularize herbal medicine. His motive in doing this was to assist the apothecaries and common folk that gathered herbs to help them understand which plants physicians wrote about in prescriptions. This action earned both himself and Nicholas Culpepper the wrath of the newly formed College of Physicians, because it allowed ordinary people to find herbal medicines in the hedgerows and fields instead of paying vastly inflated apothecaries' bills.

In 1653 **Nicholas Culpepper** wrote his book *"Complete Herbal"* . In the 18th century, essential oils were used widely in medicines. Salmon's dispensary of 1896 contains many aromatic remedies. The 19th century found that many essential oils could be produced synthetically. This was a much cheaper and easier process than using natural plants.

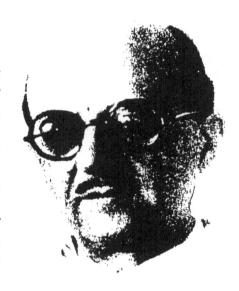

"Rene-Maurice Gattefosse" A French chemist working in his family's perfumer business, coined the term *"Aromatherapy"* in his book entitled **"Aromatherapie"**which was published in 1928. During this time he was investigating the **antiseptic properties** of essential oils. He also re-discovered the healing properties of lavender. **Two things happened** which helped to extend this interest in aromatic essential oils. **Firstly,** cosmetics often contained antiseptics and he discovered that essential oils had greater antiseptic properties than some of the antiseptic chemicals of the time. **Secondly**, one of Gattefosse's hands was badly burned when a small explosion occurred in his laboratory during an experiment. He instantly immersed it in neat **essential oil of lavender**, and was only partly surprised when he found that the burn healed at a phenomenal rate, with no sign of infection, and leaving no scar.

He also found that many essential oils when used in their entirety were more effective than using a synthetic substitutes or their isolated active ingredients. For instance, the active ingredient in eucalyptus is called *"eucalyptol" or "cineol"*. The antiseptic properties are more active when used as a whole plant in its natural form and react stronger than when separated or isolated.

Dr. Jean Valnet incorporated essential oils into his healing programme in both medical disorders and psychiatric problems. He utilized what he had learned from Rene-Maurice Gattefosse's work to treat wounded soldiers in world war two. Thanks largely to Dr. Valnet's teachings to other physicians, there are more than 1500 physicians who prescribe essential oil.

1895-1968, Madame Marguerite Maury a French biochemist helped to re-establish the reputation of aromatherapy after the second world war. She studied Dr. Jean Valnet's work and applied his research to her beauty therapy. With this knowledge she hoped to learn how to revitalize her clients by creating personal aromatic blends designed specifically for the subjects gender, temperament and particular health problems. She was probably one of the first to practice in true holistic fashion by harmonizing the physical, psychological and spiritual nature of the patient.

Introduction to Anatomy and Physiology

The following notes are subject matter relating to the amount of knowledge needed to become a therapist. Should you feel that further study would prove beneficial, then by all means feel free to do so. However, the course level of knowledge examination will be taken from material provided.

This course makes no pretence at enveloping the whole subject of anatomy and physiology, but is aimed at giving you the student a basic understanding of related anatomical parts, position and function.

Anatomy is defined as the study of the structure of the body.
Physiology is defined as being the study of the function of those parts.

For example;

▸ *The heart weighs approx. nine ounces, is pear shaped and lies tow-thirds on the left-hand side of the chest area and one third to the right.* **That is the basic anatomy.**

▸ *The heart pumps blood around the body after first oxygenating it via the lungs.* **That is the basic physiology.**

By combining the knowledge of anatomy and physiology, we are able to get a clearer picture of the organ and its relationship to the body, together with its form and composition, and so, improve our understanding of the body as a whole.

For simplicity, the body will be divided into eight main systems. Some text books divide or sub-divide into more or less systems, however, for the purpose of this course we shall look at them as follows.

1.	The Skeletal System:	Bones, structure, support, articulation and mobility.
2.	The Muscular System:	Two types of muscle, voluntary and involuntary muscles and ligaments.
3.	The Vascular System:	Including the lymphatic system, heart and blood vessels.
4.	The Neurological System:	Covers most of the nerves of the body and brain.
5.	The Digestive System:	Including related organs of digestion.
6.	The Respiratory System:	Lungs.
7.	Genito-Urinary System:	Including the reproductive and kidney system.
8.	The Endocrine System:	The glands and their effects on the body.

All professional therapists should have a basic knowledge of medical terminology, which you will need to become familiar with to assist in understanding other professionals. Although we can not teach all the terms in this short course, those which you will use the most will be taught. Understanding this terminology will make subsequent study that much easier.

HISTORICAL

It is difficult to trace the exact study of anatomy and physiology, although the Egyptians with their famous embalming process must have gained a lot of knowledge about the human body as they perfected this art. It is interesting to note that the *"R"* which European doctors write at the top of prescriptions, is in fact the **"R" symbol of the Eye of Horus,** *(the hawk headed sun god),* who lost his eye in battle and had it restored by Thoth, who was adopted as the patron God of physicians. Thoth was one of the many Gods invoked by ancient Egyptian doctors while administering their remedies.

It was with the Greeks that we learned in detail about anatomy and physiology. The first detailed accounts from this era came from **Hippocrites**, often referred to as the **Father of Medicine**.

Aristotle, is accredited as being the founder of comparative anatomy.

From the Roman era, a vast collection of surgical and dissecting instruments have been unearthed, which indicate a considerable understanding of anatomical form and function.

It was in the second century A.D. that **Galen** lived, and his name is still remembered as being one of the greatest physicians and anatomists of antiquity. His work established the foundation of European anatomy as we know it.

From the sixteenth century medical school in Italy, **Paracelsus Von Hohenheim,** graduated to become a progressive medical teacher and did much to alter the accepted ideas of his day.

In 1543, **Vesalius** published his first drawings of the structure of the human body in his book "Fabric of the Human Body", and so paved the way for modern anatomy.

Since those early times many talented doctors have contributed to expand the knowledge of anatomy in the search to uncover and simplify the complex functions of the human body.

William Harvey is linked to the role and function of the heart and the process of oxygenated blood through the lungs.

Malpighi discovered capillary circulation in 1661.

Avenbrugger of Austria discovered *"Percussion"* In the middle of the 18th century.

Rene Laennec invented the stethoscope.

1822 **Dr William Beaumont** contributed much to the understanding of the function of the digestive system.

1867 **Lister** discovered the antiseptic principles.

1877 **Pasteur** demonstrated the role of germs and disease.

1895 **Roentgen** discovered X-ray.

1904 **Baylis and Stanley** identified the first hormone.

1912 **Frederick Gowland Hopkins,** discovered vitamins.

1928 **Alexander Fleming** discovered antibiotics (*penicillin*)

1953 **James Watson** and **Francis Crick** discovered the double helix of DNA
(*Dioxyribonucleicacid*).

Anatomy and physiology are subjects of continuous study and discovery. Each year will bring new discoveries and understanding.

An Introduction to the Skeletal System

PRINCIPAL FUNCTIONS OF THE SKELETAL SYSTEM

The skeletal system provides the framework for the body, to give it **shape, support** and **locomotion.**

The two principal functions of the skeletal system are:

1/ **PROTECTION**   **e.g.**   The skull protects the brain
The rib cage protects the heart and lungs
The spinal column protects the spinal cord

2/ **LOCOMOTION**   **e.g.**   Movement.

CLASSIFICATION OF BONES

THE SKELETON COMPRISES 206 BONES.

Bone is dry, dense tissue.

Bone tissue is composed of

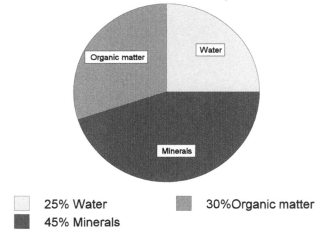

25% Water   30% Organic matter
45% Minerals

The mineral consists mainly of calcium phosphate, and a small amount of magnesium salts. These give the bone its rigidity and hardness.

The organic matter consists of fibrous material which gives the bone its toughness and resilience.

(These figures are approximate and should not be taken as literal facts.)

THERE ARE FIVE CLASSIFICATIONS OF BONES:

1) **Long Bones:** Like the femur.
2) **Short Bones:** Like the metatarsal bones.
3) **Flat Bones:** Like the frontal bone found in the skull.
4) **Irregular Bones:** Like the vertebrae.
5) **Sesamoid Bones:** These are rounded masses found in certain tendons, the best example is the kneecap *(patella)*

In addition to the two principal functions of the skeletal system, the individual bones serve other purposes, such as the attachment for tendons and muscles as well as the formation of red blood cells in the bone marrow.

To provide locomotion or movement the skeleton provides us with a number of joints or articulations.

These fall into four main categories:

1/ **BALL AND SOCKET:** Found in the hip and shoulder.

2/ **PIVOT:** Found in the radius / ulna and the axis joint.

3/ **GLIDING:** Found in the carpal and tarsal joints.

4/ **HINGE:** Found in the knee, and a partial hinge is found in the elbow joint.

Besides the four main joint articulations, there are of course two other types of joint:

SYNARTHROSES These are found in flat bones of the skull and are the fibrous joints that are thought to be fixed with **no movement at all.**

AMPHIARTHROSES These are found in joints like the spine which is a cartilaginous joint with **slight movement**.

An example of this joint is found in the spine, where the discs of fibro-cartilage separate the bones of the spine. These moveable joints are supplied with a secretion called *"synovial Fluid"*. This is a **whitish fluid,** similar in consistency to raw egg white, which acts as a lubricant between the articulating surfaces.

The **mucous bursae** are sacs containing a clear viscous fluid which acts rather like a water cushion between joints. If the **synovial membrane** becomes inflamed, this is known as *"synovitis"* (*"Tennis Elbow"* a well known European terminology). If the bursae becomes inflamed this is known as *"bursitis"*, (a well known example being *"Housemaids Knee")*.

DIAGRAM OF THE SKULL

22 BONES FORM THE SKULL:
For the purpose of this course the principal bones to remember are:

Parietal bone	Temporal bone	Sphenoid bone	Zygomatic Arch
Frontal	Maxilla	Mandible	Occipital
Mental Foramen	Mastoid process	Infra-Orbital Foramen	

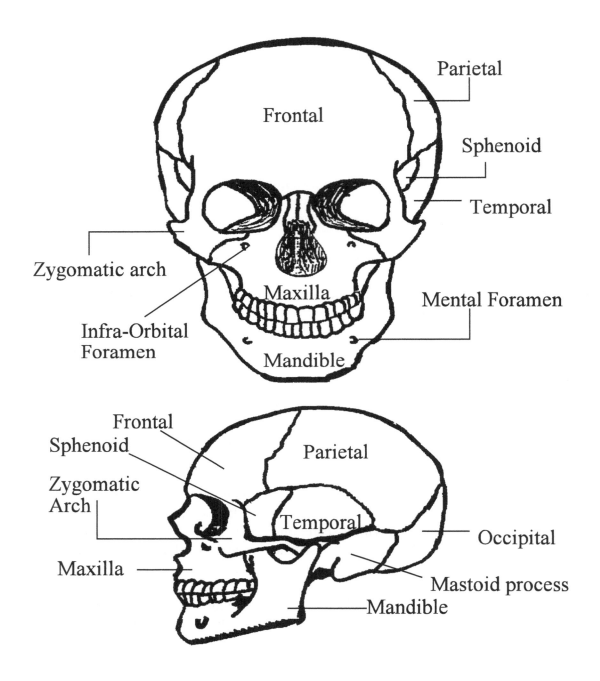

DIAGRAM OF THE VERTEBRAE

33 BONES FORM THE VERTEBRAE:

Cervical vertebrae x 7   Thoracic vertebrae x 12   Lumber vertebrae x 5
Sacrum (fused) x 5   Coccyx (fused) x 4

Separating each vertebrae is a disc of fibro-cartilage. The top two cervical vertebrae are known as the Atlas bone and the Axis bone.

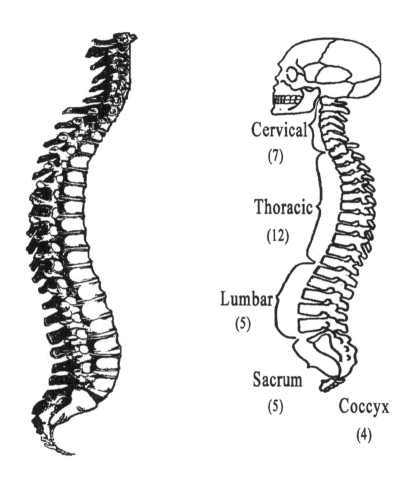

Cervical
(7)

Thoracic
(12)

Lumbar
(5)

Sacrum
(5)

Coccyx
(4)

DIAGRAM OF THE THORAX

25 BONES FORM THE THORAX: (CHEST)

The sternum, ribs x 12, *(7 pairs of true ribs and five pairs of false ribs).*
The last two pair of false ribs are known as *"floating ribs",* because they are attached at the back, but not at the front. (They are not shown on this diagram).

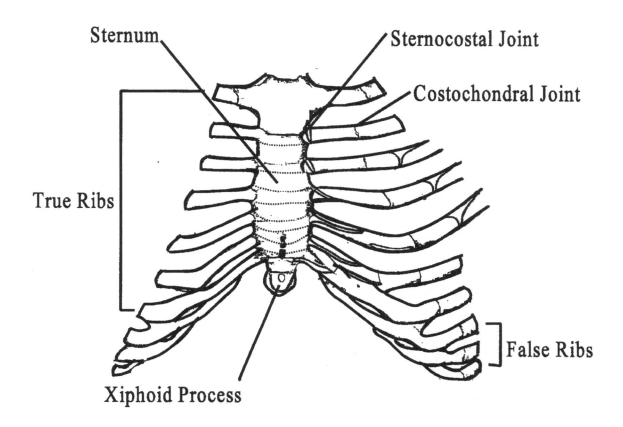

DIAGRAM OF THE UPPER LIMBS

64 BONES FORM THE UPPER LIMBS OF BOTH ARMS, 32 in each arm.
Scapula, Clavicle, Humerus, Radius, Ulna, Carpal bones x 8, Metacarpal bones x 5,
Phalanges x 14

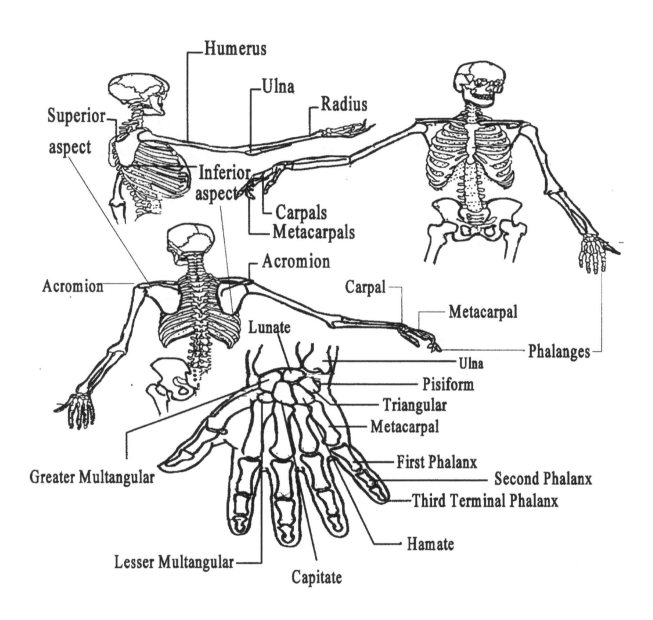

DIAGRAM OF THE PELVIS

4 BONES FORM THE PELVIS.

Right innominate bone, left innominate bone, Sacrum, Coccyx.
Each innominate bone consists of the Ilium and Pubis.

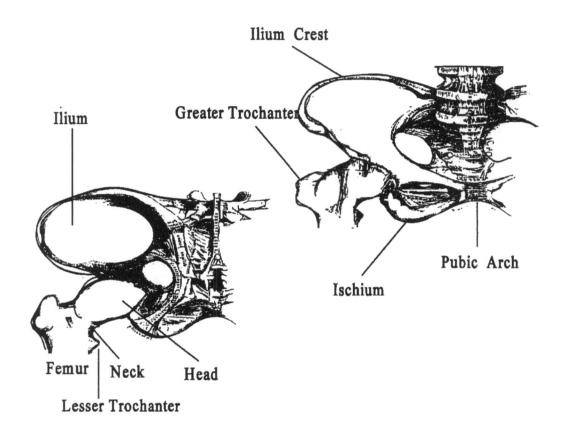

Ilium Crest

Ilium

Greater Trochanter

Pubic Arch

Ischium

Femur   Neck   Head

Lesser Trochanter

DIAGRAM OF THE LOWER LIMBS

60 BONES FORM THE LOWER LIMBS.
30 in each leg.
Femur, Patella, Tibia, Fibula,
Tarsal bones x 7,   Metatarsal bones x 5,   phalanges x 14

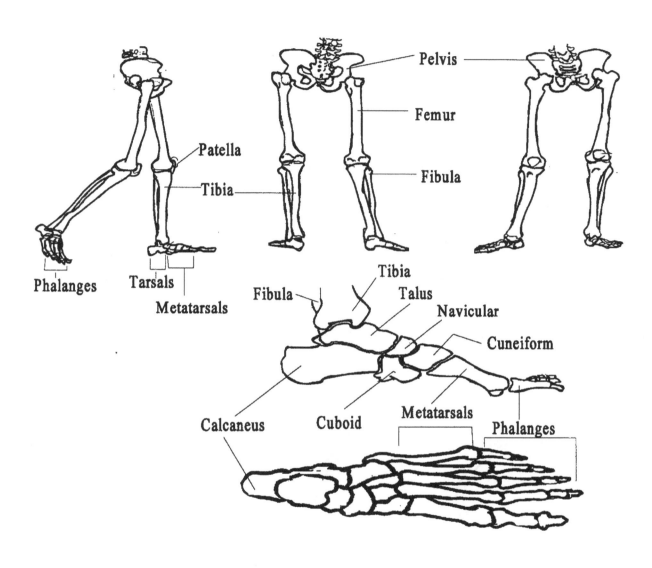

PROBLEMS RELATED TO THE SKELETAL SYSTEM

There are four main **causes** of spinal curvature:

1/ **Congenital;**   An exaggerated curvature of the spine which is present at the time of birth.

2/ **Traumatic;**   An exaggerated curvature of the spine resulting from an accident.

3/ **Environmental;**   An exaggerated curvature of the spine resulting from bad posture.

4/ **Hereditary;**   Due to a genetic weakness from one generation to another.

Exaggerated curvature of the spine falls into three categories:

1/ **Kyphosis;**   Exaggerated outward curvature of the spine in the thoracic region.

2/ **Lordosis;**   Exaggerated inward curvature in the lumbar region.

3/ **Scoliosis;**   Exaggerated lateral curvature of the spine in any area.

A classic example would be *"The Hunchback of Notre Dame"* who had **kyphosis and scoliosis of the thoracic region.**

DIAGRAM OF THE CURVATURE OF THE SPINE

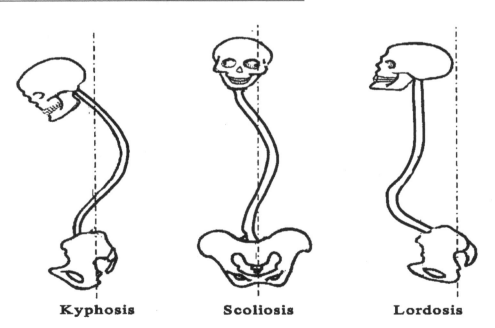

Kyphosis   **Scoliosis**   **Lordosis**

There are six main classifications of bone fractures:

1. **Compound fracture;**   When the bone is broken and protrudes through the skin.

2. **Simple fracture;**   A single break with no serious damage to surrounding tissue.

3. **Greenstick fracture;**   This is an incomplete fracture. *(as seen in children).*

4. **Complicated fracture;**   When the broken bone causes damage to surrounding tissue.

5. **Comminuted fracture;**   When the bone breaks in a number of places.

6. **Impacted fracture;**   When the broken end is driven into the other broken end.

DIAGRAM OF THE FRACTURES

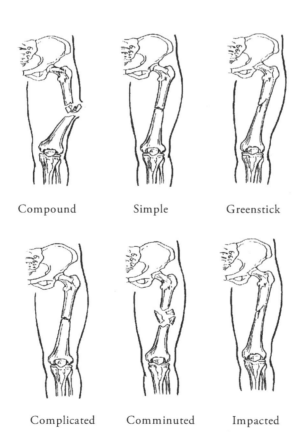

Compound   Simple   Greenstick

Complicated   Comminuted   Impacted

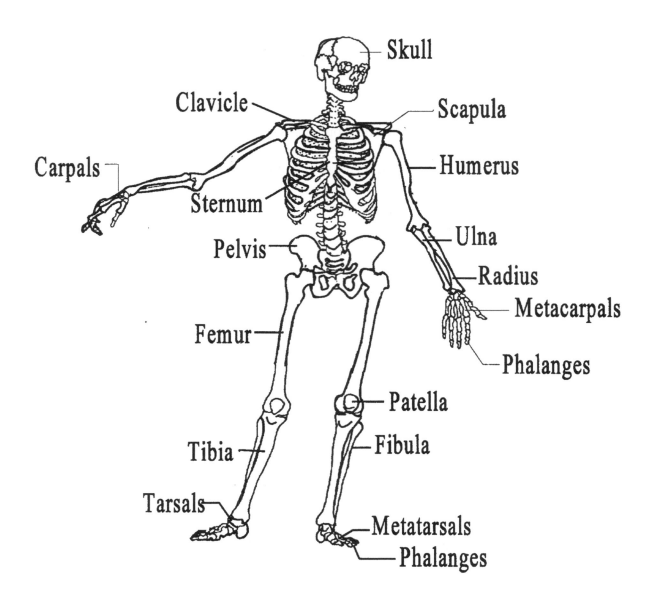

Aromatherapy For Holistic Therapists - Lesson One

Terminology

The Anatomical Position: This is the human body in the erect position with arms by the sides and the palms facing forward.

Anterior: This applies to the front of the body while in the erect position.

Appendicular Skeleton: The upper and lower limbs and their girdles.

Axial skeleton: The skeleton of the head and trunk.

Bursa: Small sac filled with fluid surrounding a joint.

Cancellous Tissue: Characterized by latticed structure as seen in the spongy tissue in bones.

Cartilage: A substance similar to bone, but not as hard. It acts as a cushion between bones and it gives shape to the nose and ears.

Dislocation: Displacement of a joint. It occurs when force is applied to the joint capsule causing the bones to separate, and applies particularly to the ball and socket joints, as the ball is forced out of the socket. When dislocated bones are returned to their proper position, it is known as *"reduction"*.

Distal: A point some distance from a given named location.

Dorsal: Anything that is related to the back. This is the term normally used when describing the back, hand or foot, eg. (back of the hand or upper part of the foot).

Foramen: Hole in a bone.

Gouty Arthritis (Gout):   Can occur in any part of the body, but is popularly associated with the big toe, resulting from urate crystals *(chalky salts of uric acid)* being deposited in and around the cartilage. This form of arthritis is much more common in men than in women.

Inferior: Situated below.

Lateral: This is to either side of the median line, eg. the outer side of the arm will be the lateral aspect while the inner side will be the median aspect.

Medial: This is an imaginary line which runs straight through the centre of the body, from the top of the head down between the two feet.

Orthopaedics:	A branch of surgery concerned with corrective treatment of the skeletal system and the study of bone disease.
Osteo:	Referring to bone.
Osteology:	The study of bones.
Osteoblasts: (Os-te-o-blasts)	When the skeleton first forms in a fetus, it consists not of bones but of cartilage and fibrous structures shaped like bones. Gradually, these cartilage "models" become transformed into real bones when the cartilage is replaced with calcified bone matrix deposited by specialized bone-forming cells called "Osteoblasts".
Palmar:	Anything that concerns the palm of the hand.
Periosteum:	A hard membrane adhering to bone and providing a protective cover. It contains blood vessels supplying blood to the bone and in its deepest layers are the bone forming cells called "Osteoblasts"
Plantar:	The underside of the foot (the sole).
Posterior:	This is the back of the body when in the erect position.
Proximal:	This is a term of comparison applied to a structure which is nearer the centre of the body or median line, eg. proximal thigh is the end of the thigh nearest to the centre of the body.
Rheumatology:	Study of muscle and joint diseases.
Sesamoid:	Small nodule of bone that often forms in the tendons at pressure points; a small rounded mass of bone, ie. Patella.
Skeleton:	Articulated bony framework of the body.
Spondylitis:	A type of arthritis which attacks the spinal vertebrae. The severest form of this disease is called "Ankylosing Spondylitis", where bone and cartilage fuse together, resulting in complete immobility.
Superior:	Above or on top.
Thorax:	Chest compartment enclosed by the ribs, backbone and diaphragm.

Common Diseases or Disorders

Disease or Disorder	ARTHRITIS
Description	An inflammation of a joint. There are several different types of arthritis, but, osteoarthritis and rheumatoid arthritis are the two you will come across most often. Osteoarthritis; a form of arthritis occurring in one or more joints which are subject to degenerative changes, causing loss of articular cartilage, and increasing bone and cartilage mass in the joint. Medically this is termed "*osteophytes*". Inflammation of the synovial membrane of the joint is common late in the disease. There are many causes that will initiate arthritis ie. Congenital or genetic defects, infection, metabolic or endocrine diseases and trauma to name but a few. Rheumatoid arthritis; A chronic, destructive and often deforming disease, characterized by inflammation of the synovial fluid leading to swelling of the joint. More commonly found in females and is variable in nature by frequent periods of remissions followed by as many periods of exacerbations. Considered by many doctors to be caused by auto-immune complications. In chronically affected joints, the delicate synovial membrane develops many villous folds and thickens because of increased numbers and size of the synovial lining cells and colonization by lymphocytes and plasma cells.
Possible Allopathic Treatment	Rest, heat pads, steroidal and non-steroidal anti-inflammatory drugs (NSAIDs) and pain killing drugs. Intra-articular corticosteroids are often used in severe cases and have the most dramatic effect short term. However, corticosteroids remain active within the body for years. Surgical intervention is often necessary. Range of motion exercises and good diet often cause improvement.
Possible Holistic Aromatherapy Treatment	Anti-inflammatory; *Caraway, Teatree, Camphor, Chamomile, Fennel, Geranium, Jasmine, Peppermint, Benzoin, Frankincense, Myrrh and Patchouli.* Analgesic (Pain-killing) oils like; *Bergamot, Cajeput, Coriander, Eucalyptus, Lemon grass, Niaouli, Black-pepper, Chamomile, Jasmine, Lavender, Marjoram, Peppermint, Rosemary and Ginger.* In some cases **Diuretic** essential oils: *Bergamot, Caraway, Eucalyptus, Lemon, Thyme, Black-pepper, Camphor, Cypress, Fennel, Geranium, Hyssop, Juniper, Lavender, Marjoram, Pine, Rosemary, Benzoin, Cedarwood, Frankincense, Patchouli and Sandalwood,* could prove useful. **Anti-depressant** essential oil like; *Basil, Bergamot, Lemon grass, Clary Sage, Geranium, Jasmine, Lavender, Melissa, Orange Blossom, Patchouli, Rose, Sandalwood and Ylang Ylang.* **Warming (Rubefacient)** essential oils like; *Bergamot, Eucalyptus, Thyme, Black Pepper, Camphor, Juniper, Lavender, Peppermint, Pine and Ginger.* **Auto-immune enhancers** like; *Cinnamon leaf, Clove bud, Frankincense.*

Disease or Disorder	OSTEOMYELITIS
Description	Infection of the bone leading to abscess formation. Inflammation of the bone marrow, usually caused by bacteria or fungi, introduced by trauma (open fractures) or contamination during surgery. The bacteria called staphylococci is the most common causative agent. The long bones in children and the spine in adults are the most common sites of infection. Persistent and severe pain and tenderness are associated with this disorder. In patients with diabetic or atherosclerotic arterial insufficiency of the lower limbs, organisms reach the bone by entering the soft tissue through a cutaneous foot ulcer. Osteomyelitis of the skull typically arises from sinus or dental infections.
Possible Allopathic Treatment	Bed rest and parenteral antibiotics or appropriate antimicrobial agents are administered, and as a last resort, surgery may be necessary to remove necrotic bone. The main indication is drainage of sub-periosteal or subcutaneous abscesses
Possible Holistic Aromatherapy Treatment	**Anti-inflammatory** essential oils; *Caraway, Teatree, Camphor, Chamomile, Fennel, Geranium, Jasmine, Peppermint, Benzoin, Frankincense, Myrrh and Patchouli.* **Analgesic** (Pain-killing) oils like; *Bergamot, Cajeput, Coriander, Eucalyptus, Lemon grass, Niaouli, Black-pepper, Chamomile, Jasmine, Lavender, Marjoram, Peppermint, Rosemary and Ginger.* In some cases **Diuretic** essential oils: *Bergamot, Caraway, Eucalyptus, Lemon, Thyme, Black-pepper, Camphor, Cypress, Fennel, Geranium, Hyssop, Juniper, Lavender, Marjoram, Pine, Rosemary, Benzoin, Cedarwood, Frankincense, Patchouli and Sandalwood* could prove useful. **Anti-depressant** essential oil like; *Basil, Bergamot, Lemon grass, Clary Sage, Geranium, Jasmine, Lavender, Melissa, Orange Blossom, Patchouli, Rose, Sandalwood and Ylang.* **Auto-immune enhancers** like; *Cinnamon leaf, Clove bud, Frankincense.*

Disease or Disorder	OSTEOPOROSIS
Description	Generalized loss of bone tissue, calcium salts and collagen in bone. This occurs during aging, and most frequently in post-menopausal women. Osteoporosis may be idiopathic or secondary to other disorders, such as thyrotoxicosis or bone demineralization caused by hyper-para-thyroidism. It is characterized by excessive loss of both calcified matrix and collagenous fibres from the bone, resulting in a dangerous pathological condition of bone degeneration, increased susceptibility to deformity of the spine and/or "spontaneous fractures". **Please note: This disorder is contra-indicated for aromatherapy treatments.** Great care must be extended when dealing with this disorder: do not exert pressure on any joint. The school does not suggest that you attempt to treat this disorder.
Possible Allopathic Treatment	Treatment should involve preventative measures by assessing the risk factors, ie. Postmenopausal women may be given estrogen replacement therapy. Estrogen may arrest or decrease disease progression. Calcium supplements may show increased bone density under certain dietary conditions.
Possible Holistic Aromatherapy Treatment	**Anti-inflammatory** essential oils; *Caraway, Teatree, Camphor, Chamomile, Fennel, Geranium, Jasmine, Peppermint, Benzoin, Frankincense, Myrrh and Patchouli.* **Analgesic** (Pain-killing) oils; *Bergamot, Cajeput, Coriander, Eucalyptus, Lemon grass, Niaouli, Black-pepper, Chamomile, Jasmine, Lavender, Marjoram, Peppermint, Rosemary and Ginger.* In some cases **Diuretic** essential oils: *Bergamot, Caraway, Eucalyptus, Lemon, Thyme, Black-pepper, Camphor, Cypress, Fennel, Geranium, Hyssop, Juniper, Lavender, Marjoram, Pine, Rosemary, Benzoin, Cedarwood, Frankincense, Patchouli and Sandalwood* could prove useful. **Anti-depressant** essential oil; *Basil, Bergamot, Lemon grass, Clary Sage, Geranium, Jasmine, Lavender, Melissa, Orange Blossom, Patchouli, Rose, Sandalwood and Ylang Ylang.* **Warming (Rubefacient)** essential oils; *Bergamot, Eucalyptus, Thyme, Black Pepper, Camphor, Juniper, Lavender, Peppermint, Pine and Ginger.* **Auto-immune enhancers;** *Cinnamon leaf, Clove bud, Frankincense.*

Disease or Disorder	OSTEOSCLEROSIS
Description	An abnormal increase in the density of bone tissue with thicker, harder bone. This is sometimes due to a congenital disorder. It is commonly associated with ischemia *(a decreased oxygenated supply of blood to an organ)*, chronic infection or tumour formation, and may also be caused by faulty bone reabsorption as a result of some abnormality involving the osteoclasts *(growth and repair during bone healing)*.
Possible Allopathic Treatment	Treatment is symptomatic, requiring rest and relief from pain.
Possible Holistic Aromatherapy Treatment	**Anti-inflammatory** essential oils; *Caraway, Teatree, Camphor, Chamomile, Fennel, Geranium, Jasmine, Peppermint, Benzoin, Frankincense, Myrrh and Patchouli.* **Analgesic** (Pain-killing) oils like; *Bergamot, Cajeput, Coriander, Eucalyptus, Lemon grass, Niaouli, Black-pepper, Chamomile, Jasmine, Lavender, Marjoram, Peppermint, Rosemary and Ginger.* In some cases **Diuretic** essential oils: *Bergamot, Caraway, Eucalyptus, Lemon, Thyme, Black-pepper, Camphor, Cypress, Fennel, Geranium, Hyssop, Juniper, Lavender, Marjoram, Pine, Rosemary, Benzoin, Cedarwood, Frankincense, Patchouli and Sandalwood* could prove useful. **Anti-depressant** essential oil; *Basil, Bergamot, Lemon grass, Clary Sage, Geranium, Jasmine, Lavender, Melissa, Orange Blossom, Patchouli, Rose, Sandalwood and Ylang Ylang.* **Warming (Rubefacient)** essential oils; *Bergamot, Eucalyptus, Thyme, Black Pepper, Camphor, Juniper, Lavender, Peppermint, Pine and Ginger.* **Neurological stimulators**: *Basil, Bergamot, Camphor wood, Chamomile (m), Cinnamon, Clary sage, Coriander, Cypress, Frankincense, Marjoram Sweet, Neroli, Nutmeg, Peppermint, Petitgrain, Pine, Rose Otto, Rosemary.* **Auto-immune enhancers**; *Cinnamon leaf, Clove bud, Frankincense.*

Disease or Disorder	ANKYLOSING SPONDYLITIS
Description	There are two types; 1. **spondylitis** and 2. **ankylosing spondylitis** Ankylosing spondylitis is the most severe form of arthritis of the spine. Similar to rheumatoid arthritis in symptoms, but different in that males are affected more than females. The articulating cartilage is destroyed, fibrous adhesions develop, and eventually **bone fusion occurs** with calcification of the intra vertebral discs. This condition often occurs in the sacroiliac joints and spreads slowly upward.
Possible Allopathic Treatment	Joint discomfort is relieved by pain killing drugs, nonsteroidal anti-inflammatory drugs (NSAIDs), exercise and other supportive measures by suppressing articular inflammation, pain, and spasm. As a last resort, surgery may be required.
Possible Holistic Aromatherapy Treatment	**Anti-inflammatory** essential oils; *Caraway, Teatree, Camphor, Chamomile, Fennel, Geranium, Jasmine, Peppermint, Benzoin, Frankincense, Myrrh and Patchouli.* **Analgesic** (Pain-killing) oils; *Bergamot, Cajeput, Coriander, Eucalyptus, Lemon grass, Niaouli, Black-pepper, Chamomile, Jasmine, Lavender, Marjoram, Peppermint, Rosemary and Ginger.* In some cases **Diuretic** essential oils: *Bergamot, Caraway, Eucalyptus, Lemon, Thyme, Black-pepper, Camphor, Cypress, Fennel, Geranium, Hyssop, Juniper, Lavender, Marjoram, Pine, Rosemary, Benzoin, Cedarwood, Frankincense, Patchouli and Sandalwood* could prove useful. **Anti-depressant** essential oil; *Basil, Bergamot, Lemon grass, Clary Sage, Geranium, Jasmine, Lavender, Melissa, Orange Blossom, Patchouli, Rose, Sandalwood and Ylang Ylang.* **Warming (Rubefacient)** essential oils; *Bergamot, Eucalyptus, Thyme, Black Pepper, Camphor, Juniper, Lavender, Peppermint, Pine and Ginger.*

Essential Oils

GINGER

Latin name: *zingiber officinale*   **Botanical Family**:   *Zingiberaceae*

Three main areas where this oil can help:
1.   **Digestive problems**
2.   **Immune enhancer during illness**
3.   **Rheumatic pain**

Properties	Uses
Analgesic	Arthritis, rheumatism, aches and pains, angina, indigestion
Expectorant	Bronchitis, sinusitis, colds, influenza
Digestive Stimulant	Constipation, flatulence, indigestion, nausea, loss of appetite, travel/motion sickness or morning sickness
Tonic	Fatigue, impotence, immune-stimulant *(increases phagocyte action)*
Stimulant	Promotes circulation, memory loss *(clears mind)*, lowers high cholesterol, helps with varicose veins, muscle fatigue

Place of Origin

Being a native to Asia it was grown originally in the coastal regions of **India**. It arrived in Europe in the middle ages and was introduced into South America by the Spaniards. For commercial purposes it is also grown in the West Indies, China and Africa.

Ginger is a perennial herb and has been used for thousands of years in the preparation of foods as well as a medicinal spice. It is one of the most highly respected spices from the Middle Ages, growing to a height of approximately 2 feet. To describe it, the leaves look long and narrow, almost reed-like grown from a stemming tuber.

Method of Extraction

The essential oil of ginger is obtained through **steam distillation** from the unpeeled, dried, ground root or tuber (rhizomes). It is a pale yellow, amber or greenish liquid with a warm, spicy fresh scent.

Traditional Uses

The Chinese have long valued ginger for its ability to promote strength and ensure a long life. They used it in cooking to break up phlegm and strengthen the heart.

The Romans used it for cooking and medicinally for the treatment of advanced cataracts. A ginger preparation was made up and applied onto the eyes several times a day. **Dioscorides** recommended it as a stomachic to help a sluggish system and aid as a digestive stimulant.

> (Please note that this preparation was not essential oil of ginger.
> Never apply essential oils neat or diluted on or near the eyes.)

Herbal Medicine

Fresh ginger is commonly used as a digestive aid. Its spicy taste, soothes the digestive system and helps to calm internal spasms. It is often used to quell nausea.

In baths, it can help improve circulation while decreasing muscular aches and pains.

Aromatherapy

In Traditional Chinese Medicine, ginger is used in many conditions where the body is not coping effectively with moisture *(damp)* whether the damp pathology originates from within or without.

A tonic to the digestive system, essential oil of ginger is effective in dealing with digestive complaints like flatulence, indigestion, diarrhea and constipation. For those who suffer from slow digestion, ginger will increase the action to assist with the problem. For those who experience nausea or travel sickness, this is an excellent way to relieve the discomfort. Apply in a blend to the abdomen using circular clockwise motions.

A stimulant to many systems, ginger will increase circulation thereby warming conditions such as, cold feet and chilblains. The analgesic effect will assist problems such as muscle fatigue, rheumatism and arthritic pain. Apply as a topical application.

The stimulating properties to the immunological system will benefit from use and will help fight against influenza, viral infections and colds. When you take into consideration the warming and tonifying qualities, this essential oil will help clear the damp mucous conditions that so often occur in the lungs especially if there is a white mucous present.

For those suffering from poor memory, the action of ginger will help clear the mind. It will assist memory while combatting fatigue that is commonly found today.

Warning: May irritate sensitive skins. Do not apply neat onto the skin. Always use this oil diluted.

ORANGE, BITTER OR SWEET

Latin name: *Bitter orange* *citrus aurantium var. amara* Botanical Family: *Rutaceae*
Sweet orange *citrus sinensis*

Three main areas where this oil can help:
1. Digestive problems
2. Liver tonic & detoxification
3. Antidepressant

Properties	Uses
Antidepressant	Anxiety, depression
Digestive	Constipation, diarrhea, colic, indigestion, appetite stimulant
Nervine	Irritability, insomnia, nervous tension, palpitations, to help relax or calm
Tonic	Detoxifies, cleansing, high blood pressure
Stimulant	Liver stimulant, lymphatic stimulant, water retention, oedema, cellulite

Place of Origin
The orange tree is native to the far East, China and India and it was believed to have been brought to Europe in around the 17th Century. Today it is most commonly found in the Mediterranean region, Israel and America *(California and Florida)*.

The orange tree is an evergreen that can grow up to 10 metres high. Compared to the sweet orange, bitter oranges have fruits that are smaller and darker and the leaf stalk is broader with a heart shape. Bitter orange trees are well known for its resistance to disease while the sweet orange variety is less hardy. The essential oil can be obtained from both the sweet orange and the bitter orange.

Method of Extraction
Essential oil of orange is obtained through pressing the fresh orange rinds. Often today, it may also be obtained from steam distillation of the same parts. An inferior essential oil is sometimes steam distilled from the fruit pulp, a by-product of orange juice manufacture. The oil is yellow-orange or dark orange liquid with a fresh fruity scent. The steam distilled version has a paler yellow hue than that of the pressed version.

Traditional Uses
Although the orange originated in China and by the Middle Ages, it was commonly used by Arabian physicians. In the 16th Century, in China, sweet orange was used to increase bronchial secretions and the bitter orange was used for its expectorant properties.

Herbal Medicine

Today, the Chinese still used the orange in herbal medicine. The fruit is used to stimulate digestion, while helping to improve constipation.

It is calming to the nervous system, and moves stagnant Qi *(energy)*. It is useful in cases such as anxiety and shock. Coughs, *(especially when there is thick, yellow phlegm present)* will benefit from the fruit of the orange, again for its known expectorant properties.

Aromatherapy

The primary effect of orange is on the liver and digestive system. It will help decongest both the liver and the spleen. Most people today require a cleansing action when it relates to the liver, due to the types of food we consume and the environment we live in.

Diarrhea, constipation or other digestive complaints that seem to stem from a nervous disorder will benefit from the application of orange essential oil due to the tonic action it has. It helps encourage peristalsis. It is also a bile stimulant and could assist in the digestion of fats. It has been said to be an appetite stimulant.

Varicose veins and cellulite benefit from orange essential oil. It has astringent properties with cleansing and detoxifying properties. The lymphatic system also benefits because of the draining effect of fluids and wastes that accumulate within the lymph.

The essential oil of orange is uplifting and helps dispel irritability while encouraging a positive outlook. Although there is no proof, sweet orange seems psychologically more cheering and uplifting than the bitter orange variety.

Due to the high content of Vitamin C, use of orange helps with the formation of collagen and therefore could be useful for the growth and repair of body tissues such as skin *(aged, wrinkled dermatitis),* bone *(broken bones or rickets)* and muscles and cellular repair.

Warning: As with most citrus oils, orange oil is considered photo toxic. However, it is known that bitter orange oil is more likely to provoke phototoxicity than the sweet variety. Either oil may irritate sensitive skin.

IMMORTELLE

Latin name: *helichrysum angustifolium*   Botanical Family: *Compositae*
         (also known as helichrysum, everlasting)

Three main areas where this oil can help:
1.   Skin problems
2.   Arthritis/rheumatism
3.   Immune enhancing

Properties   Uses

Properties	Uses
Anti-inflammatory	Thrombophlebitis, varicose veins, rheumatism, arthritis, allergies, bruising
Cytophylactic	Scarring, boils, abscesses, dermatitis, eczema, skin care
Nervine	Depression, lethargy, anxiety, stress, tension, irritability
Expectorant	Coughs, colds, flu, asthma, bronchitis, sinusitis
Stimulant	Liver, gallbladder, spleen stimulant, regulates bile secretions, detoxifies lymph, cleanses blood

Place of Origin
Closely related to the sunflower, this wild plant may also be known as Helichrysum or *"Italian Everlasting"*. It is found growing in the Mediterranean area, and Italy, with France and Yugoslavia being the main areas that produce this essential oil.

Method of Extraction
Steam distillation of the flowering tops is used to obtain this essential oil. If steam distillation occurs within 24 hours after harvesting, a high quality essential oil will be yielded. However, it can be easily damaged if the steam gets too hot during the distillation process. If this occurs, the quality of the oil will not be as high therapeutically. An alternative method, solvent extraction is commonly carried out in France, resulting in an absolute.

Immortelle has a woody scent yet remaining warm and spicy. It is a pale yellow with a red hint to it when produced through steam distillation. A thick yellow-brown liquid is the result when in an absolute form. Should you obtain an absolute, remember to gently warm the bottle in your hands to obtain a thinner consistency. Some of the chemical constituents found in Helichrysum angustifolium are geraniol, linalool, nerol, neryl acetate, pinene, and beta-caryophyllene.

Traditional Uses
In Europe, Immortelle is used for respiratory complaints in the form of an infusion. Common disorders such as coughs, bronchitis and asthma respond favourably. Eczema, psoriasis as well as other skin conditions

show improved responses as do headaches and liver problems.

Herbal Medicine
This herb has been used to expel intestinal worms. Homeopathy tinctures are made from the fresh plant and prescribed for both gallbladder disorders and lumbago.

Aromatherapy

A cell regenerating oil in general, whether dealing with the skin *(scars, acne, dermatitis, etc.)* or tissues. Wounds, burns, bruises, eczema and other skin conditions will benefit from the cytophylactic, antiseptic and astringent properties. It is said to be an excellent tonic and stimulant for many organs. It is stimulating and energizing for the liver, spleen, gallbladder and pancreas as well as the whole endocrine system. It will aid in the detoxification and cleansing process via the lymph glands. Aids in the process of lymphatic drainage and strengthens the immune system.

Immortelle, considered hepatic in property, will help reduce liver and spleen congestion. On occasion, the use of immortelle on people with diabetes has allowed some individuals to reduce their intake of insulin by regulating the pancreas.

By its action of breaking down mucous, this essential oil is a benefit to the respiratory system in general. It will soothe problems such as coughs, sinusitis, bronchitis, influenza and allergic reactions. Its antiviral properties will help contribute in the fight against many infections.

Rheumatism, arthritis and general aches and pains will be eased with the use of Immortelle due to its antispasmodic and anti-inflammatory properties.

Psychologically, this base note has a relaxing and elevating effect on the mind. It encourages deeper breathing which, like frankincense can be used to induce relaxed states, with higher consciousness which is ideal for meditation. It is also said to increase dream activity.

VETIVER

Latin name: *vetiveria zizanoides*   Botanical Family: *Gramineae*

The three main areas where this oil can help are:
1.   **Immune stimulant**
2.   **Stress related illness**
3.   **Skin care**

Properties   Uses

Properties	Uses
Nervine	Anxiety, insomnia, depression, tension, mental exhaustion
Anti-inflammatory	Aches and pains, rheumatism, arthritis, eczema
Immune-stimulant	Low immunity, debility
Circulatory stimulant	Poor circulation, anaemia

Place of Origin
This tropical grass native to India, Indonesia and Sri Lanka has historically been used as an insect repellant. Vetiver, *vetiveria zizanoides, or Andropogon muricatus* and widely known as "khus khus", and has been used in the East since antiquity for perfume.

Method of Extraction
The essential oil is steam distilled from the roots. A higher quality essential oil will produced when distilled from older roots. This oil also improves with age. For the perfumery business, a resinoid is produced by solvent extraction. Vetiver is similar in therapeutic properties to lemongrass, citronella and even palmerosa. Instead of a citrus scent, it possesses more of a deep musky, earthy scent with a slight lemon overtone.

Principal chemical constituents include: benzoic, furfurol, vetiverol, vetivone and vetivene

Traditional Uses
Vetiver has been used in the East for centuries for its fragrance. The roots are woven into aromatic matting and screens. This plant has always been in high demand by perfumers as a base note in their blends.

Herbal Medicine
Most of the uses for the aromatic root is non medical, but a tea is made from the root for a general stimulation/tonic type drink. Vetiver has also been used as an insect repellant.

Aromatherapy

A circulatory and immune stimulant due to its ability to strengthen the red blood corpuscles, vetiver will increase the blood flow. This rubefacient would be beneficial for such conditions as arthritis, rheumatism, fibromyalgia and muscular aches and pains. It possesses anti-inflammatory as well as anti-spasmodic properties

Mental and physical exhaustion responds well with the use of vetiver. This soothing, sedative oil works when dealing with disorders of the nervous system. Any type of stress-related illness will benefit from its balancing effect on the central nervous system. Its ability to promote sleep will help those with insomnia or sleep disorders and may even aid those who are presently on medication or tranquillizers. Its tonic properties will aid in restoring the body back to health.

Depression, nervous exhaustion and debility especially that stems from stress will improve.

One of the many essential oils indicated for skin care, vetiver is beneficial for its ability to penetrate deeply and help plump up any thin and sagging skin. Again, due to its action of increasing blood circulation, the skin would become healthier by aiding cellular regeneration, which in turn would help skin conditions such as cuts, wounds and even acne. It helps balances sebum (oil) secretion on the skin. For seniors suffering from poor circulation, topical application would be applicable.

Question and Answer Sheets

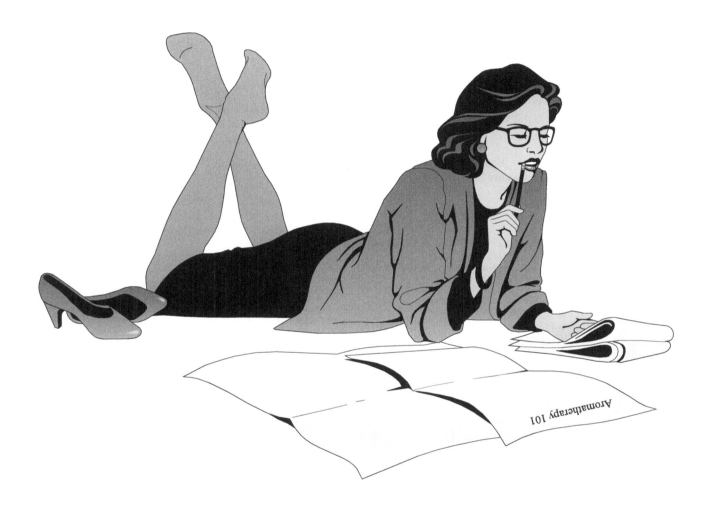

Please keep the questions for review.
Circle the correct answer/s on the Answer Sheets at the back of the book and
return these sheets only to your instructor.

Questions - Lesson #1

1. Which Chinese Emperor in 3,000 B.C. wrote a book on herbal medicine and what was his book called?
a. Huang Ti, The Yellow Emperor's Classic of Internal Medicine
b. Huang Ti, The Ti Dynasty Classic of Internal Medicine
c. Li Chiu, the Yellow Emperor's Classic of Internal Medicine
d. Lascaux, the Chinese Emperor's Classic of Herbal Medicine

2. Why was perfume so important to the ancient Egyptians?
a. used as a disinfectant in public bathing
b. it was firmly linked to politics
c. it was firmly linked to religion
d. it was a sign of chastity.

3. How many years did the Egyptian priests forecast that their embalmed bodies would last?
a. forever
b. 5,000 years
c. 2,000 years
d. 3,000 years

4. Which traces of herbs in use today were found in the bandages of Egyptian mummies.
a. galbanum resin, cedar, myrrh
b. lavender, galbanum resin and garlic
c. nutmeg, rosemary and cumin
d. galbanum, clove, garlic

5. Most aromatherapy books claim that the Egyptians distilled which oils for themselves?
a. cinnamon, clove and nutmeg
b. aniseed, cedar, garlic and cumin
c. none, they imported them
d. cedar, cinnamon, clove and galbanum

6. Which traditional Indian medicine (from India), dating back some 3,000 years incorporated essential oils in their healing potions?
a. Brahman
b. Ayur Veda
c. Mohameddan
d. Garam Masalla

7. Which race took over the knowledge of medicinal herbs and oils from the Egyptians?
a. Babylonians
b. Arabs
c. Greeks
d. Romans

8. Greek soldiers carried into battle, which essential oil in the form of an ointment for the treatment of wounds?
a. frankincense
b. lavender
c. galbanum
d. myrrh

9. Who wrote a treatise on herbal medicine which included the effects of 300 plants and their uses?
a. Hippocrates
b. Galen
c. Marcus Aurelius
d. Dioscorides

10. Which Greek surgeon and physician to the Emperor Marcus Aurelius of Rome, started out as a surgeon to a school of gladiators.
a. Hippocrates
b. Galen
c. Marcus Aurelius
d. Dioscorides

11. Who wrote "De Materia Medica" in 50 AD.?
a. Hippocrates
b. Galen
c. Marcus Aurelius
d. Dioscorides

12. Who is credited with the invention of distillation of essential oils?
a. Ali Ibn Sina
b. Galen
c. Ali Baba
d. Dioscorides

13. How did the knowledge of herbal medicine arrive in Europe from the Mediterranean area in those ancient times?
a. the spice trade routes
b. the Crusaders
c. the salt road
d. the explorers

14. During the seventeen century which oils were burned to ward off the Bubonic Plague?
a. rosemary and thyme
b. parsley and sage
c. frankincense and pine
d. rosemary and pine

15. **Which industrial workers were virtually immune to the Bubonic Plague?**
a. the herbalists
b. the medical suppliers
c. the squires
d. the perfumers

16. **Up until the nineteenth century, medical practitioners carried a little cassoulet filled with aromatics on top of their walking sticks. Why?**
a. to act as a personal antiseptic
b. to scent the air
c. to cover the smell of unwashed bodies
d. to act as a personal perfume

17. **What was William Turner known as, and what was different about his books on herbs?**
a. the Father of Botany, his books had floral pictures in them
b. the Father of Botany, his books were in English
c. the first English author on plants and herbs
d. the father of British Homeopathy, his books were in English

18. **Who wrote "The Complete Herbal" in 1653?**
a. William Turner
b. Nicholas Salmon
c. Nicholas Culpepper
d. Rene-Maurice Gattefosse

19. **Who coined the term "Aromatherapy" which is still used today.**
a. William Turner
b. Nicholas Salmon
c. Nicholas Culpepper
d. Rene-Maurice Gattefosse

20. **What two things happened to the author of the book "Aromatherapie" that helped to extend his interest in aromatic essential oils?**
a. he discovered that essential oils were more antiseptic than synthetics
b. he discovered that essential oils could be produced synthetically
c. a major burn on his hand healed without problems after being dipped in essential oil of lavender
d. he discovered essential oils helped preserve the mummies

21. **What was the book called that was written by Rene-Maurice Gattefosse?**
a. Aromatherapie
b. Ye old book of herbal recipes
c. Aromatherapy of beginners
d. Essential oils and their uses

22. **What does the following term mean; dorsal.**
a. used to describe the upper aspect of the hand and the foot.
b. used to describe the side of the body.
c. used to describe the middle of the body.
d. used to describe the underside of the hand or foot.

23. **What does the following term mean; lateral.**
a. to describe the upper aspect of the hand and the foot.
b. used to describe the side of the body.
c. used to describe the middle of the body.
d. describe the underside of the hand/ foot.

24. **What does the following term mean; appendicular skeleton**
a. skeleton of the upper limbs and their girdles.
b. skeleton of the upper and lower limbs and their girdles.
c. skeleton of the lower limbs and their girdles.
d. skeleton of the feet and hands and their appendages.

25. **What does the following term mean; cartilage.**
a. used to describe part of the bone that contains marrow.
b. used to describe the ears.
c. a substance similar to bone, but harder.
d. a substance similar to bone but not as hard.

26. **What does the following term mean: dislocation.**
a. displacement of a joint, normally associated with a ball and socket joint
b. hyper-extension of a limb
c. transplanting a bone to a different body area
d. used to describe the movement of a group of people from one place to another.

27. **What does the following term mean: spondylitis.**
a. used to describe pain in the neck.
b. severe arthritis causing the spine to fuse.
c. arthritis of the hands or feet.
d. arthritis of the spine.

28. **What does the following term mean: rheumatology.**
a. chronic arthritis characterized by loss of cartilage and spur formation.
b. a study of arthritis found only in men.
c. acute arthritis associated with geriatrics.
d. a study of chronic joint disease.

29. What does the following term mean: gout.
a. chronic arthritis characterized by loss of cartilage and spur formation.
b. form of arthritis found mainly in men.
c. acute arthritis associated with geriatrics.
d. chronic arthritis found only in the knees.

30. What is the periosteum?
a. part of the pelvic cavity
b. the hard outer membrane of the bone
c. bone cancer
d. a latticed structure found deep within the bone

31. What are the two principal functions of the skeleton?
a. locomotion and protection
b. movement and support
c. mobility and frame
d. shape and movement

32. How many bones make up the adult human skeleton?
a. 527
b. 206
c. 302
d. 157

33. What is the composition of bones?
a. water, calcium and organic matter
b. calcium, organic matter, magnesium and phosphorus
c. water, organic matter and mineral
d. organic matter, mineral and calcium

34. What are the five classifications of bones? Name and give one example of each.

BONE TYPE	EXAMPLE
a. long bones	1. metacarpals
b. short bones	2. knee cap
c. skinny bones	3. vertebrae
d. flat bones	4. femur
e. fat bones	5. hyoid
f. irregular bones	6. ribs
g. sesamoid bones	7. frontal

35. Name the four main categories of joint articulation and give one example.

JOINT TYPE	EXAMPLE
a. ball and socket	1. knee
b. hinge	2. hip
c. mobile	3. elbow
d. pivot	4. carpal
e. gliding	5. radius/ulna

36. What is a synarthroses?
a. a fixed joint with no movement
b. a cartilaginous joint with limited movement
c. slight movement at right angles
d. no movement at right angles

37. What are the four main causes of spinal curvature?
a. environmental
b. congenital
c. traumatic
d. hereditary
e. surgery

38. What are the three categories of exaggerated spinal curvature? Name and describe each one.

CATEGORY	DESCRIPTION
a. kyphosis	1. exaggerated lateral curvature of the spine
b. lordosis	2. exaggerated inward curvature of the lumbar region
c. mordosis	3. exaggerated curvature of the thoracic region
d. scoliosis	4. exaggerated inward curvature of sonorosis the lumbar region
e. sonorosis	5. exaggerated outward curvature of the thoracic region
f. cervicosis	6. exaggerated outward curvature of the cervical region

39. What disorder, according to history, did the Hunchback of Notre Dame suffer from?
a. kyphosis & scoliosis of the thoracic region
b. kyphosis & scoliosis of the lumbar region
c. mordosis & lordosis of the thoracic/cervical regions
d. scoliosis & lordosis of the lumbar region

40. Label the diagram of the spine.
(SEE ANSWER SHEET FOR DIAGRAM)

41. Label the diagram of the skull.
(SEE ANSWER SHEET FOR DIAGRAM)

42. Label the diagram of the skeletal system.
(SEE ANSWER SHEET FOR DIAGRAM)

43. What does the following term mean; arthritis.
a. infection of a joint.
b. inflammation of a joint.
c. inflammation on a bone.
d. painful swelling causing itching.

44. What types of essential oils would you use for arthritis?
a. anti-inflammatory
b. anti-depressant,
c. auto-immune enhancers
d. analgesic
e. diuretic
f. rubefacient,
g. neurological stimulators

45. What is osteomyelitis?
a. infection of the muscle leading to cancer
b. infection of a nerve leading to nerve damage
c. infection of a joint
d. infection of the synovial fluid
e. infection of the bone leading to abscess formation

46. What types of essential oils would you use for osteomyelitis?
a. anti-inflammatory
b. anti-depressant,
c. auto-immune enhancers
d. analgesic
e. diuretic
f. rubefacient,
g. neurological stimulators

47. What is osteoporosis?
a. generalized loss of bone tissue
b. generalized loss of nerve tissue
c. generalized loss of joint tissue
d. generalized loss of synovial fluid
e. generalized loss of lymph tissue

48. What types of essential oils would you use for osteoporosis?
a. anti-inflammatory
b. anti-depressant,
c. auto-immune enhancers
d. analgesic
e. diuretic
f. rubefacient,
g. neurological stimulators

49. What is osteosclerosis?
a. an abnormal increase in the muscle density
b. an abnormal increase in the nerve density
c. an abnormal increase in the bone density
d. an abnormal increase in the synovial fluid
e. an abnormal increase in the abscess formation

50. What types of essential oils would you use for osteosclerosis?
a. anti-inflammatory
b. anti-depressant
c. auto-immune enhancers
d. analgesic
e. diuretic
f. rubefacient,
g. neurological stimulators

51. What is ankylosing spondylitis?
a. severe form of infection of the muscle
b. infection of a nerve leading to nerve damage
c. infection of a joint
d. severe form of arthritis of the spine
e. severe form of synovial fluid infection

52. What types of essential oils would you use for ankylosing spondylitis?
a. anti-inflammatory
b. anti-depressant
c. auto-immune enhancers
d. analgesic
e. diuretic
f. rubefacient,
g. neurological stimulators

53. Name the three main uses for essential oil of ginger?
a. digestive problems
b. skin problems
c. rheumatic pain
d. immune enhancer
e. reduces fevers & stimulates appetite

54. What do you have to be careful of when using ginger?
a. effects patients with rheumatism adversely
b. skin irritant
c. arthritis inflammation
d. neurological over-stimulation
e. raises fevers & diminishes appetite

55. Name the three main uses for essential oil of orange?
a. rheumatism or arthritis
b. digestive problems
c. depression, anxiety
d. liver tonic
e. immune enhancer

56. What two things do you have to be careful of when using orange?

a. effects patients with rheumatism adversely

b. skin irritant

c. arthritis inflammation

d. neurological over-stimulation

e. photo-toxic

57. Name the three main uses for essential oil of immortelle?

a. digestive stimulant

b. sudorific

c. rheumatism & arthritis

d. immune enhancer

e. skin problems

58. What do you have to be careful of when using immortelle?

a. effects patients with rheumatism adversely

b. no known adverse effects

c. arthritis inflammation

d. neurological over-stimulation

e. raises fevers & diminishes appetite

59. Name the three main uses for essential oil of vetiver?

a. digestive disorders

b. skin care problems

c. immune stimulant

d. neurological and stress disorders

e. reduces fevers & stimulates appetite

60. What do you have to be careful of when using vetiver?

a. effects patients with rheumatism adversely

b. skin care irritation

c. arthritis inflammation

d. neurological over-stimulation

e. none of the above

Answer Sheet - Lesson #1

(Keep the questions for review. Circle the correct answer/s and return these sheets only to your instructor.)

1.   A   B   C   D

2.   A   B   C   D

3.   A   B   C   D

4   A   B   C   D

5.   A   B   C   D

6.   A   B   C   D

7.   A   B   C   D

8   A   B   C   D

9.   A   B   C   D

10.   A   B   C   D

11.   A   B   C   D

12.   A   B   C   D

13.   A   B   C   D

14.   A   B   C   D

15.   A   B   C   D

16.   A   B   C   D

17.   A   B   C   D

18.   A   B   C   D

19.   A   B   C   D

20.   A   B   C   D

21.   A   B   C   D

22.   A   B   C   D

23.   A   B   C   D

24.   A   B   C   D

25.   A   B   C   D

26.   A   B   C   D

27.   A   B   C   D

28.   A   B   C   D

29.   A   B   C   D

30.   A   B   C   D

31.   A   B   C   D

32.   A   B   C   D

33.   A   B   C   D

34.   Draw a line from a letter to a matching number

        A   B   C   D   E   F   G

        1   2   3   4   5   6   7

35.   Draw a line from a letter to a matching number
        A   B   C   D   E

        1   2   3   4   5

36.   A   B   C   D

37.   A   B   C   D   E

38.   Draw a line from a letter to a matching number
        A   B   C   D   E   F

        1   2   3   4   5   6

39.   A   B   C   D

40.   Please label the diagram of the spine

Name the section of the spine and give the number of vertebrae in each section

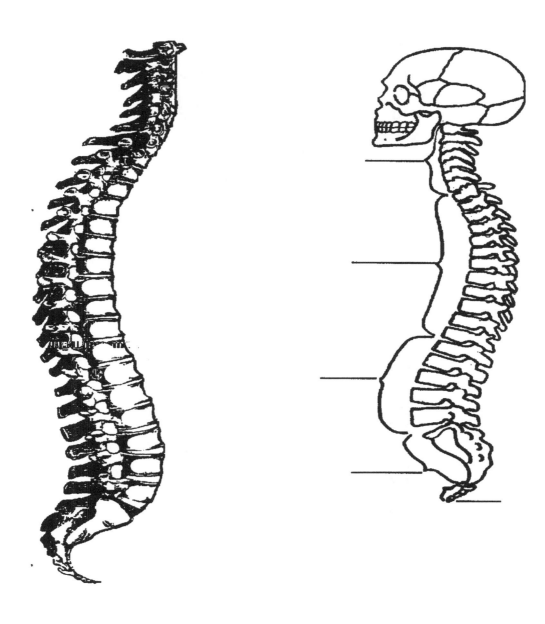

41.   Label the diagrams of the skull

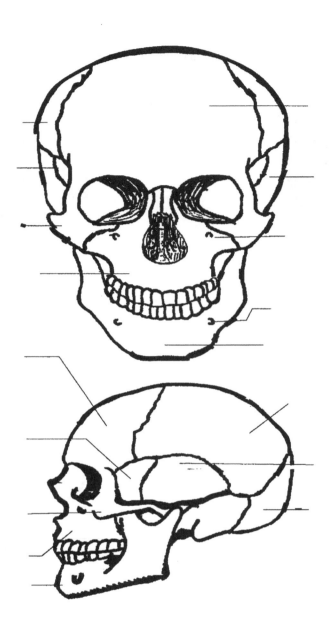

42.   Label the skeletal system

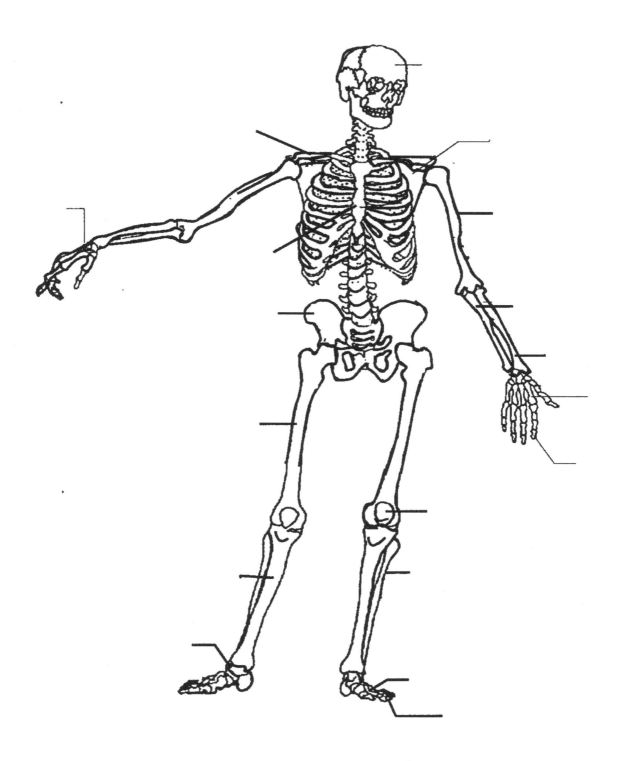

43.	A	B	C	D

44.	A	B	C	D	E	F	G

45.	A	B	C	D	E

46.	A	B	C	D	E	F	G

47.	A	B	C	D	E

48.	A	B	C	D	E	F	G

49.	A	B	C	D	E

50.	A	B	C	D	E	F	G

51.	A	B	C	D	E

52.	A	B	C	D	E	F	G

53.	A	B	C	D	E

54.	A	B	C	D	E

55.	A	B	C	D	E

56.	A	B	C	D	E

57.	A	B	C	D	E

58.	A	B	C	D	E

59.	A	B	C	D	E

60.	A	B	C	D	E

LESSON TWO

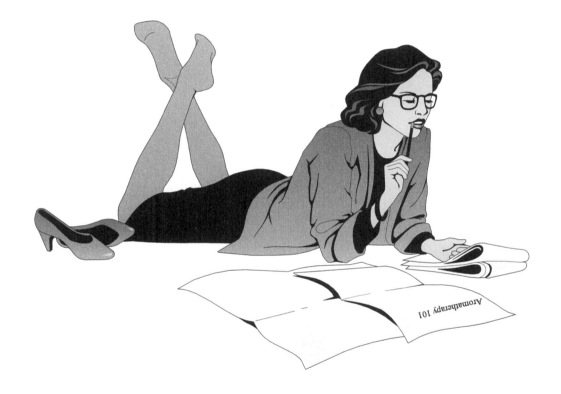

Lesson #2

Table of Contents

An Introduction to the Muscular System

Definition: Kinesiology - *"the scientific study of movements"* When referring to the skeletal system or the muscular system we must also study the movements of muscles as well as the anatomical structure and position of this system.

HISTORICAL

The history of this system goes back many years. Philosophers and scientists like Hippocrates, Aristotle and Galen and other gifted men supplied many important texts on this subject. Artists like DaVinci, Galvani and Vesalius have depicted and illustrated many incredibly accurate drawings that have captured the imagination causing such a fascination that even to this day, modern anatomy teachers frequently use their work to emphasize a point.

WHAT IS A MUSCLE

Muscles are composed of highly specialized cells that can generate a focused force or produce skeletal movement. Skeletal muscle cells are responsible for all voluntary actions that range from speaking to moving the limbs. Cardiac and smooth muscles are involuntary muscles that maintain the functions of the cardiovascular, respiratory, digestive, gastrointestinal, and genito-urinary systems. Muscles are responsible for up to 50% of the total body weight. Their function is to permit movement of the skeleton.

There are two types of muscle: 1. Voluntary muscles   2. Involuntary muscles

1. Voluntary Muscle

These are muscles that are under conscious control. Muscles attached to the skeleton are called voluntary muscles. This means that they are anatomically and mechanically arranged in parallel, to allow the cells to function independently of one another. The total force exerted will equal the sum of the force generated by each cell. Voluntary muscles are striated in appearance (cross banded) and a typical striated muscle is composed of thousands of muscle fibres enclosed in bundles surrounded by a sheath of fibrous tissue called a *"fascia"*. At either end of this muscle is a whitish coloured, noncontractile fibrous tendon which serves to attach the muscle to the bone, cartilage, ligament or other tendinous structure.

There are four types of structure of striated muscle:

▸ Fusiform: The fibre bundles lie almost parallel to the long axis or *"line of push or pull"* of the muscle, but they are slightly curved, so that the muscle tapers at each end.

▸ Unipenniform: The muscles bundles are parallel to each other but the fibres lie obliquely and converge, like the plumes of a medieval quill pen, to one side of a tendon.

▸ Bipenniform: Similar to unipenniform but with a larger number of fibres that runs down both sides of the muscle with a tendon that runs the complete length of the muscle down the centre, similar in appearance to a feather. An example would be the rectus femoris.

▸ Multipenniform: Similar to bipenniform but with an even larger number of fibres. These fibres are arranged in the curved bundles in one or more planes as found in sphincter muscles.

2. Involuntary Muscle

These are muscles that operate without conscious control, and are responsible for the life- preserving functions of the body. e.g. heart, respiration, digestion, etc. These muscles must be capable of not only generating force and movement, like skeletal muscle cells, but of also maintaining organ dimensions against applied loads, ie. vascular smooth muscles must bear the load imposed by the blood pressure to regulate blood flow.

3. Cardiac Muscle

There is however, a third category or type of muscle which is a mixture of the two. This is known as the "cardiac muscle". A cross section of the cardiac muscle shows that while it is an involuntary muscle, it displays characteristics which bear a superficial resemblance to a voluntary muscle, although the striation is not as well defined.

Points of attachments:

The term "*the point of origin*" is meant to convey its fixed or central point of attachment.

The term " *the point of insertion*" is meant to convey the moveable point to which the force of the muscle is directed. As a rule, the *origin* is the end of the muscle proximal to the centre of the body and the *insertion,* distal to the body.

Muscle consists of a number of contractile or elastic fibres bound together in bundles. These are contained in a thick band which is usually spindle shaped and always contained in a sheath. The sheath extends to form strong fibrous bands known as tendons, and it is the tendons that attach the muscle to the bone. These bundles are termed "m*yofibrils*".

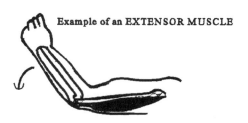

Example of an EXTENSOR MUSCLE

TRICEPS An extensor extends a limb

In order to maintain muscle tone, the muscles receive a stimulus through a chemical called noradrenaline. This is one of the chemicals produced by the autonomic nervous system in nerve transmission to the muscle from motor nerves.

Muscles always work in pairs. The one that contracts is known as the "synergist" and is the prime mover , while the muscle that extends is known as the "antagonist".

This action and reaction between the synergist and the antagonist means that the muscles are never completely at rest. They are either slightly under tension or slightly under contraction. This tension and contraction is called muscle tone.

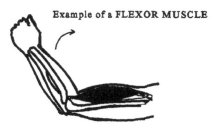

Example of a FLEXOR MUSCLE

BICEPS A flexor flexes a limb

When we bend our forearm the biceps contract (*synergist*),

while the triceps extend (*antagonist*). However, to straighten the arm, the biceps then become the antagonist and the triceps become the synergist.

How muscles move:
Skeletal muscle movement is initiated by a chemical called *"acetylcholine"*. One of the major achievements of the 20th-century is the discovery of what makes a muscle work. The process involves a chemical reaction and an exchange of nerve signals. For instance, when your arm dangles by your side, the biceps muscle appears thin, and stringy. But if you clench your fist, and flex your forearm, the biceps muscle becomes tense and bulges out.

To help you understand how muscles work, use your imagination and envision a block of stone that needs to be raised up on a small pyramid. 100 people are above the stone pulling on a rope which is attached to the stone, as it slowly rises it needs to be guided into place. To facilitate this smoothly, we need 50 people holding on to another rope attached on the other side of the stone to prevent the stone from going too far or too fast. The end result is the stone glides smoothly into place. The bicep and tricep work in a similar manner. The bicep contracts, causing the arm to bend. The tricep tries to prevent the bicep from contracting and acts as a brake to prevent the bicep from contracting too fast and causing you injury, it also gives you more control to offer fine motor control to perform delicate tasks. The chemical messenger "acetylcholine" acts on the muscle to instigate muscle movement in much the same way as a foreman on the pyramid controls the movements of the labourours.

The point where the message-bearing nerve-fibre links with the muscle fibre is called the "motor end plate". This activating mechanism lies within the muscle fibre. When a message reaches the end plate, the plate secretes the powerful chemical called acetylcholine, which passes into the muscle fibre and produces jolting electrical charges that get the muscle action under way.

There are some 640 named muscles in the body, but there are thousands of muscles that are unnamed. When a muscle contracts, energy is required. This involves a breaking down of glucose, glycogen and fat, which in turn liberates the energy required for contraction or extension. Whenever energy is used during this process, there will always be waste products excreted from the muscles to be taken away by the venous system.

Should the activity produce more waste products than the venous or lymph systems are able to cope with, (these waste products being "lactic acid, carbon dioxide, heat and water"), then the waste remains in the muscle fibres and gives a feeling of stiffness. During this increased activity, the heart rate quickens to increase the flow of blood to the muscles to take away these metabolites and to help dissipate the heat generated.

Muscles are put into groups depending on the function they perform.
- ▸ An adductor bends a limb towards the median line.
- ▸ An abductor takes a limb away from the median line.
- ▸ A sphincter surrounds and closes an orifice or opening.
- ▸ A supinator turns a limb to face upwards.
- ▸ A pronator turns a limb to face downwards.
- ▸ A rotator rotates a limb.

The following is a short list of some of the principal muscles of the body. This is not a comprehensive list of all muscles, only those most commonly used and named. However, the student is encouraged to study this subject in greater depth at a later date.

DIAGRAM OF THE MUSCLES OF THE BODY

Anterior view   Posterior view

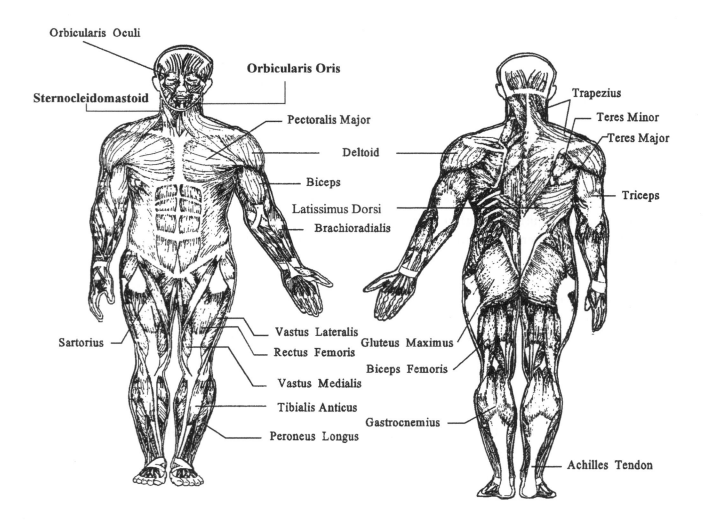

MUSCLES OF THE BODY

Head and Neck

FRONTALIS *(OR EPICRANEAS)*	Elevates eyebrows and draws scalp
ORBICULARIS OCCULI	Closes eyelids.
ORBICULARIS ORIS	Puckers mouth.
MASSETER	Muscle of mastication.
BUCCINATOR	Compresses cheeks and retracts the angle of the mouth.
STERNOCLEIDOMASTOID	Flexes head and turns head from side to side.
PLATYSMA	Muscle of facial expressions.

Trunk of Body

TRAPEZIUS	Rotates inferior angle of scapula laterally, raises shoulder, draws scapula backwards.
SPINALIS *(OR SPINATUS)*	Extends vertebral column.
LATTISSIMUS DORSI	Adducts the shoulder and draws the arm back and down.
SERRATUS MAGNUS	Draws the scapula forward.
GLUTEUS MAXIMUS	Extends to assist in raising body from sitting position.
PSOAS	Flexes hip joint and trunk on lower extremities.
PECTORALIS MAJOR	Flexes shoulder joint, depresses shoulder adducts and rotates humerus.
ABDOMINIS OBLIQUES	Supports abdominal viscera and flexes vertebral *(internal and external oblique)* column.
ABDOMINIS TRANSVERSALIS	As above
ABDOMINIS RECTUS	As above

Arms and Legs

DELTOID	Abduction of the humerus to right angles.
BICEPS BRACHIALIS	Flexes and supinates forearm.
TRICEPS BRACHIALIS	Extends elbow joint.
BRACHIALIS ANTICUS	Flexes elbow joint.
CORACO BRACHIALIS	Flexes and adducts humerus.
BRACHIO RADIALIS *(supinator longus)*	Flexes elbow joint.
PRONATOR TERRES *(Pronator radii terres)*	Pronates forearm.

Arms and Legs *(continued)*

SUPINATOR *(Supinator radii breves)*	Supinates forearm.
FLEXOR CARPI RADIALIS	Flexes wrist joint.
RECTUS FEMORIS,	Extends knee joint
VASTUS LATERALIS,	Extends knee joint
VASTUS MEDIALIS *(Quadriceps)*	Extends the knee joint.
SARTORIUS	Flexes hip and knee joints and rotates femur.
ADDUCTOR MAGNUS,	Adduct thigh.
LONGUS,	Adduct thigh
AND BREVIS	Adduct thigh
BICEPS FEMORIS *(Ham strings)*	Flexes knee joint.
SEMI-TENDINOSUS, *(Ham strings)*	Flexes knee joint and extends hip joint.
SEMI-MEMBRANOSUS *(Ham strings)*	Flexes knee joint and extends hip joint.
GRACILLIS	Adducts femur and flexes knee joint.
GASTROCNEMIUS	Flexes ankle and knee joint.
TIBIALIS ANTICUS	Flexes and inverts foot.
PERONEUS LONGUS	Inverts and flexes foot and supports arches
FLEXOR DIGITORUM LONGUS	Flexes toes
EXTENSOR DIGITORUM LONGUS	Extends toes
TENDON ACHILLES	Assists in flexion of the foot.

Terminology

atony: loss of muscle tone

atrophy: muscle wasting or a reduction of muscle size

ganglion: a cystic swelling of a joint or tendon sheath commonly found on the back of the wrist

myositis: a term used to indicate muscle inflammation

sprain: an injury to a ligament

strain: an injury to a muscle or tendon

Common Diseases or Disorders

Disease or Disorder	FIBROSITIS
Description	Inflammation of the fibrous connective tissue, usually characterized by a poorly defined set of symptoms. It is caused by a build up of urea and lactic acid. It usually includes pain and stiffness of the neck, shoulder and upper body. Fibrositis usually develops in middle age. The person is often tense, leading to the belief of a psychosomatic or psychogenic origin (stress).
Possible Allopathic treatment	Salicylates, sedatives, tranquillizers, muscle relaxants and intra-articular injections of a local anaesthetic may be prescribed in treatment
Possible Holistic Aromatherapy treatment	Anti-inflammatory essential oils; *Caraway, Teatree, Camphor, Chamomile, Fennel, Geranium, Jasmine, Peppermint, Benzoin, Frankincense, Myrrh and Patchouli.* Pain-killing analgesic oils; *Bergamot, Cajeput, Coriander, Eucalyptus, Lemon-grass, Niaouli, Black-pepper, Chamomile, Jasmine, Lavender, Marjoram, Peppermint, Rosemary and Ginger.* In some cases Diuretic essential oils: *Bergamot, Caraway, Eucalyptus, Lemon, Thyme, Black-pepper, Camphor, Cypress, Fennel, Geranium, Hyssop, Juniper, Lavender, Marjoram, Pine, Rosemary, Benzoin, Cedarwood, Frankincense, Patchouli and Sandalwood* could prove useful.

Disease or Disorder	LUMBAGO (LOW BACK PAIN)
Description	Fibrocystic inflammatory condition occurring in the lumbar region, often referred to as lumbago. It can be acute or chronic in nature. Inflammation causes the muscle to spasm which in turn immobilises the lumbar vertebrae causing more pain and often radiating sciatica. With movement or exercise these symptoms are intensified and exacerbated. Often related to overuse or microtrauma causative factors. More common in males than females and may be caused or intensified by stress. Men often show or develop localized pain due to occupational or recreational strain.
Possible Allopathic treatment	In milder cases this disorder may remit spontaneously with the reduction of stress. Stretching exercises may help, better sleep patterns, local application of heat and gentle massage. Low doses of tricyclic agents at night (amitriptyline) will improve sleep, and aspirin to help manage pain. Painful areas may respond to injections of a 1% Lidocaine solution or hydrocortisone acetate. Even antidepressant drugs at a very low dose may prove useful.
Possible Holistic Aromatherapy treatment	Anti-inflammatory essential oils; *Caraway, Teatree, Camphor, Chamomile, Fennel, Geranium, Jasmine, Peppermint, Benzoin, Frankincense, Myrrh and Patchouli.* Pain-killing analgesic oils; *Bergamot, Cajeput, Coriander, Eucalyptus, Lemon-grass, Niaouli, Black-pepper, Chamomile, Jasmine, Lavender, Marjoram, Peppermint, Rosemary and Ginger.* Anti-depressant essential oil; *Basil, Bergamot, Lemongrass, Clary Sage, Geranium, Jasmine, Lavender, Melissa, Orange Blossom, Patchouli, Rose, Sandalwood and Ylang Ylang.* Warming (Rubefacient) essential oils; *Bergamot, Eucalyptus, Thyme, Black Pepper, Camphor, Juniper, Lavender, Peppermint, Pine and Ginger.*

Disease or Disorder	TORTICOLLIS
Description	Fibrositis of the neck muscles *(Sternocleidomastoid muscle)*. The head takes up an abnormal position due to the neck muscles being in a state of contraction. Believed to be associated with injury to the sternocleidomastoid muscle on one side at birth. In adult life it is normally the result of trauma or a secondary disorder associated with disorders like Tardive Dyskinesia, hyperthyroidism, basal ganglia disease etc.
Possible Allopathic treatment	Normally treatable but neurological and idiopathic processes are more difficult to treat. The spasm responds well to physiotherapy. Drugs are effective for pain (ie. anticholinergics) muscle relaxants (ie. caclofen) or tricyclic antidepressants (ie. amitriptyline). Multiple injections of botulinum toxin type A (oculinum) into the dystonic muscles of the neck may improve the position of the head or reduce painful muscle spasm. On a surgical approach, selective denervation of the neck muscles shows the most success.
Possible Holistic Aromatherapy treatment	Anti-inflammatory essential oils; *Caraway, Teatree, Camphor, Chamomile, Fennel, Geranium, Jasmine, Peppermint, Benzoin, Frankincense, Myrrh and Patchouli.* Anti-spasmodic essential oils; *Aniseed, Basil, Bergamot, Black Pepper, Cajeput, Chamomile, Clary-sage, Coriander, Cypress, Fennel, Ginger, Hyssop, Jasmine, Juniper, Lavender, Marjoram, Melissa, Orange, Peppermint, Patchouli, Pettitgrain, Rosemary, Thyme.* Mixed with Pain-killing analgesic oils; *Bergamot, Cajeput, Coriander, Eucalyptus, Lemon-grass, Niaouli, Black-pepper, Chamomile, Jasmine, Lavender, Marjoram, Peppermint, Rosemary and Ginger.* Anti-depressant essential oil; *Basil, Bergamot, Lemongrass, Clary-sage, Geranium, Jasmine, Lavender, Melissa, Orange Blossom, Patchouli, Rose, Sandalwood and Ylang Ylang.* Warming (Rubefacient) essential oils; *Bergamot, Eucalyptus, Thyme, Black Pepper, Camphor, Juniper, Lavender, Peppermint, Pine and Ginger.*

Disease or Disorder	CRAMP
Description	A localized painful area effecting one or more of the muscle groups. The most common cause being either vigorous exercise or certain metabolic disorders. e.g. when there is a sodium or water depletion. Severe cramps normally occur in striated muscle, resulting from excessive exertion and/or high ambient temperatures causing sweating. Although cramps are often the results of excessive loss of sodium and occasionally potassium and magnesium during strenuous activity at high atmospheric temperatures (38C), the onset is often abrupt, affecting the muscles of the extremities first. Severe pain and carpopedal spasm (a spasm of the hand or foot) may temporally incapacitate the muscles of the hands or feet. Often sporadic, the cramping makes the muscles feel like hard knots. Vital signs are usually normal. The skin may be either hot and dry or clammy and cool.
Possible Allopathic treatment	In most instances, cramps are prevented or are rapidly relieved by drinking fluids or eating foods containing sodium chloride (salt). If the patient cannot take food or drink orally, 0.9% sodium chloride IV may be necessary in extreme circumstances. Sodium chloride tablets are often used as a preventative measure, but may cause stomach irritation, and an overdose may lead to oedema. Awareness of the problem is usually sufficient to prevent it.
Possible Holistic Aromatherapy treatment	Sometimes just standing up will relieve cramping spasm and alleviate the spasm on the lower extremities. By applying Anti-spasmodic essential oils; *Aniseed, Basil, Bergamot, Black Pepper, Cajeput, Chamomile, Clary-Sage, Coriander, Cypress, Fennel, Ginger, Hyssop, Jasmine, Juniper, Lavender, Marjoram, Melissa, Orange, Peppermint, Patchouli, Pettitgrain, Rosemary, Thyme.* Pain-killing analgesic oils; *Bergamot, Cajeput, Coriander, Eucalyptus, Lemon-grass, Niaouli, Black-pepper, Chamomile, Jasmine, Lavender, Marjoram, Peppermint, Rosemary and Ginger.*

Disease or Disorder	FIBROMYALGIA
Description	Fibromyalgia, also known as myofascial pain syndrome, is a disorder characterized by aches, pains and stiffness with persistent fatigue. The pain can be either widespread, or it may be limited to certain locations of the body often localised around areas of tendon insertions. There is normally no inflammation present. Fibro, means fibrous tissues that include muscles, tendons, ligaments, and other *"white"* connective tissues and myalgia means, muscular pain. This condition is more common in females and is made worse by damp or cold conditions, physical or mental stress and sleeping disturbances. Symptoms can be exacerbated by physical or emotional stress.
Possible Allopathic treatment	Myalgia has been known to remit spontaneously in mild cases, but will become chronic if stress is not dealt with. Stretching exercises will help, sleeping pills are often prescribed, heat pads will offer some relief as will gentle massage. Low doses of tricyclic drugs like amitriptyline will help with sleep, Aspirin may help with pain. Incapacitating local areas of pain may be injected with 1% lidocaine solution or hydrocortisone acetate suspension
Possible Holistic Aromatherapy treatment	Anti-inflammatory essential oils; *Caraway, Teatree, Camphor, Chamomile, Fennel, Geranium, Jasmine, Peppermint, Benzoin, Frankincense, Myrrh and Patchouli.* Mixed with Pain-killing analgesic oils; *Bergamot, Cajeput, Coriander, Eucalyptus, Lemon-grass, Niaouli, Black-pepper, Chamomile, Jasmine, Lavender, Marjoram, Peppermint, Rosemary and Ginger.* Anti-depressant essential; *Basil, Bergamot, Lemongrass, Clary Sage, Geranium, Jasmine, Lavender, Melissa, Orange Blossom, Patchouli, Rose, Sandalwood and Ylang Ylang.* Warming (Rubefacient) essential oils; *Bergamot, Eucalyptus, Thyme, Black Pepper, Camphor, Juniper, Lavender, Peppermint, Pine and Ginger.* Anti-spasmodic essential oils; *Aniseed, Basil, Bergamot, Black Pepper, Cajeput, Chamomile, Clary-Sage, Coriander, Cypress, Fennel, Ginger, Hyssop, Jasmine, Juniper, Lavender, Marjoram, Melissa, Orange, Peppermint, Patchouli, Pettitgrain, Rosemary, Thyme.*

Disease or Disorder	BURSITIS
Description	Acute/chronic inflammation of the bursae, also involving the connective tissue and surrounding structure of a joint. Severe pain is the chief symptom, particularly during movement of the afflicted limb.
Possible Allopathic treatment	Pain control with drugs and maintenance of joint motion is the main concern. A popular measure used for pain relief is intrabursal injections of adrenocorticosteroid, analgesics, anti-inflammatory agents, ice or cold pads and immobilization of the inflamed joint.
Possible Holistic Aromatherapy treatment	Anti-inflammatory essential oils; *Caraway, Teatree, Camphor, Chamomile, Fennel, Geranium, Jasmine, Peppermint, Benzoin, Frankincense, Myrrh and Patchouli.* Pain-killing analgesic oils; *Bergamot, Cajeput, Coriander, Eucalyptus, Lemon-grass, Niaouli, Black-pepper, Chamomile, Jasmine, Lavender, Marjoram, Peppermint, Rosemary and Ginger.* In some cases Diuretic essential oils: *Bergamot, Caraway, Eucalyptus, Lemon, Thyme, Black-pepper, Camphor, Cypress, Fennel, Geranium, Hyssop, Juniper, Lavender, Marjoram, Pine, Rosemary, Benzoin, Cedarwood, Frankincense, Patchouli and Sandalwood* could prove useful. Anti-depressant essential oil; *Basil, Bergamot, Lemongrass, Clary Sage, Geranium, Jasmine, Lavender, Melissa, Orange Blossom, Patchouli, Rose, Sandalwood and Ylang Ylang.* Warming (Rubefacient) essential oils; *Bergamot, Eucalyptus, Thyme, Black Pepper, Camphor, Juniper, Lavender, Peppermint, Pine and Ginger.*

Disease or Disorder	MUSCULAR DYSTROPHY
Description	Muscular dystrophy (MD) refers to a genetically transmitted disease characterized by a progressive atrophy of skeletal muscle groups without evidence of degeneration of neural tissue (unlike MS). Frequently found in young boys aged 3-7 yrs, the disease is characterised by loss of strength, disability and even deformity. The cause is still unknown but evidence leads us to believe that it is linked to an inborn error of metabolism. The pelvic girdle is effected first and then the shoulder girdle. There are two main types of MD, *"pseudohypertrophic"* (duchenne) limb-girdle muscular dystrophy and *"facioscapulohumeral"* (landouzy-dejerine) characterized by weakness of the facial muscles.
Possible Allopathic treatment	Diagnostic confirmation is made by muscle biopsy, electromyography and genetic pedigree. Treatment consists of physiotherapy and orthopaedic procedures to minimize deformity. The added burden of obesity should be avoided. Prednisone may improve functional capabilities.
Possible Holistic Aromatherapy treatment	Pain-killing analgesic oils; *Bergamot, Cajeput, Coriander, Eucalyptus, Lemon-grass, Niaouli, Black-pepper, Chamomile, Jasmine, Lavender, Marjoram, Peppermint, Rosemary and Ginger.* Anti-depressant essential oil; *Basil, Bergamot, Lemongrass, Clary Sage, Geranium, Jasmine, Lavender, Melissa, Orange Blossom, Patchouli, Rose, Sandalwood and Ylang Ylang.* Warming (Rubefacient) essential oils; *Bergamot, Eucalyptus, Thyme, Black Pepper, Camphor, Juniper, Lavender, Peppermint, Pine and Ginger.* Neurological stimulators: *Basil, Bergamot, Camphor, Chamomile (m), Cinnamon, Clary sage, Coriander, Cypress, Frankincense, Marjoram Sweet, Neroli, Nutmeg, Peppermint, Pettitgrain, Pine, Rose Otto, Rosemary.* Auto-immune enhancers; *Cinnamon leaf, Clove bud, Frankincense.*

Disease or Disorder	ANKLE SPRAINS
Description	Sprains are an injury to a ligament. Ankle sprains can be classified according to the extent of soft tissue damage. grade 1: Mild, no ligament tearing, tender area with minimum swelling. grade 2: Moderate, partial or incomplete tearing, painful and walking with difficulty, obvious swelling. grade 3: Severe, complete tear of the ligament, swelling, internal haemorrhaging, walking is out of the question, very painful.
Possible Allopathic treatment	grade 1: strapping with elastic bandages, ice and elevation of the limb. grade 2: a walking-cast to immobilize the ankle for three weeks. grade 3: cast immobilization or surgery. Surgery is controversial because the extreme fragmentation of ligaments makes repair difficult. Some surgeons cast solitary anterior talofibular ruptures but recommend surgical repair if the fibulocalcaneal ligament is torn.
Possible Holistic Aromatherapy treatment	Ice-packs to reduce swelling and inflammation. Anti-inflammatory essential oils; *Caraway, Teatree, Camphor, Chamomile, Fennel, Geranium, Jasmine, Peppermint, Benzoin, Frankincense, Myrrh and Patchouli.* Pain-killing analgesic oils; *Bergamot, Cajeput, Coriander, Eucalyptus, Lemon-grass, Niaouli, Black-pepper, Chamomile, Jasmine, Lavender, Marjoram, Peppermint, Rosemary and Ginger.* In some cases Diuretic essential oils: *Bergamot, Caraway, Eucalyptus, Lemon, Thyme, Black-pepper, Camphor, Cypress, Fennel, Geranium, Hyssop, Juniper, Lavender, Marjoram, Pine, Rosemary, Benzoin, Cedarwood, Frankincense, Patchouli and Sandalwood* could prove useful. Anti-depressant essential oil; *Basil, Bergamot, Lemongrass, Clary Sage, Geranium, Jasmine, Lavender, Melissa, Orange Blossom, Patchouli, Rose, Sandalwood and Ylang Ylang.*

Disease or Disorder	STRAIN
Description	A strain is an injury to a muscle or its tendon. It is caused by exerting physical force resulting in injury to the muscle or tendon.
Possible Allopathic treatment	Strap with elastic bandages. Apply ice, if bruising is present and elevate the limb. Healing is rapid. Generally it will take 2-4 days if rest is observed.
Possible Holistic Aromatherapy treatment	Anti-inflammatory essential oils; *Caraway, Teatree, Camphor, Chamomile, Fennel, Geranium, Jasmine, Peppermint, Benzoin, Frankincense, Myrrh and Patchouli.* Pain-killing analgesic oils; *Bergamot, Cajeput, Coriander, Eucalyptus, Lemon-grass, Niaouli, Black-pepper, Chamomile, Jasmine, Lavender, Marjoram, Peppermint, Rosemary and Ginger.* In some cases Diuretic essential oils: *Bergamot, Caraway, Eucalyptus, Lemon, Thyme, Black-pepper, Camphor, Cypress, Fennel, Geranium, Hyssop, Juniper, Lavender, Marjoram, Pine, Rosemary, Benzoin, Cedarwood, Frankincense, Patchouli and Sandalwood* could prove useful. Anti-depressant essential oil; *Basil, Bergamot, Lemongrass, Clary Sage, Geranium, Jasmine, Lavender, Melissa, Orange Blossom, Patchouli, Rose, Sandalwood and Ylang Ylang.*

Essential Oils

CLARY SAGE

Latin name: *salvia sclarea*   Botanical Family: *Labiatae*

The three main areas where this oil can help are:
1.   Muscle relaxant
2.   Asthma
3.   Stomach cramps and menstrual problems

Properties	Uses
Antispasmodic	Menstrual cramps, lumbago, muscle strain, asthma & labour pains
Sedative	Anxiety, tension, insomnia, hyperactivity, panic, colic, PMS
Antidepressant	Depression, post natal depression, nervous tension, frigidity, impotence
Tonic	Kidney disorders, high blood pressure, debility, fatigue
Nervine	Epilepsy, stress *(calms parasympathetic system)*, convulsions

Place of Origin
The plant is native to Italy, Syria and southern France, but will grow wherever the soil is dry enough, as damp soil will rot the roots. It grows to the height of 2-3 feet, with tall flower spikes rising above the hairy leaves. Its flowers are blue and slightly smaller than the sage plant.

Clary shares many of the properties of sage, but contains a far lower proportion of thujone and so does not present the risks of toxicity associated with the high level of thujone in sage. The essential oil is almost clear, with a straw colouring and has a wonderfully woody aroma.

Due to its similarity in flavour to muscatel wine in Germany, many a dishonest wine merchants would use clary sage to adulterate cheaper wines to make them taste like true muscatel wine. Unfortunately, this produces an exaggerated state of drunkenness followed by an equally exaggerated hangover. Amusing though this may seem, it is important to warn anybody using clary sage essential oil not to take alcohol, as it will produce dramatic if not unpleasant or colourful dreams.

Method of Extraction
The essential oil of clary sage is distilled from the flowers and flowering tops. It contains borneol, salviol, cineol, sclareol, salvene and salvone. It is cultivated for use as an aromatherapy oil in France and Russia.

Traditional Uses
The name clary sage is obtained from the name *"sclarea"*. This is derived from the Latin name *"clarus"* meaning clear. It was shortened to clary meaning *'clear eye'*. An infusion was created from the seeds and used on those

suffering from symptoms such as blurred vision, or tired and strained eyes.

Skin inflammations and abscesses were treated by crushing the seeds into a thick paste *(mucilage)* and applied over the affected area.

Herbal Medicine
Some herbalists recommend using clary sage as a remedy to assist in the removal of debris from the eye. The well known antispasmodic properties of this plant are used in an infusion form to aid digestive upsets and as a tonic to the kidneys. The juice of the herb helps relieve menstrual problems by regulating the menstruation periods.

Aromatherapy
The effects of clary sage are euphoric to some and will make others very relaxed or drowsy. For this reason, this essence is a good choice to use for all kinds of stress and tension. Clary sage is a powerful muscle relaxant, and it is especially useful where muscular tension arises from mental or emotional stress.

Asthma responds well to clary as it both relaxes spasms in the bronchial tubes, and helps the anxiety and emotional tension often found in asthma sufferers. The same properties seem to be potentially useful for migraine sufferers. Because of its relaxing, warming and antispasmodic properties, it is also useful for digestive problems, especially cramps or griping colicky pains where a hot compress of clary is very comforting.

Menstrual cramps respond well to this method as the antispasmodic action of clary will quite quickly stop the uterine contraction that causes pain, as well as regulate scanty or missing periods. If the cramps are accompanied by heavy menstrual flow, it is suggested to avoid clary since it may increase the flow.

Clary will act as a tonic, which is useful in convalescence, especially after the 'flu when people feel very lethargic; during depression and the post-natal recovery period. Excessive sweating can be prevented by using this oil on an illness where fever or high temperatures are present. It will also reduce excessive production of sebum, especially on the scalp, and can be put in a final rinsing water after shampooing for people with very oily hair or dandruff.

As an aphrodisiac, the action of the many properties has proved useful for couples who are experiencing a *"bad patch"* in their relationship.

It effects on the nervous system are sedative, anti-convulsive and tonic. In the area of stress-related illness, this oil is probably one of the most powerful relaxants known to us in aromatherapy. If used with care, it can help with the ever growing number of people whose suffering arises from the anxiety created by twentieth century life.

Warning: *It should not be used during pregnancy, since it can have an emmenagogue* *action.*
          Clary sage may increase the flow of a heavy menstrual cycle.
          This oil is very sedative and can make concentration difficult.
          Not to be taken with alcohol.

BLACK PEPPER

Latin name: *piper nigrum*   Botanical Name: *Piperaceae*

The three main areas where this oil can help are:
1.   Colds and influenza
2.   Arthritis
3.   Muscle problems

Properties	Uses
Digestive	Constipation, indigestion, diarrhea, loss of appetite, heartburn, sluggish digestion, nausea, flatulence
Stimulant	Debility, fatigue, paralysis, poor circulation, rheumatism, arthritis
Expectorant	Bronchitis, coughs, colds
Analgesic	Sore throats, toothaches, aches and pains, head cold

Place of Origin
Black pepper *(piper nigrum)* is cultivated in Malabar, Java, Sumatra and Penang. Where the plant grows naturally to a height of twenty feet or more, but is usually pruned to a maximum of twelve feet for convenience. The red berries from the plant are picked before they are ripe and placed in the sun to dry, which turns them black. Hence the name *"Black Pepper"*.

White peppercorns are from the same plant but the berries are not pocked until they are fully ripe, and the pericarp *(outer layer)* is removed before drying.

Method of Extraction
The essential oil is extracted by means of steam distillation from the unripe berries that have been dried in the sun. Oil of black pepper is a light amber colour and smells very much like clove oil, but has more of a pleasant, refined scent.

Traditional Uses
The word pepper originates from the Latin *"piper"* which in turn comes from the Sanskrit *"pippali"*. Pepper, like cinnamon and clove, is one of the oldest recorded known spices. It has been known as both a medicinal plant and a culinary spice in the far east and was being used in and around India over 4,000 years ago.

Of all the spices, this is one of the oldest. It was also extensively used in ancient Greece and Rome. Three thousand years ago black pepper had already become an important article of commerce. Its value was recorded as more expensive than gold. As a point of interest, *"Attila the Hun"* is reputed to have demanded 3,000 pounds of Pepper as part of the ransom for the city of Rome.

A strengthener of the body in general, it was used for digestive, circulatory, muscle and nerve disorders.

Herbal Medicine
Incorporate into pills and powders taken in doses of 5-15 grains which is 325-975 mgs for digestive stimulant and anti flatulent remedy. It is also, according to Culpeper *"it dissolves the wind in stomach or bowels, provokes urine, helps cough and other chest diseases".*

Aromatherapy
In rural areas of India, powdered black pepper is given as an inhalation in cases of fainting and hysteria. Some aromatherapists use it for flatulence, congestive chills and fevers.

Because it exerts a great influence over the muscles, it is often used for muscle tone problems. As a rubefacient and stimulant it is sometimes successful in cases of rheumatoid arthritis or paralysis, but must always be used with discretion.

Due to its stimulating and tonic properties, it is a useful oil to include in a synergistic blend for dancers and athletes, when used before a training period or a performance. It helps prevent pain and stiffness and may even improve the performance. When combined with rosemary just before running, it has been reported by marathon runners to have improved their time and produced less muscle fatigue and pain. This should be followed up by a treatment massage as soon as possible afterwards with a variety of oils like lavender and marjoram.

Black pepper is a hot, warming oil as well as slightly stimulating as an aphrodisiac. Like all warming oils, Black Pepper is used for colds and influenza and it can also be used to bring down high temperatures or fevers, when used in small amounts. It has a pronounced stimulating action on the circulation or digestive tract which means that it could be used to assist sluggish digestion, without causing griping pains. Because of its antispasmodic action it'll soothe muscles as well as restoring tone to smooth muscles for problems like prolapsed colon, uterus, etc.

Black pepper has proved most useful as an antitoxic agent with regard to some types of food poisoning.

CHAMOMILE

Latin name: German Chamomile *matricaria chamomilla*   Botanical name: *Compositae*
Roman Chamomile   *anthemis nobilis*
Moroccan Chamomile   *ormenis multicaulis*

The three main areas where this oil can help are:

1.   German Chamomile -   Skin disorders
                             Anti-inflammatory for muscle and joint disorders
                             Arthritis

2.   Roman Chamomile -   Analgesic and muscle relaxant
                             Depression
                             Insomnia

3.   Moroccan Chamomile -   Analgesic & relaxing
                             Muscles complaints
                             Joint disorders

Properties	Uses
Analgesic	neuralgia, headaches, migraines, toothache muscular pain
Anti-inflammatory	allergies, acne, eczema, skin disorders, arthritis, sprains, bruises, nephritis
Antispasmodic	pms, menstrual cramps, colic, flatulence, dyspepsia
Nervine Antidepressant	anxiety, tension, anger, irritability, promotes relaxation
Stomachic	diarrhea, colitis, gastritis, flatulence, peptic ulcers

Place of Origin
There are a number of species growing in Europe, North Africa, Hungary, South America, France, Bulgaria, Yugoslavia and the more temperate regions of Asia.

German chamomile *"matricaria chamomilla"*
This oil is found in the more eastern parts of Europe, despite its herbal name. It is similar in appearance to Roman chamomile, but has a smaller flower with fewer petals. This species is used for chamomile tea. Four species of chamomile are found growing wild in England, but only one is used in medicine and aromatherapy. This is Roman chamomile, or *"anthemis nobilis"*. It grows to about a foot in height with fine feathery leaves with a white petalled flower that has a distinctive yellow centre.

Chamomile Maroc, *"ormenis multicaulis"* is native to North West Africa, Southern Spain, and now in Israel. It is given its name because it is distilled in Morocco. This is not a true chamomile, but does possess similar properties to the German and Roman variety.

Although the cost of this essential oil is not inexpensive, it is less costly than either Roman or German chamomile.

Method of Extraction

Steam distillation from the flowers and the leaves. Its main constituents include chamazulen, coumarin, heterosides, flavonics, camphor, terpenes, and various esters. The exact chemical composition varies between the different types of chamomiles

The colour or the essential oils will vary from a deep blue found in German Chamomile to the very light blue with that of the Roman Chamomile.

German Chamomile is very concentrated, thick and sticky in consistency and gradually turns green with age. Interest in chamomile has recently been revived because of the fact that it contains azulene, a fatty substance that is formed during the distillation process. It is an excellent anti-inflammatory agent that possesses both calming and soothing properties, even when used in very small quantities. It is now being used in a number of pharmaceutical preparations as well as in the beauty and skin care industry.

Azulene is present in both German and Roman chamomile, but varies greatly in the amount present in each oil. German chamomile contains about 25% azulene, hence its dark blue colour, while Roman chamomile contains about 1%.

Traditional Uses

Chamomile has long been part of may pharmacopoeias. In the tea form, chamomile has a history of use for digestive and stomach upsets, relaxation and cystitis. Today it is still recommended by the British Herbal Pharmacopoeia for nervous dyspepsia, restlessness and irritability in children.

Known to the Saxons as *"may then"*, chamomile is one of the oldest known English medicinal herbs. Along with lavender and peppermint, it is one of the principal oil-producing herbs grown in this country. The Greeks gave it its name called *'Kamai-Melon'* which means *"ground apples"* because of the fragrance the flower produces. It is also called *"the plants physician"* as it is believed to keep other plants healthy if grown amongst them.

Herbal Medicine

Commonly used in tea form for nerves and menstrual cramps. Chamomile helps promote a natural hormone, like thyroxine, which helps rejuvenate the texture of the skin and hair. A soothing sedative with no harmful

---

effects. Safe and useful for babies and children for the treatment of colic and stomach problems.

Aromatherapy

Anti-inflammatory in nature, this oil is useful for a wide variety of problems both internal and external, including problems like arthritis, bursitis, sprains and bruises. Cold compresses are used when the swelling is a result of an injury. Do not massage in these situations. However, combining the analgesic and anti-inflammatory actions of this essential oil with massage when dealing with muscular pain is an excellent remedy. Hot compresses are ideal for situations such as abscesses, boils, infections, splinters and more. Internal inflammatory conditions, especially those resulting from a nervous origin such as colitis, colic, peptic ulcers, diarrhea and gastritis will benefit from the application.

The pain relieving properties of chamomile make this essential oil beneficial in the treatment of many complaints including pms, cramps, aches and pains, cystitis *(effective due to the combination with its disinfectant properties)*, headaches, toothaches and ear aches.

I have found that with an ear infection if one drop of Roman chamomile diluted oil is placed in the ear and a small wad of cotton inserted inside. Any remaining essential oil can be applied with gentle massage around the outside of the ear. The results are spectacular to say the least.

Often used in the treatment of skin care, chamomile is particularly effective where the skin is very sensitive, red or dry. One of the most important application is in the treatment of allergies such as eczema, rashes, irritation, urticaria and all dry flaky and itchy conditions. German chamomile is often used in many skin and beauty creams due to the high azulene content, although Roman chamomile is effective as well and has the ability to dissolve sebum.

Chamomile is calming on the mental and emotional level. Historically it has been used for hysterical and nervous conditions. It is very calming on the mental and emotional level and can be seen to parallel its physical effects. It is a soothing antidepressant and particularly helpful where stress and anxiety are inclined to make a person irritable or nervous, by promoting relaxation.

Marjoram (Sweet)

Latin name: *origanum marjorana*   Botanical family: *Labiatae*

The three main areas where this oil can help are:
1.   Anti-inflammatory for arthritis
2.   High blood pressure
3.   Detoxifying muscles

Properties   Uses

Properties	Uses
Anti-inflammatory	Arthritis, rheumatism
Vasodialator	High blood pressure, narrowing of the arteries, bruises, detoxifier
Expectorant	Colds, bronchitis, asthma, respiratory problems
Nervine/Sedative	Insomnia, hysteria, nervous tension, anxiety, stress, hyperactivity
Digestive	Flatulence, indigestion, constipation, colic
Analgesic	Headaches, migraines, aches and pains

Place of Origin

The plants thrive on sunny hillsides and are indigenous to the Mediterranean, Yugoslavia and parts of Hungary and Iran.

The Latin name for marjoram *"origanum marjorana"* is derived from the word *"major"* meaning greater. This is not because the plant has a smaller relative, but it was thought in ancient times to grant longevity, hence a greater life span.

Method of Extraction

Essential oil of marjoram is steam distilled from the flowering tops of the plant. It is yellowish, darkening to brown as it ages. Its active components include: borneol, camphor, origanol, pinene and sabinene. The aroma is warm and penetrating.

Traditional Uses

Nicholas Culpepper says *"it helpeth all diseases of the chest which hinder the freeness of breathing"*. British monks in the thirteen century, were using sweet marjoram in infusion for nervous disorders and it was widely thought that marjoram would antidote poison.

Herbal Medicine

The herb is used as an infusion one ounce of leaves to one pint of boiling water. The dose being two fluid ounces three to four times a day. The fresh plant simmered in grapeseed oil for rheumatic complaints. External uses of marjoram are applied to stiff joints, varicose veins, afflicted rheumatic as well as swollen areas. Internally it is used as a tea to help with digestive problems or sore throats. As a tonic, taken with an equal part of chamomile and taken as an infusion.

Aromatherapy

Marjoram is an essential oil with a wide variety of uses. Commonly used for its sedative properties, marjoram is able to stimulate the parasympathetic system *while reducing the effects of the sympathetic system*, resulting in general vasodialation. Narrowing of the arteries, high blood pressure and bruises will benefit from this action on the blood vessels. The same action on the tiny capillaries just beneath the skin produces a feeling of local warmth when marjoram is used. This is one of the reasons it is a valuable oil to be utilized when dealing with the aches and pains after a strenuous workout. The increase in circulation will help remove any toxic products such as lactic and uric acid that are a residue of exercise. Combined with its anti-inflammatory properties, people suffering with arthritis and rheumatism or other joint disorders that cold and stiffness are associated with, will find relief with the use of Marjoram.

Stomach pains, constipation, indigestion, flatulence are helped through the soothing action of marjoram on the digestive system. It is carminative and laxative and is valuable in the treatment of bloating and will help increase peristalsis.

Marjoram should not be used in large amounts as it can dull the senses, reduce libido and can cause drowsiness. Although in smaller amount it is an ideal remedy for insomnia or sleep disorders.

Psychologically this essential oil is not only warming on a physical level, but also on an emotional level. It is comforting and calming for those suffering from psychological trauma such as grief, loneliness, nervous tension and anxiety. However, it should not be overused, or for any extended periods of time as it can have a numbing or deadening effect on the emotions. By this same action, in lessening both the emotional response and the physical sensation, marjoram has the effect of being an anti-aphrodisiac and has been used in the past, particularly in religious institutions, for this same reason where the promotion of celibacy is required.

Warning: *Marjoram is best avoided during pregnancy.*

LAVENDER

Latin name: *lavandula angustifolia*   Botanical name: *Labiatae*

The four main areas where this oil can help are:
1.   Burns and skin problems
2.   Viral infections
3.   Muscular aches and pains
4.   Headaches

Properties	Uses
Analgesic	Headaches, migraines, arthritis, rheumatism, muscular aches and pains
Antiviral/ Antiseptic	Colds, influenza, throat infections, laryngitis, catarrh, asthma, bronchitis, whooping cough
Sedative	Insomnia, nervous tension, depression, colic, hysteria
Cicatrisant	Acne, boils, burns, eczema, psoriasis, wounds, dermatitis, insect bites
Nervine	Epilepsy, hypertension, heart palpitations

Place of Origin

Lavender *"lavandula angustifolia"* comes from the Latin *"lavare"* which means *"to wash"*. This flower has been used widely for personal bath and for the cleansing of wounds.

There are several vanities of lavender in cultivation which are of use for its medicinal purposes. The common lavender, which is the most important medicinally is known as *"lavandula angustifolia"*, *"lavandula officinalis"* or sometimes *"lavendula vera"*. This is the most delicately scented lavender.

Lavender is a native of the Mediterranean area. It flourishes all over Europe, and is extensively cultivated in England, France and Yugoslavia.

Method of Extraction

Essential oil of lavender is distilled from the flowers and the stalks of the plant. The active constituents include the ethers of linalyl and geranyl, geraniol, linalol, cineol, d-borneol, limonene, 1-pinene, caryophyllene, the esters of butyric and valerianic acid and coumarin.

Traditional Uses

One of the oldest English perfumes is now widely used in the art of aromatherapy for its vast range of healing properties. It's well known properties have been used for centuries. Historically the Romans used lavender to bath and cleanse wounds, as well as for a preparation for childbirth. Its affinity for the skin and the powerful healing properties was discovered by French chemist Rene Maurice Gattefosse early this century.

Herbal Medicine

Common herbal uses include lavender as an insect repellant. Used as a stimulant and applied topically, it has been proved useful in the treatment of neuralgic pain, rheumatism, sprains, bruises, bites and general aches and pains. An infusion made from the powdered flowers 1 teaspoon to one pint of boiling water and sipped prevents fainting and nausea.

Aromatherapy

Essential oil of lavender is probably the most versatile essential oil to date. Its useful and therapeutic properties make it invaluable in any aromatherapists repertoire. It is an excellent normaliser and balancer. Lavender, when mixed with another essential oil will not only enhance its own action, but will heighten the action of any other oil mixed with it.

The analgesic action of lavender works by lowering the reaction to pain within the central nervous system while simultaneously reducing the pain locally. Any muscular pain, whether arising from tension or from muscle fatigue, arthritis, rheumatism, headaches or migraines will find enormous relief through the use of this oil.

Soothing, anti-inflammatory and calming *(it calms cerebrospinal activity)*, skin conditions will respond with the application of this oil. Acne shows improvement through use due to the inhibition of bacteria that causes the skin infection, while soothing the skin and helping to balance the over-secretion of oil. An extremely strong cellular regenerator, it has a pronounced healing effect on burns *(apply one drop directly onto the afflicted area)*, eczema, psoriasis, boils, scars and wounds. Because of its antidepressant and sedative effects, lavender will act on emotional factors which may underlie the physical manifestations of many skin related disorders.

Insomnia, nervous tension, hysteria and colic will also respond to the actions of lavender. The oil has a sedative action on the heart and will lower blood pressure, and relieve palpitations.

The insect repellant and insecticide properties of lavender have been known for centuries. Lavender, especially combined with other essential oils, will aid in the elimination of not only mosquitoes, but also lice and scabies

Question and Answer Sheets

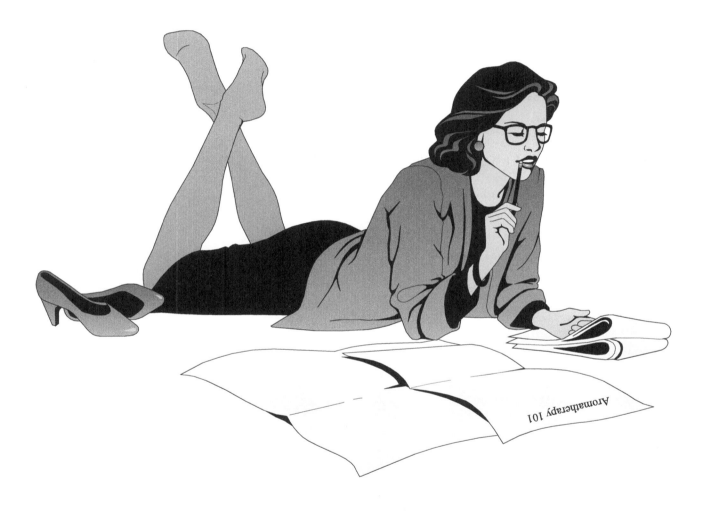

Please keep the questions for review.
Circle the correct answer/s on the Answer Sheets at the back of the book and
<u>return these sheets only</u> to your instructor.

Questions - Lesson #2

1.   What percentage of total body weight do the muscles make up?

a. up to 30%

b. up to 25%

c. up to 50%

d. up to 40%

2.   What is the function of the muscles?

a. the support the body

b. to permit movement of the skeleton

c. to prevent injury to internal organs

d. to keep the skin in place

3.   What are the two main types of muscles and what do they control?

a. voluntary muscles are under conscious control

b. involuntary muscles are without conscious control

c. cardiac muscles are controlling circulation

d. contractile muscles are controlling movement

4. Which chemical initiates voluntary muscle movement?

a. acetylcholine

b. noradrenaline

c. synergist

d. antagonist

5.   Muscles always work in pairs, what is this pair called?

a. acetylcholine

b. noradrenaline

c. synergist

d. antagonist

6.   What is muscle tone?

a. the measurement of fitness of a muscle

b. the tension and contraction of the muscle

c. the electronic energy generated by a muscle

d. the amount of strength a muscle has

7.   When bending the forearm, which muscle contracts; which muscle extends; which is the synergist; which is the antagonist?

a. the triceps extends and is the synergist

b. the biceps contracts and is the synergist

c. the triceps contracts and is the antagonist

d. the triceps extends and is the antagonist

e. the biceps extends and is the antagonist

8.   When muscles contract, energy is required.   This involves a breaking down of what body chemicals?

a. water

b. glucose

c. sugar

d. fat

e. lactic acid

f. glycogen

g. carbon dioxide

9.   When muscle contraction occurs, what waste products are excreted?

a. water

b. glucose

c. sugar

d. fat

e. lactic acid

f. glycogen

g. heat

h. carbon dioxide

10 What removes these waste products?

a. the venous system

b. the arterial system

c. the lymph system

d. the circulatory system

---

11. If the waste product is not removed from the muscle, what is the result?

a. bulky muscles

b. strained muscles

c. stiffness and pain

d. swollen muscles

12. What does an adductor do?

a. bends a limb toward the median line

b. takes a limb away from the median line

c. turns a limb to face upwards

d. turns a limb to face downwards

13. What does an abductor do?

a. bends a limb toward the median line

b. takes a limb away from the median line

c. turns a limb to face upwards

d. surrounds and closes an orifice or opening

14. What is a sphincter muscle?

a. bends a limb toward the median line

b. turns a limb to face upwards

c. surrounds and closes an orifice or opening

d. rotates a limb

15. What does a supinator do?

a. bends a limb toward the median line

b. turns a limb to face upwards

c. surrounds and closes an orifice or opening

d. rotates a limb

16. What is atony?

a. reduction in size of a muscle or muscles

b. a cystic swelling of a joint or tendon sheath

c. an abnormally low degree of muscle tone

d. an injury to a ligament

17. What does atrophy mean?

a. reduction in size of a muscle or muscles

b. a cystic swelling of a joint or tendon sheath

c. an abnormally low degree of muscle tone

d. an injury to a ligament

18. What is a ganglion?

a. reduction in size of a muscle or muscles

b. a cystic swelling of a joint or tendon sheath

c. an abnormally low degree of muscle tone

d. an injury to a muscle or its tendon

19. What does the term myositis mean?

a. a term used to indicate inflammation of muscle

b. a term used to indicate an injury to a ligament

c. to indicate an injury to a muscle or its tendon

d. a term used to indicate viral infection in a muscle

20. What is a sprain?

a. a term used to indicate inflammation of a muscle

b. a term used to indicate an injury to a ligament

c. to indicate an injury to a muscle or its tendon

d. a term used to indicate viral infection in a muscle

21. What is a strain?

a. a term used to indicate inflammation of a muscle

b. a term used to indicate an injury to a ligament

c. to indicate an injury to a muscle or its tendon

d. a term used to indicate an abnormally low degree of muscle tone

22. Where would you find the trapezius? What is its function?

a. across the shoulder area, it rotates inferior angle of scapula laterally, raises the shoulder, draws scapula backwards

b. across the front of the neck, it flexes the head and turns the head from side to side

c. across the buttocks and upper back of thigh, it extends to assist in raising the body from sitting position

d. across the lower back, it contracts to maintain upright, homosapien posture

23. Where would you find the sternocleido-mastoid muscle? What is its function?

a. across the shoulder area, it rotates inferior angle of scapula laterally, raises the shoulder, draws scapula backwards

b. across the front of the neck, it flexes the head and turns the head from side to side

c. across the buttocks and upper back of thigh, it extends to assist in raising the body from sitting position

d. across the lower back, it contracts to maintain upright, homosapien posture

24. Where would you find the gluteus maximus? What is its function?

a. across the top of the arm, it abducts the humerus to right angles

b. across the front of the neck, it flexes the head and turns the head from side to side

c. across the buttocks and upper back of thigh, it extends to assist in raising the body from sitting position

d. across the lower back, it contracts to maintain upright, homosapien posture

25. Where would you find the deltoid muscle? What is its function?

a. across the top of the arm, it abducts the humerus to right angles

b. across the front of the neck, it flexes the head and turns the head from side to side

c. across the back of the arm, it extends the elbow joint

d. across the side of the face, it compresses cheeks and retracts the angle of the mouth

26. Where would you find the:

a. biceps   A. back of the calf

b. triceps   B. front of the upper arm

c. vastus lateralis   C. side of the back

d. sartorius   D. back of the upper arm

e. gastrocnemius   E. front of the thigh

f. latissimus dorsi   F. outer side of front of the thigh

G. from medial knee to lateral thigh

H. along the spine

27. What does the term fibrositis mean?

a. inflammation of soft fibrous connective tissue

a. inflammation of the muscles of the neck

c. inflammation of the fibrous muscles of the abdomen

d. inflammation of the nerves of the legs

28. What is lumbago?

a. inflammation of soft tissue

b. inflammation of the muscles of the neck

c. inflammation of the muscles in the lumbar region

d. inflammation of the fibrous abdominal muscles

29. What is torticollis?

a. inflammation of soft tissue

b. inflammation of the muscles of the neck

c. inflammation of the muscles in the lumbar region

d. inflammation of the nerves of the legs

30. What is fibromyalgia

a. an inflammatory muscle disorder

b. muscular aches and pains

c. atrophy of soft connective tissue

d. an autoimmune disorder

31. Label the muscles of the body.

(SEE ANSWER SHEET FOR DIAGRAM)

32. How is essential oil of clary sage extracted?

a. distillation

b. pressing

c. enfleurage

d. maceration

33. Name three things that the essential oil of clary-sage can help?

a.   reduces drunkenness when added to alcohol

b.   muscle relaxant

c.   asthma

d.   stomach cramps

e.   respiratory problems

34. What do you have to be careful of when using clary sage?

a.   pregnancy

b.   can increase menstrual flow

c.   do not use with alcohol

d.   all of the above

e.   none of the above

35. How is essential oil of black pepper extracted?

a. distillation

b. pressing

c. enfleurage

d. maceration

36. Name three things that the essential oil of black pepper can help?

a. muscular problems

b. arthritis

c. acne skin care problems

d. anti-fungal agent

e. respiratory problems

37. Name three things that the essential oil of Roman chamomile can help?

a.   depression

b.   analgesic and muscle relaxant

c.   insomnia

d.   stimulates the production of red blood cells

e.   stimulate peristalsis during constipation

38. Name three types of essential oil of chamomile?

a.   Roman chamomile

b.   Chamomile Moroc

c.   Chamomile blue

d.   German chamomile

e.   English chamomile

39. Which chamomile is better suited for disorders resulting from mental stress?

a.   Roman chamomile

b.   Chamomile Moroc

c.   Chamomile blue

d.   German chamomile

e.   English chamomile

40. Which chamomile is better suited for nervous or musclar tensions?

a.   Roman chamomile

b.   Chamomile Moroc

c.   Chamomile spanish

d.   German chamomile

e.   English chamomile

41. Which chamomile is the cheapest because it is not a true chamomile?

a.   Roman chamomile

b.   Chamomile Moroc

c.   Chamomile blue

d.   German chamomile

e.   English chamomile

42. Name three things that the essential oil of marjoram can help?

a.   lowers the parasympathetic nervous function and raises the sympathetic function.

b.   increases sexual response

c.   anti-inflammatory for arthritis

d.   high blood pressure

e.   detoxifying muscles

43. What do you have to be careful of when using marjoram?

a.   skin irritant

b.   epilepsy

c.   pregnancy

d.   no known contra-indications

44. Name four things that the essential oil of lavender can help?

a.   burns and other skin problems

b.   virus infections

c.   muscular aches and pains

d.   headaches

e.   toothache

f.   weakens contractions and delays labour

Answer Sheet - Lesson #2

(Keep the questions for review. Circle the correct answer/s and return these sheets only to your instructor.)

1   A   B   C   D

2.   A   B   C   D

3.   A   B   C   D

4.   A   B   C   D

5.   A   B   C   D

6.   A   B   C   D

7.   A   B   C   D   E

8.   A   B   C   D   E   F   G

9.   A   B   C   D   E   F   G   H

10.   A   B   C   D

11.   A   B   C   D

12.   A   B   C   D

13.   A   B   C   D

14.   A   B   C   D

15.   A   B   C   D

16.   A   B   C   D

17.   A   B   C   D

18.   A   B   C   D

19.   A   B   C   D

20.   A   B   C   D

21.   A   B   C   D

22.   A   B   C   D

23.   A   B   C   D

24.   A   B   C   D

25.   A   B   C   D

26.   a. biceps   A   B   C   D   E   F   G   H
        b. triceps   A   B   C   D   E   F   G   H
        c. vastus lateralis A   B   C   D   E   F   G   H
        d. sartorius   A   B   C   D   E   F   G   H
        e. gastrocnemius   A   B   C   D   E   F   G   H
        f. latissimus dorsi A   B   C   D   E   F   G   H

27.   A   B   C   D

28.   A   B   C   D

29   A   B   C   D

30.   A   B   C   D

31.   Label the following diagram.

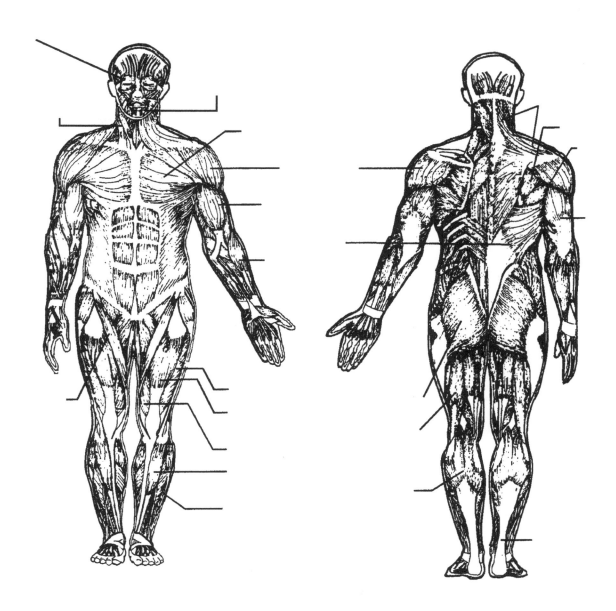

32.   A   B   C   D

33.   A   B   C   D   E

34.   A   B   C   D   E

35.   A   B   C   D

36.   A   B   C   D   E

37.   A   B   C   D   E

38.   A   B   C   D   E

39.   A   B   C   D   E

40.   A   B   C   D   E

41.   A   B   C   D   E

42.   A   B   C   D   E

43.   A   B   C   D

44.   A   B   C   D   E   F

LESSON
THREE

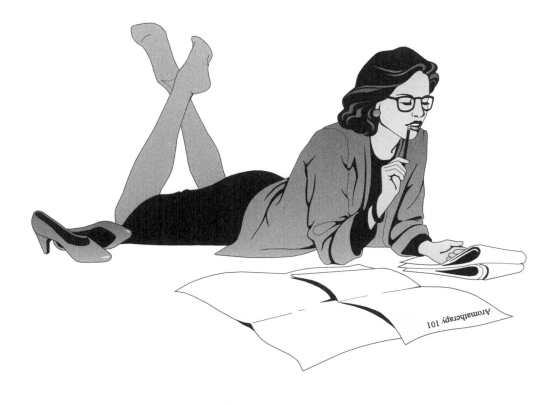

Lesson #3
Table of Contents

Bibliography:

The Simon & Schuster, Anatomy & Physiology by Dr. James Bevan.

Aromatherapy A to Z by Patricia Davis.

Aromatherapy Workbook by Shirley Price

Introduction to Essential Oils

WHAT ARE ESSENTIAL OILS

Essential oils could be described as being a highly volatile liquid, with various mixtures of natural chemical compounds obtained from plants. All essential oils are of natural origin and contain the odorific constituents of the plant which has been grown organically.

These constituents break down as follows:
terpenes, alcohols, phenols, aldehydes, acids, esters, oxides and lactones.

Essential oils, although given the name of oil are not actually oil, and are not to be confused with fixed or carrier oils. Essential oils do not stain clothing (There are a few exceptions to this rule)

There are three main industries that use essential oils besides the aromatherapist. They are;
1. Food Industry: for flavour
2. Pharmaceutical industry: for use as medicines and anti-bacterial agents.
3. Perfume industry: for cosmetics.

When matched with these industrial giants, the humble aromatherapist will only use a small proportion by comparison. It is because of this fact, that the difficulty of obtaining pure good quality essential oil is difficult.

The quantities used by each one of these industries would be many times the amount used by the aromatherapy practitioner at any given time. An appropriate scale of comparison would be; Many years ago I asked one of these industries for a sample of a particular oil, to my surprise I received a 4 litre container. Unfortunately, the oil was useless to an aromatherapist due to adulteration with additives and fixatives to give it a longer shelf life and an unvaried strength.

The fact that all three of these industries just can not afford to have an oil of unknown constituent proportion or strength, which would vary from crop to crop, is well known. For instance, if you were to purchase a particular perfume and next year you purchased the same perfume and it smelled different, the perfume factory that produced and marketed that perfume would soon be in trouble and possibly go out of business.

Plants do not grow to order, because they are at the mercy of ecological and environmental changes. The weather could be warm, hot, cool or cold. It may rain a lot or not long enough. The ground conditions may vary from year to year with the use of crop fertilizer or pesticides that may be needed to save a crop from a resilient bug or two, and lastly the airborne pollution which will effect the crop.

All of these variables taken into consideration will mean that a given crop with a high measure of terpenes as one of its constituents one year, could yield a low measure of terpenes the next year. This could dramatically alter the taste, smell or viscosity of the oil as well as the amount of oil obtained from the plant.

Standardization is a necessity in the fragrance field and there are required dilutions and concentrations in manual set out by the pharmaceutical industry. These standards unfortunately have nothing to do with the quality or purity of the product. Because of this, the chemist will lower the standard of the oil as it is not set out that the changes are done through either an artificial or natural means. This is done by corrupting the oil with an additional compound, that will not detract from the required result, be it taste or smell. This unfortunately makes commercially bought oil useless to the aromatherapist, because its therapeutic properties are no longer present, as the practising aromatherapist will require, only a pure unadulterated essential oil to work with.

The difficulty of obtaining high quality pure essential oils to aromatherapists, is because many distillers just do not want to be bothered with the problems of supplying what may seem to them as insignificant quantities. The distiller will not supply them because they are not required in large quantities commercially therefore, not a viable commodity to market for a profit. Until aromatherapy has grown significantly we will have to contend with high prices from the existing independent organic farm distillers who produce essential oils solely for aromatherapy practitioners.

Oils are obtained from different parts of the plant. e.g.
Leaves (*eucalyptus*), twigs or berries (*juniper*), bark (*cinnamon*),
wood (*sandalwood*), roots (*sassafras*), flowers (*orange blossom*), fruits (*lemon*), rhizomes (*ginger*).

Oils sometimes come from different parts of the same plant, for example:
- Orange oil comes from the orange fruit,
- Petitgrain comes from the orange leaf,
- Neroli comes from the orange blossom.
- Bitter or Seville orange tree gives Neroli Bigarade.
- Sweet orange tree gives Neroli Portugal.

Essential oils used in aromatherapy, are the result of the collective knowledge gained over thousands of years from many contributing countries. Their marvellous therapeutic properties together with their medicinal capabilities, are known and recognized all over the world. All essential oils are anti-bacterial and many of them are anti-viral or posses fungicidal qualities. Besides being one of the oldest therapies with a proven track record, it is also very simple to administer. This ancient form of treatment was able to help people in the past; even to this day, aromatherapy is able to compete with modern treatments like steroids, without any of the harmful side effects offered by contemporary medicine.

Aromatherapists achieve the best results by using only the purest natural essential oils available, nothing is taken away from or added to the oil. Essential oils could be described as pro-biotic, which is the opposite of anti-biotic (strengthens living tissue whilst killing bacteria). This means that we can use natural essential oils on living tissue without the risk of side effects, which can be so disastrous in the case of their synthetic substitutes. It's interesting to note that the body may accustom itself to the effects of the chemical syntheses which leads to increased dosages to maintain the same effect. But this is not the case when using essential oils which retain their effectiveness in respect to repeated applications and can actually strengthen the living tissue while killing off the bacterial germ or virus.

There are two essential oils that are of animal origin: Musk and Ambergris.
These expensive oils are used in perfumery, but are not used in any way for aromatherapy.

Some Properties of Essential Oils

1.   Essential oils are highly volatile and evaporate quickly.
2.   Essential oils are soluble in alcohol and ether, but only 20% soluble in water.
3.   Essential oils are soluble and mix well with all carrier oils.
4.   Essential oils become useless therapeutically in soaps. (Synthetic substitute oils are normally used to give the allusion and smell of aromatherapy to help sell the product).
5.   Some essential oils may be safe to take internally, but we do not advocate that you do so.
6.   All essential oils are hypo-allergenic.

All of the essential oils come under one of three categories:

1.   Top Notes: Light fragrant oils that are often used for acute problems and evaporate quickly.

2.   Middle Notes: Are calming and stimulating. In other words - balancing.

3.   Base Notes :   Heavy, stronger smelling oils that are often used for chronic problems and evaporate slowly.

Essential Oils, Latin and Family Name
For Information Only

ESSENTIAL OIL	LATIN NAME	FAMILY
BASIL	Ocimum Basilicum	Labiatae
BERGAMOT	Citrus Bergamia	Rutaceae
BLACK PEPPER	Piper Nigrum	Piperaceae
CAJUPUT	Melaleuca Leucodedron	Myrtaceae
CHAMOMILE GERMAN	Matricaria Chamomilla	Compositae
CHAMOMILE MOROCCAN	Ormenis Multicaulis	Compositae
CHAMOMILE ROMAN	Anthemis Nobilis	Compositae
CAMPHOR	Cinnamomum Camphora	Lauraceae
CARAWAY	Carum Carvi	Umbelliferae
CEDARWOOD East African	Cedrus Atlantica	Coniferae
CINNAMON Leaf or Bark	Cinnamonum Zeylanicum	Lauraceae
CLARY SAGE	Salvia Sclarea	Labiatae
CLOVE Bud	Eugenia Caryophyllata	Myrtaceae
CORIANDER	Coriandrum Sativum	Umbelliferae
CYPRESS	Cupressus Sempervirens	Coniferae
EUCALYPTUS	Eucalyptus Globulus	Myrtaceae
FENNEL	Foeniculum Vulgare	Umbelliferae
GERANIUM	Pelargonium Graveolens	Geraniaceae
GINGER	Zingiber Officinale	Zingiberaceae
HYSSOP	Hyssopus Officinalis	Labiatae
IMMORTELLE	Helichrysum Angustifolium	Asterceae compositae
JUNIPER Berry	Juniperus Communis	Coniferae
LAVENDER	Lavendula Officinalis	Labiatae
LEMON	Citrus Limonum	Rutaceae
LEMON GRASS	Cymbopogon Citratus Gramineae	
LINDEN BLOSSOM	Tilia eropaea	Tiliaceae
MARJORAM	Origanum Marjorana	Labiatae
MARIGOLD TAGETES	Tagetes Glandulifera T. Patula	Compositae
MELISSA	Melissa Officinalis	Labiatae
MYRTLE	Myrtus Communis	Myrtaceae
NIAOULI	Melaleuca Viridiflora	Myrtaceae
NUTMEG	Myristica Fragrans	Myristicaceae
ORANGE SWEET PORTUGAL	Citrus Sinensis	Rutaceae
ORANGE Bitter Bigarade	Citrus Aurantium	Rutaceae
ORIGANUM	Origanum Vulgare	Labiatae
PATCHOULI	Pogostemom Cablin	Labiatae
PEPPERMINT	Mentha Piperita	Labiatae
PETITGRAIN	Citrus Aurantium	Rutaceae
PINE NEEDLE	Pinus Sylvestris	Pinaceae
ROSEMARY	Rosemarinus Officinalis	Labiatae

ESSENTIAL OIL	LATIN NAME	FAMILY
SAGE	Salvia Officinalis	Labiatae
SANDALWOOD	Santalum Album	Santalaceae
SAVORY	Satureia Montana	Labiatae
TARRAGON	Artemisia Dragunculus	Compositae
TI or TEA TREE OIL	Melaleuca Alternifolia Myrtaceae	
THYME White	Thymus Vulgaris	Labiatae
YLANG YLANG	Cananga Odorata	Anonaceae

ABSOLUTES	LATIN NAME	FAMILY
JASMINE	Jasminum Officinale	Jasminaceae
	Or Jasminium Grandiflorum	
NEROLI ORANGE BLOSSOM	Citrus Aurantium v. Amara	Rutaceae
ROSE	Rosa Centifolia or	Rosaceae
	R Damascena	

RESINOIDS	LATIN NAME	FAMILY
BENZOIN	Styrax Benzoin	Styraceae
FRANKINCENSE	Boswellia Carterii	Burseraceae
OLIBANUM	Boswellia Carterii	Burseraceae
MYRRH	Commiphora Myrrha	Burseraceae
	Or Commiphora Molmol	

THE PURITY OF ESSENTIAL OILS

Quality is an important consideration when purchasing or using essential oils, as you want to make sure you are using a naturally complete, pure healing essential oil. Only genuine essential oils can guarantee the anticipated healing effect.

Oils that are grown organically are more expensive, but their quality makes them worth the price. To give an example of the quality and price of essential oils, let us take a look at jasmine oil. Millions of blossoms are needed to obtain one pound of pure essential oil of jasmine. A single plant does not contain much essential oil. *The blossoms are harvested during the early morning at sunrise, as the essential oil gathers in the blossom at night.* During the day, oil moves to the stalks and leaves, but these cannot be harvested because that would destroy the plant. Once the blossoms are harvested, the process of production is costly. An inexpensive oil of jasmine can never be genuine, pure or authentic.

"Caveat emptor" (Latin for *"buyer beware"*). If you purchase essential oils from shops or in the catalogues, you may well find the best price does not necessarily mean the best essential oil. Bear in mind, however, that all over the world there are suppliers whose goal is to make as much profit as possible by using the minimal amount of pure essential oil. They adulterate the oil with similar oils, vegetable oils, or alcohol, and possibly synthetic oils are also used as substitutes. These synthetics have no therapeutic healing properties at all. Although they smell good, and may serve a slight effect on the psychological plane, your body does not recognize them as healing agents, and you will experience none of the effects you might expect, since these substances have no life force. They simply smell pleasant. Diluted oils do not have the total healing properties of pure oils. You can never be sure which substances the dilution contains, unless the label states that an absolute oil is a diluted oil with a high quality vegetable oil additive.

When buying essential oils, it is important to know your supplier. Try not to buy essential oils unless recommended by another person whom you trust. Once you have a good and worthy supplier, you will find that their knowledge about the oil extends beyond just selling the oil; they are aware of the botanical family, the Latin name, the country of origin and the year it was distilled. This might seem like a lot of useless information, but when your reputation is on the line, you will be glad you have the support of your supplier and the confidence to order oils without fear of dishonesty.

THE METHODS OF OBTAINING ESSENTIAL OILS

A variety of methods are used to obtain essential oils from whole plants, leaves, blossoms, roots, barks, resins, or fruit peels. The basic process is to break the cell's wall, thereby releasing the essential oil.

STEAM DISTILLATION
Distillation is the main method by which essential oils are extracted from the plants. There are two methods of distillation:

1.   DIRECT
The *DIRECT* method of distillation involves placing the plant material in water which is then heated and brought to boil.

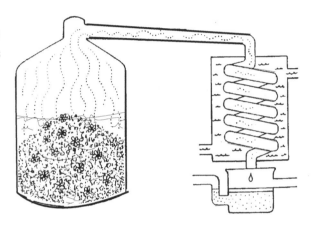

2.   STEAM
The *STEAM* method of distillation is the process of placing the plant material on a rack or grid and heating the water above or beneath it. The steam passes through the plant matter, causing the aromatic essence held within the plant to be released.

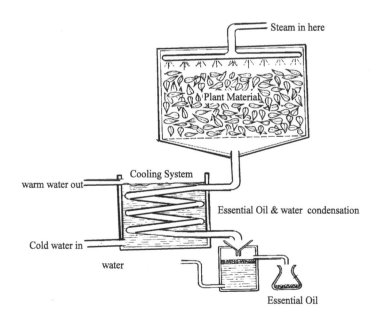

In either method, the heat and steam cause the walls of plant cells to break down and release the essence in the form of vapour. This vapour, together with steam, is gathered into a pipe which passes through cooling tanks. This causes the mixed vapours to return to liquid form so that they can be collected in vats at the end of the process. The steam condenses into a watery distillate while the essence from the plant becomes an essential oil. This oil, being lighter than water, collects in the upper part of the vat and can easily be separated. In some cases, the water is sold as flower or herbal water.

MACERATION

There are two methods used in the maceration process. One method is the preparation of aromatic plants by prolonged soaking in warm water or oil creating an infusion. The plant material is filtered from the liquid; the resulting liquid containing the essential oil. In the case of water being used, it is used as "a wash". If oil is used to soak the plant matter, it is used as an infusion oil, i.e. calendula oil.

In the second case, the blossoms are dipped into hot oil until the walls of the cells break apart and the hot oil absorbs the essence. Later, the oil and the essence are separated. This is an old-fashioned and expensive method rarely used today.

PRESSING

Essences of citrus fruits, such as oranges, lemons, grapefruits and tangerines, are obtained by pressing the unpolluted, natural peels of the fruit. The peel is pressed between two pieces of wood, one of which has a sponge attached to it. The pressed oil is then released and absorbed by the sponge. The oil is then collected by wringing out the sponge. This type of essence is of high quality and may be suitable for internal use.

ENFLEURAGE / EXTRACTION   (To produce an absolute)

Some of the finest flower absolutes are produced by means of solvent extraction. Extraction is reserved for plants with a low concentration of essential oil like Jasmine. These oils usually have a finer fragrance. There are two methods used to extract the essential oil:

1.   In the first, the blossoms are spread on perforated metal sheets and washed continuously with the same water until all essential oils are dissolved. Afterwards, the essential oils are separated from the water by distillation.

2.   In the second method, both enfleurage and maceration depend on the physical fact that fat will absorb the essential oils found within the plant. A sheet of glass is placed onto a wooden frame and coated with a thin layer of fat, freshly picked flowers are then spread over the fat.

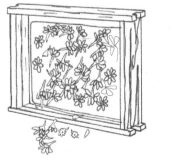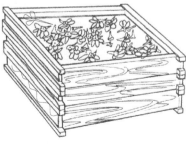

Wooden frames used in enfleurage method

After 24 hrs the flowers will have given up all their oils to the fat, the frames are turned upside-down to remove the dried and withered flowers ready to begin the process all over again. The process is repeated for up to three months. When the fat has been completely saturated with the essential oil the fat is then collected and cleared of any debris; the resulting mixture is known as a *pomade*. The essential oils of the flowers are isolated from the pomade with a solvent, such as petrol ether. After the solvent has evaporated, a paste called a "concrete" remains. This paste also contains waxes and chlorophyll, and is only partly soluble in alcohol. The paste is mixed with alcohol, heated to 120 degrees Fahrenheit, cooled again and filtered. The remaining alcohol is removed through evaporation. Finally, an oily residue remains called an *"absolute"* and it is totally soluble in alcohol.

If not separated, the fats are used for cosmetics such as high quality creams, called *"huiles francaises"*. The essential oils obtained in this manner are called Absolute oils. They are not suitable for internal use. The pomade is then diluted in alcohol and shaken vigorously for twenty-four hours to separate the fat from the essential oils. The alcohol absorbs the essential oil from the fat. This alcohol is then evaporated, leaving a very concentrated essential oil. A large number of flowers are needed to produce a small amount of essential oil. It takes 1000 pounds of petals to make approximately two pounds of rose oil, this equates to 30 roses to make one drop of essential oil. This is a very costly, time consuming process, which accounts for the high price of these oils or absolutes. *Absolute oils* are not suitable for internal use as they always contain trace residues of the solvents.

To avoid the high prices of true, natural and pure absolute oil, some companies will often offer these absolute oils that are diluted with up to 90% vegetable oil. This does not affect or damage the healing properties and the scent is still strong since these oils are highly concentrated. In fact, it is recommended to use them diluted.

CARBON DIOXIDE EXTRACTION
A modern extraction process used today. This method utilizes gas with a lower temperature setting (30 degrees C) than steam distillation. With high pressure, the carbon dioxide is put into another state where it displays qualities of both a liquid and a gas. It is very expensive to process essential oils by this method. The equipment is costly, although the quality and the fragrance of the essential oils extracted are of excellent purity due to the oils only come into contact with the carbon dioxide.

SOLVENT EXTRACTION

This process is commonly used for gums and resins as well as flowers. Flowers are treated with petroleum, ether or benzine. Resins and gums are treated with acetone. The plant material is placed in a glass container and saturated with a solvent, which is then heated electrically causing the odour bearing molecules to evaporate, and is then filtered.

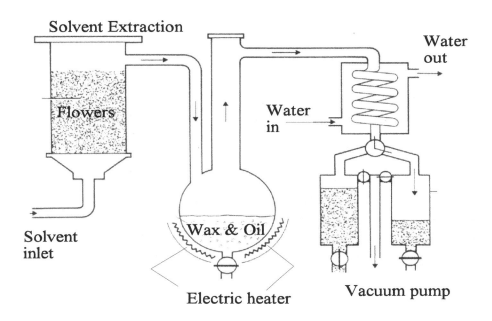

PHYTOL PROCESS

Developed in England by a large pharmaceutical company, this phytonic process uses a special gas called *"non-CFC's"* (non-chlorofluorocarbons). This gas, that can now produce essential oils, has been commonly used in inhalers. The benefits of this process is the ability to extract the essential oils at a lower temperature than carbon dioxide extraction can currently do with a much gentler process. The result are oils that are as close to their natural form as possible. Melissa essential oil is commonly extracted through this process.

An Introduction to the Digestive System

The digestive system could be described as an assembly line that works in reverse, because it takes in whole food products and breaks them down into their chemical components. The food you eat is broken down by digestive juices into small, easily absorbable nutrients that generate the energy required to maintain a healthy body.

For a healthy and efficient working body to be maintained, the food content needs to be both balanced and nutritious. We are to a greater or lesser degree responsible for our own basic health; the old saying *"we are what we eat"* is true in many cases. Because of this, we need to have at least a basic understanding of the process involved with digestion and to understand some of the ways in which it can go wrong.

The body requires raw material to grow and repair itself as well as for heat and energy. These raw materials are supplied in the form of food that comes in a variety of packages that we ingest and convert to compounds which generate and sustain life.

It takes about three to six hours for a meal to be converted from solids to semi-liquids in the stomach. The rate at which the stomach moves food along is controlled primarily by the duodenum. The sphincter releases hormones that control the muscle movements of the stomach regulates the rate of digestion. As a result, the duodenum receives the chyme gradually, in just the right amount for optimum digestion and absorption. When the stomach is full, it signals for the release of the hormone gastrin, which speeds up digestion.

The average adult has a digestive tract that is about thirty feet long from one end to the other, it could be described as a strong muscular continuous tube, starting at the mouth and passing through the larynx, oesophagus, stomach, small and large intestine and ending at the rectum.

Associated with this system are the accessory organs;

     a)   the tongue
     b)   teeth
     c)   salivary glands.
     d)   liver
     e)   pancreas

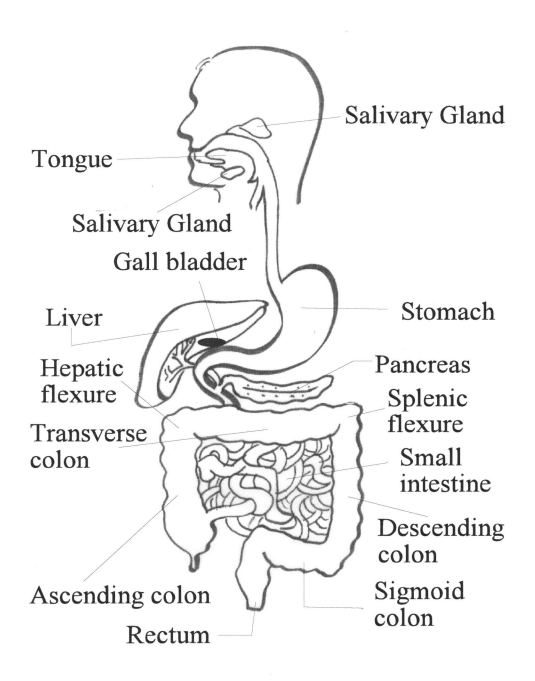

Salivary Gland

Tongue

Salivary Gland

Gall bladder

Liver

Stomach

Hepatic
flexure

Pancreas

Splenic
flexure

Transverse
colon

Small
intestine

Descending
colon

Ascending colon

Sigmoid
colon

Rectum

Let's start at the beginning.

THE MOUTH

is the body's first line of defence for the digestive system. The mouth has at least four functions.

1. To break up food by chewing
2. To lubricate with saliva
3. To assist in regulating the body temperature
4. To consciously initiate swallowing

THE TONGUE

The tongue is an immensely mobile mass of muscle which helps the teeth to tear food to pieces by forcing it against the bony top plate of the roof of the mouth, and then form the crushed and moistened particles into a ball, or bolus ready for swallowing. When the tongue moves up and back, pressing against the hard palate, it propels the bolus to the back of the mouth and into the oesophagus. It also gives warning of possible injury by registering pain when foods are too hot, and revulsion when they are spoiled. It consists of striated voluntary muscle and it is attached mainly to the mandible and hyoid bones.

The upper surface of the tongue is covered with papillae, of which there are three forms;

1. The filiform papillae, found chiefly on the dorsal aspect of the tongue.
2. The fungiform, found mainly on the sides and tip of the tongue.
3. The vallate, which is the largest of the papillae in a "v" formation at the back of the tongue. Taste-buds are found in the walls of the vallate papillae.

On a healthy tongue, the papillae are usually pinkish-white and velvety smooth, and are crossed by slits or fissures that reveal the red tongue beneath.
Although they combine to make a myriad of different flavours, there are believed to be only four primary tastes; sweet, sour, bitter and salty.

Various parts of the tongue have taste buds that are especially sensitive to one of the basic sensations of taste. You taste salty and sweet mainly on the front of the tongue, sour on the sides and bitter at the back. The middle of the tongue registers almost no taste. As a matter of interest, there is a substance that will register sweet on the tip of the tongue and bitter by the time it reaches the back, this is *"saccharin"*.

Taste is highly individual. This means that different people will be attracted to different foods and flavour, part of the explanation being heredity. Some genes make the receptors for bitterness especially sensitive. In these people, saccharin is likely to produce a strong sensation of bitterness. Each person's saliva has its own special taste, which in turn effects the taste of the food. If, for example, your saliva has a low sodium content, food containing a given amount of salt would taste saltier to you than to another person whose saliva is high in sodium.

THE TEETH

There are thirty-two permanent teeth in the adult human body. Deciduous teeth start to appear at about six months, by the age of three the child has about twenty teeth. Between the ages of six and twelve the deciduous teeth are shed and replaced by permanent teeth. A further six teeth and molars will appear. By the age of 25 a total of 32 teeth should be present. 8 Incisors, 4 canine, 8 premolars (or bicuspids) and 12 molars.

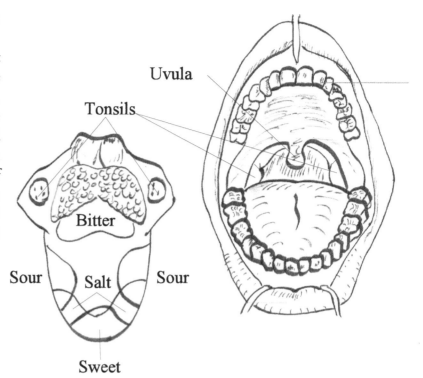

The tooth consists of three parts:

The crown:
This consists of a dense mineral or enamel surrounding the hard dentine, which has a soft centre called *"the pulp"*. This is filled with blood vessels, lymphatics and the nerves, which reach it through the root canal.

Neck:
The neck adheres to the gum.

The root:
The root penetrates the bone, where it is held in place by a ligament and cementum.

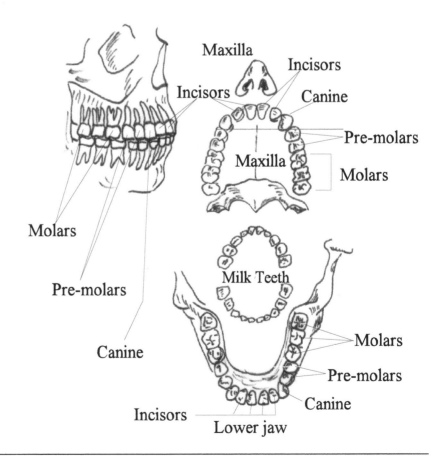

SALIVARY GLANDS

There are three pairs of salivary glands;

1.   The parotid glands, found in front of and a little below the ears. You may have become familiar with this gland when you were a child as these were the glands that swelled when you had mumps, swollen or not these are the largest salivary glands.

2.   The sublingual glands, situated just below the tongue, are smaller than the parotid glands, about the size of a walnut.

3.   The submandibular glands, situated below the mandible, are the smallest of the salivary glands.

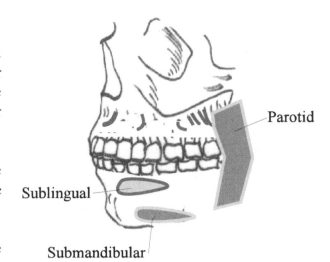

The salivary glands produce secretions containing the starch-reducing enzyme, ptyalin which helps in the digestion of cooked starches.

To help you get a clear picture of what saliva does, try chewing on a piece of dry bread, paying attention to the way it tastes. When it develops a sweet flavour, you will know that your saliva has begun to convert the complex starch molecules in the bread to a mixture of simple sugars, glucose and maltose. This is accomplished by a digestive enzyme known as salivary amylase, or ptyalin. Of course, saliva does a lot more than just break down starches into sugars, because without saliva you would find it very difficult to swallow. The mucus in saliva adheres to food and moistens it during chewing to enable it to slide easily down the oesophagus. Another function of saliva is to help keep the mouth healthy because it is also mild germicide, saliva kills bacteria, especially the kind that causes so much tooth decay.

From the mouth the food then passes into the pharynx which is a muscular tube with seven openings. These are:

1.   The mouth
2.   The oesophagus
3.   The larynx
4 & 5.   Two posterior apertures of the nose
6 & 7.   Two auditory (eustachian) tubes from the ear

From the pharynx the food passes into the oesophagus, which is a muscular tube lined with mucous membrane and covered with fibrous tissue. From here, the food passes into the stomach.

THE STOMACH

The stomach is a muscular sac. Its size and shape varying with its contents and muscular tone. When it has no food in it, it is shaped like a "j"; when it is full, it takes the shape of a boxing glove. When filled to capacity, the average stomach can hold up to 1.5 litres of food.

The stomach presents two curvatures, the greater and lesser curvature and for the purpose of description, is divided into three parts;

1. The cardiac portion
2. The body
3. The pyloric

The openings into the stomach are guarded by circular bands of muscle, like purse strings. The cardiac sphincter muscles at the top end, and the pylorus sphincter muscle at the other end. The cardiac sphincter prevents acid and ingested food from backing up and the pylorus sphincter muscle prevents food from leaving the stomach prematurely.

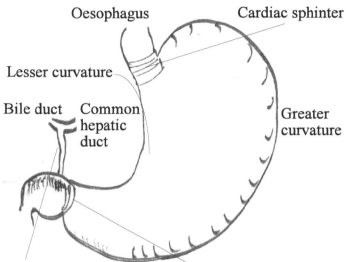

Each ball of food, or bolus, enters the part of the stomach called the fundus and pushes food previously eaten down and out towards the stomach walls.

The fundus and the main body of the stomach serve as a storage area, holding food until it is time for it to move along to the antrum and the duodenum pronounced "*du-o-dee-num*".

The stomach has three coats or coverings;
     1. The outer coat of serous membrane
     2. The middle muscular coat
     3. The inner mucous membrane

The inner mucous membrane is arranged in folds or rugae, which disappear when the stomach is distended. The membrane is lined with glands which produce gastric juice. This contains the enzymes pepsin (responsible for protein digestion) and rennin (responsible for the curdling of milk) as well as hydrochloric acid.

The middle layer contains a network of blood vessels that nourish the structure, as well as nerves that activate glands and muscles.

The outer or third layer are the muscles that move food, and in certain parts of the system, soften it and mix it with chemicals. This last layer is also a protective covering.

The hydrochloric acid the stomach secretes is corrosive enough to dissolve a razor blade or annihilate living cells. Sometimes it actually eats into the stomach itself and creates ulcers. Usually, however, the stomach remains impervious to attack.

First, the gastric lining is coated with mucus, which forms a barrier between the acid and the stomach and the stomach walls. The mucus, somewhat alkaline, neutralises the acid and thus helps to keep the stomach from digesting itself. Furthermore, the stomach lining sheds cells at the rate of half a million a minute and replaces them so rapidly that the stomach has what amounts to a new lining every three days. Even if hydrochloric acid does damage the cells, the stomach makes repairs automatically.

SMALL INTESTINE

From the stomach the food passes into the small intestine, the first part of this being the duodenum which is about ten inches long and shaped like a letter "c". As food enters the duodenum from the stomach, it stimulates four different organs to release the chemicals needed to finish digestion. There are:

1. The small intestine pours forth mucus to protect the duodenum from damage by gastric acid. It also produces hormones that stimulate the liver, pancreas and gall bladder to release digestive substances.
2. The gallbladder stores and releases bile.
3. The pancreas produces an alkaline juice to neutralize acid.
4. The liver, described later in this lesson.

The remainder of the small intestine comprises the "jejunum", pronounced *"je-joo-num"*, which is about eight feet long and the ilium which is about twelve feet long. The inner coat of the small intestine is comprised of mucous membrane arranged in folds known as valvulae conniventes, and unlike the rugae of the stomach these folds do not disappear with the distension of the intestines.

The mucous membrane is covered with minute finger-like projections known as villi, each villi contains a lacteal for the absorption of fat, and a capillary loop for the absorption of sugar and protein.

This mucous membrane also contains intestinal glands which produce a secretion known as succus entericus which contains enzymes for the digestion of proteins and sugars. The mucous membrane is studded with lymphatic nodes and in the latter part of the small intestine, which is known as the ilium, groups of these nodules are found and are known as peyers patches.

The function of these peyers patches is to fight infection. The small intestine then merges with the large intestine which although wider than the small intestine, is much shorter, being in total, 5-6 feet long.

THE LARGE INTESTINE

For the purpose of this description, the large intestine is divided into nine parts. Starting with the caecum into which the ilium opens, the opening being guarded by the ileo-caecal valve which allows on-flow but prevents back-flow of intestinal contents.   Then we have the vermiform appendix, which is about three inches in length and terminates in a blind end.

Next, there is the ascending colon which passes up the right side of the abdomen to bend sharply at the right hepatic flexure to the transverse colon, the left splenic flexure and the descending colon which goes down the left side of the abdomen to the sigmoid colon *(flexure);* and the rectum which is five to six inches long, the exit of which, guarded by two sphincter muscles, known as the anus.

<u>DIAGRAM OF THE LARGE INTESTINE</u>

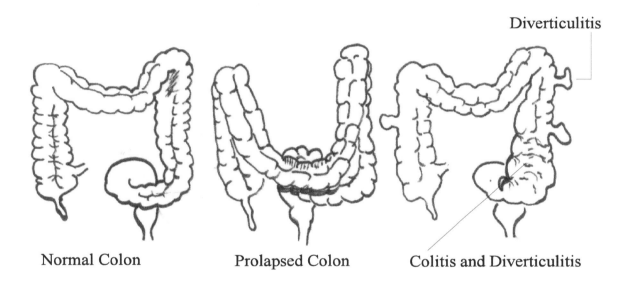

Diverticulitis

Normal Colon   Prolapsed Colon   Colitis and Diverticulitis

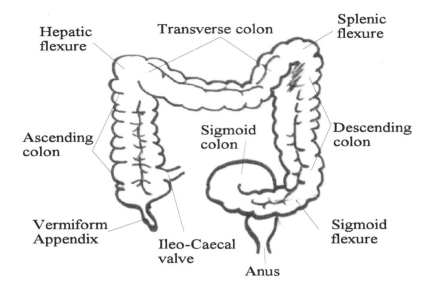

Hepatic flexure

Transverse colon

Splenic flexure

Ascending colon

Sigmoid colon

Descending colon

Vermiform Appendix

Ileo-Caecal valve

Anus

Sigmoid flexure

Having examined the alimentary canal it is necessary to look at the supporting organs of digestion.

THE LIVER

The liver is situated in the right hand side of the body just below the diaphragm. This is really a gland and is the largest organ in the body. It measures about ten to twelve inches across and six to seven inches from back to front, weighing approximately three and a half pounds. Protected by the rib cage, it is divided into two lobes, the large right lobe and the smaller left lobe overlaying the stomach where it joins the oesophagus.

DIAGRAM OF THE LIVER

The right lobe is much larger than the left, and is subdivided into three sections. The liver can function even if as much as 90% of it was removed. If the liver were destroyed by disease, the only hope for survival would be a liver transplant. Because of its many functions, it is unlikely that a machine could do all of its work. The liver is one of the few organs capable of repairing itself to be fully functional again, given time and a change in lifestyle.

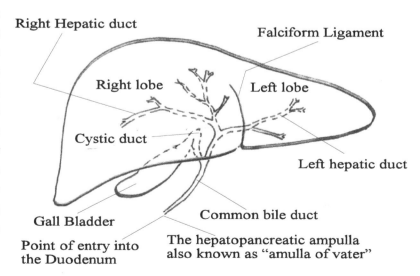

Right Hepatic duct

Falciform Ligament

Right lobe

Left lobe

Cystic duct

Left hepatic duct

Gall Bladder

Common bile duct

Point of entry into the Duodenum

The hepatopancreatic ampulla also known as "amulla of vater"

The liver has many functions, one of these is the formation of bile, which it produces up to two pints a day. This passes along to the gall bladder which is a muscular pear shaped sac about three inches long. Its function is to store bile and to concentrate it, which it does by eight to ten times, then as and when required , the bile passes out of the gall bladder into the duodenum. The Vitamins A, B, E, and K are stored in the liver. All but the "B" vitamins are soluble in fats and are therefore absorbed into the body with fatty materials.

The detergent action of bile in the small intestine breaks down these fats, along with the vitamins, into suspended globules that are absorbed through the intestinal wall and get into the blood via lymph vessels. Without bile, the body would be deficient in its vital stockpile of vitamins.

It's worth noting that a healthy liver removes a yellow pigment called "bilirubin" from the blood, converts it to a form which can be excreted into bile, and eliminates it from the body. A diseased liver, however, cannot do that, so the pigment remains in the bloodstream, and the skin and the whites of the eyes take on the yellowish tinge called "jaundice". It's interesting to note that when people talk about *"yellow jaundice"*, they are repeating themselves, because the term *"jaundice"* is derived from the word that means "yellow". Bilirubin is a waste product from the destruction of worn-out red blood cells. Under normal conditions, it gives the stool its characteristic colour. When a person has jaundice, the urine and the tears darken, but the stool becomes lighter.

It has already been seen that the liver manufactures bile but it has a variety of other functions. It is a powerful detoxifying organ, breaking down many kinds of toxic molecules and rendering them harmless. It is a reservoir for blood, a storage organ for some vitamins and particularly for digested carbohydrates in the form of glycogen which it releases to sustain blood and sugar levels. It manufactures enzymes, cholesterol, proteins, vitamin *"A"* from carotene, blood coagulation factors and other elements.

Bile is a complex fluid containing amongst other things bile salts and bile pigments. The pigment is derived from the disintegration of red blood cells and it is these which give the yellow brown colour to faeces which is excreted, while the bile salts are reabsorbed and reused. The salts promote efficient digestion of fats by a detergent action which gives very fine emulsification of fatty materials.

PANCREAS

The *Greek* name pancreas, means *"all flesh" or "all meat"* the pancreas is a cream coloured gland, 6-8 inches long and about 1 ½ inches wide. Resembling a fish, with a large head and a long tail, the pancreas extends across the body, behind the stomach, in the upper left side of the abdomen. The larger end of it rests next to the duodenum. The function of the pancreas is to secrete enzymes and hormones, including insulin, that are needed for the digestion and absorption of food. Insulin is manufactured by cells known as the islets of langerhans, which are scattered like little islands throughout the pancreas.

The pancreas is sometimes described as two organs in one:
- ▸ The exocrine cells of the pancreas secrete digestive enzymes into the duodenum;
- ▸ The endocrine cells release two hormones, glucagon and insulin, into the blood.

Glucagon acts in exactly the opposite way to insulin. While both hormones govern the level of glucose in the blood stream, glucagon is secreted in response to glucose deficiency. If there is insufficient response by this hormone, the result is hypoglycaemia.

Insulin regulates the utilization of glucose in the body. All body tissues except the brain require insulin for the absorption of glucose. If the pancreas fails to produce insulin, or secretes it in insufficient quantities, the result is a serious disease called diabetes mellitus.

A duct running the length of the organ, collects pancreatic juice and passes it to the duodenum at the same point that the common bile duct passes in bile.

The islets of langerhans are specialised cells of the pancreas which produce insulin. This passed into the general circulation and controls carbohydrate metabolism.

During the process of digestion, the larger particles of protein, carbohydrates, and fats must be reduced in size and converted into simpler substances to enable them to be absorbed through the walls of the digestive tract and into the blood stream. Proteins are converted to peptones and polypeptides which are then converted into amino acids.

Similarly, carbohydrates must be reduced, the large particles, starches or polysaccharides, are reduced to disaccharides which in turn are reduced to monosacharides. Fats are split into their component parts, fatty acids and glycerine. It should be noted that with one or two exceptions, there is no absorption of food elements until they reach the intestine where fatty acids and glycerine pass into the lacteals of the villi and amino acids into the capillary blood vessels. Fatty products are conveyed into the lymphatic system entering the systemic circulation via the thoracic duct. Amino acids and simple sugars are carried by the portal veins to the liver.

The movement of food along the digestive tract is made possible by wave-like muscular contractions known as peristalsis, the action is from the outside of the digestive tubes inwards and downwards, so that the food is forced further along the tube.

The stomach, being a muscularly controlled sac, is always on the move. It might be compared with an old fashioned milk churn where the food is pushed around and around until it is well and truly mixed with gastric juice which is a mixture of enzymes in hydrochloric acid.

As we have already seen, the stomach has a pyloric valve at the point where it merges with the small intestine. The function of this valve is to control the releases of the partially digested food material into the small intestine. Watery foods, such as soup, leave the stomach quite quickly whilst fats remain in the stomach longer. On average, an ordinary mixed diet meal is emptied from the stomach in 3-6 hours.

Terminology

Ampulla of vater: Point at which the common bile and pancreatic ducts enter the duodenum.

Amylase: Enzyme that converts starch into maltose.

Anal sphincter: Circular muscle at the end of the digestive tract.

Appendix: Small finger-like protuberance from the caecum.

Bile duct: Conveys bile from the cystic and hepatic ducts to the bile duct and into the duodenum at the ampulla of vater.

Bile-pigments: Dark-coloured substance formed by the breakdown of red blood cells.

Bile salts: Complex salts excreted by the liver that help in the emulsification of intestinal fats.

Bilirubin: Principal bile pigment.

Enterogastrone: Hormone secreted by the duodenum to slow down the gastric action.

Erepsin: Duodenal enzyme to break peptones into amino-acids.

Gastrin: Hormone produced by the stomach to maintain the gastric secretions.

Glycogen: Simple form of starch that can be broken down into glucose.

Glycogon: Hormone secreted in response to low glucose level of blood.

Ileo-caecal valve: Valve that allows the chyme to pass from the terminal ileum into the caecum but not return.

Insulin: Glucose-controlling hormone secreted by the pancreas.

Maltase: Duodenal enzyme to reduce sugar to glucose.

Pepsin: Gastric enzyme that splits protein into peptones.

Rennin: Gastric enzyme that curdles milk.

Trypsin: Pancreatic enzyme that splits peptones and proteins into amino-acids.

Urea: Nitrogen containing substance formed from ammonia by the liver.

Common Diseases or Disorders

Disease or Disorder	APPENDICITIS
Description	This is an acute inflammation of the vermiform appendix. A distended and inflamed appendix may rupture, in which case it produces toxic materials and can cause peritonitis which is an acute inflammation of the abdomen. The inflammation is caused by an obstruction such as a hard mass of faeces or a foreign body in the lumen of the appendix, fibrous disease of the bowel wall, an adhesion, or a parasitic infestation. The most common symptom is constant pain in the lower right quadrant of the abdomen. The patient often feels intermittent pain in the mid-abdomen and gets relief by bending the knees and waist into the fetal position. Vomiting and a low-grade fever of 99degs.-102degs., an elevated white blood count, rebound tenderness, and a rigid abdomen are accompanying symptoms.
Possible Allopathic Treatment	Appendectomy, within 24 - 48 hours of the first symptoms, delay may result in rupture and peritonitis as faecal matter is released. The fever will rise sharply once peritonitis begins.
Possible Holistic Aromatherapy Treatment	Seek medical attention immediately, if after treatment or surgery and hospitalization is not required, but if symptoms persist try - Anti-spasmodic essential oils like; *Aniseed, Basil, Bergamot, Black Pepper, Cajeput, Chamomile, Clary-Sage, Coriander, Cypress, Fennel, Ginger, Hyssop, Jasmine, Juniper, Lavender, Marjoram, Melissa, Orange, Peppermint, Patchouli, Pettitgrain, Rosemary, Thyme.* Anti-inflammatory essential oils like; *Caraway, Teatree, Camphor, Chamomile, Fennel, Geranium, Jasmine, Peppermint, Benzoin, Frankincense, Myrrh and Patchouli.* Mixed with Pain-killing analgesic oils like; *Bergamot, Cajeput, Coriander, Eucalyptus, Lemon-grass, Niaouli, Black-pepper, Chamomile, Jasmine, Lavender, Marjoram, Peppermint, Rosemary and Ginger.* In some cases Auto-immune enhancers like; *Cinnamon leaf, Clove bud, Frankincense.*

Disease or Disorder	PERITONITIS
Description	An inflammation of the peritoneum often produced by either bacteria or an irritating substance introduced into the abdominal cavity via a penetrating wound or perforation or rupture of an organ in the Gastro-Intestinal tract or the reproductive tract. The most common cause is a rupture of the veriform appendix or perforations in the Colon due to diverticulitis. Secondary causes are peptic ulcers, gangrenous gallbladder, gangrenous obstructions of the small bowel, ruptures of the spleen, liver, ovarian cyst, or fallopian tube.
Possible Allopathic Treatment	The patient is hospitalised and placed in a bed in a semi-Fowler's position with knees flexed to facilitate breathing and localize pus in the lower abdomen. Oxygen, parenteral fluids with electrolytes, antibiotics and emetics are administered as ordered. Surgery is usually delayed until the patient is stabilized. Patients who respond to antibiotics receive a liquid diet.
Possible Holistic Aromatherapy Treatment	Only after conventional allopathic treatment has been attempted should holistic treatment be considered... Anti-spasmodic essential oils like; *Aniseed, Basil, Bergamot, Black Pepper, Cajeput, Chamomile, Clary-Sage, Coriander, Cypress, Fennel, Ginger, Hyssop, Jasmine, Juniper, Lavender, Marjoram, Melissa, Orange, Peppermint, Patchouli, Pettitgrain, Rosemary, Thyme.* Anti-inflammatory essential oils like; *Caraway, Teatree, Camphor, Chamomile, Fennel, Geranium, Jasmine, Peppermint, Benzoin, Frankincense, Myrrh and Patchouli.* Mixed with Pain-killing analgesic oils like; *Bergamot, Cajeput, Coriander, Eucalyptus, Lemon-grass, Niaouli, Black-pepper, Chamomile, Jasmine, Lavender, Marjoram, Peppermint, Rosemary and Ginger.* In some cases Diuretic essential oils could prove useful: *Bergamot, Caraway, Eucalyptus, Lemon, Thyme, Black-pepper, Camphor, Cypress, Fennel, Geranium, Hyssop, Juniper, Lavender, Marjoram, Pine, Rosemary, Benzoin, Cedarwood, Frankincense, Patchouli and Sandalwood.* Anti-depressant essential oil like; *Basil, Bergamot, Lemongrass, Clary Sage, Geranium, Jasmine, Lavender, Melissa, Orange Blossom, Patchouli, Rose, Sandalwood and Ylang Ylang.* Warming (Rubefacients) essential oils like; *Bergamot, Eucalyptus, Thyme, Black Pepper, Camphor, Juniper, Lavender, Peppermint, Pine and Ginger.* Auto-immune enhancers like; *Cinnamon leaf, Clove bud, Frankincense.*

Disease or Disorder	CIRRHOSIS OF THE LIVER
Description	Cirrhosis of the liver is the breakdown of normal liver tissue that leaves non-functioning scar tissue surrounding areas of functioning liver tissue. There are several types of cirrhosis of the liver but portal cirrhosis is by far the most common. This is also referred to gin drinkers liver, or alcoholic liver. It is usually caused by exposure to poison which can include such substances as carbon tetrachloride and phosphorous but, by far the most common cause is the ingestion of alcohol. This makes the liver leathery and produces on its normally smooth surface, nodules varying in size from a pin head to a bean which gives it a hobnailed appearance. Other common causes are nutritional deprivation and hepatitis. The symptoms are nausea, fatigue, anorexia, weight loss, ascites, varicosities and spider angiomas.
Possible Allopathic Treatment	Treatment depends on the etiology. The liver has remarkable regenerator abilities, but recovery is slow.
Possible Holistic Aromatherapy Treatment	Anti-inflammatory essential oils like; *Caraway, Teatree, Camphor, Chamomile, Fennel, Geranium, Jasmine, Peppermint, Benzoin, Frankincense, Myrrh and Patchouli.* Mixed with Pain-killing analgesic oils like; *Bergamot, Cajeput, Coriander, Eucalyptus, Lemon-grass, Niaouli, Black-pepper, Chamomile, Jasmine, Lavender, Marjoram, Peppermint, Rosemary and Ginger.* In some cases Diuretic essential oils could prove useful: *Bergamot, Caraway, Eucalyptus, Lemon, Thyme, Black-pepper, Camphor, Cypress, Fennel, Geranium, Hyssop, Juniper, Lavender, Marjoram, Pine, Rosemary, Benzoin, Cedarwood, Frankincense, Patchouli and Sandalwood.* Anti-depressant essential oil like; *Basil, Bergamot, Lemongrass, Clary Sage, Geranium, Jasmine, Lavender, Melissa, Orange Blossom, Patchouli, Rose, Sandalwood and Ylang Ylang.* Warming (Rubefacients) essential oils like; *Bergamot, Eucalyptus, Thyme, Black Pepper, Camphor, Juniper, Lavender, Peppermint, Pine and Ginger.* Auto-immune enhancers like; *Cinnamon leaf, Clove bud, Frankincense.*

Disease or Disorder	JAUNDICE
Description	Jaundice is normally evidenced by the yellowness of the skin, mucus membranes and sclerae of the eyes, caused by an excess of bile pigments known as bilirubin in the circulatory system. It may occur when the outflow of the bile has been blocked and when the liver becomes obstructed. A large portion of the bile which is produced by the liver is absorbed directly into the blood stream, as it cannot flow normally out of the bile duct into the duodenum. Persons with jaundice may also experience nausea, vomiting, abdominal pain and dark urine. Jaundice is a symptom of many disorders related to the liver.
Possible Allopathic Treatment	Useful diagnostic procedures include a clinical evaluation of the signs & symptoms, tests of liver function, and techniques for direct or indirect visualization ie. X-Ray, Cat scan, Ultra-sound, endoscopy or exploratory surgery and biopsy.
Possible Holistic Aromatherapy Treatment	Seek medical attention straight away, to assist allopathic treatment during recovery try... Anti-inflammatory essential oils like; *Caraway, Teatree, Camphor, Chamomile, Fennel, Geranium, Jasmine, Peppermint, Benzoin, Frankincense, Myrrh and Patchouli.* Mixed with Pain-killing analgesic oils like; *Bergamot, Cajeput, Coriander, Eucalyptus, Lemon-grass, Niaouli, Black-pepper, Chamomile, Jasmine, Lavender, Marjoram, Peppermint, Rosemary and Ginger.* In some cases Diuretic essential oils could prove useful: *Bergamot, Caraway, Eucalyptus, Lemon, Thyme, Black-pepper, Camphor, Cypress, Fennel, Geranium, Hyssop, Juniper, Lavender, Marjoram, Pine, Rosemary, Benzoin, Cedarwood, Frankincense, Patchouli and Sandalwood.* Anti-depressant essential oil like; *Basil, Bergamot, Lemongrass, Clary Sage, Geranium, Jasmine, Lavender, Melissa, Orange Blossom, Patchouli, Rose, Sandalwood and Ylang Ylang.* Auto-immune enhancers like; *Cinnamon leaf, Clove bud, Frankincense.*

Disease or Disorder	ACUTE PANCREATITIS
Description	If the pancreas protein-digesting enzymes are activated while in the pancreas, they are powerful enough to digest the pancreas itself. This condition, known as acute pancreatitis, can occur if the pancreatic duct is obstructed and the digestive enzymes are forced to accumulate in the pancreas. When this happens, the substances that normally inhibit the activation of the enzymes are overwhelmed, and the pancreas may be damaged or even destroyed by its own juices. Acute pancreatitis is generally the result of damage to the biliary tract, such as by alcohol, trauma, infectious disease, or certain drugs. Characterized by severe abdominal pain radiating to the back, fever, anorexia, nausea and vomiting.
Possible Allopathic Treatment	Treatment includes nasogastric suction to remove gastric secretions. To prevent stimulation of the pancreas, nothing is given by mouth. Intravenous fluids and electrolytes are administered and nonmorphine derivatives are given to relieve pain.
Possible Holistic Aromatherapy Treatment	Seek medical attention first, to aid in recovery try... Anti-spasmodic essential oils like; *Aniseed, Basil, Bergamot, Black Pepper, Cajeput, Chamomile, Clary-Sage, Coriander, Cypress, Fennel, Ginger, Hyssop, Jasmine, Juniper, Lavender, Marjoram, Melissa, Orange, Peppermint, Patchouli, Pettitgrain, Rosemary, Thyme.* Anti-inflammatory essential oils like; *Caraway, Teatree, Camphor, Chamomile, Fennel, Geranium, Jasmine, Peppermint, Benzoin, Frankincense, Myrrh and Patchouli.* Mixed with Pain-killing analgesic oils like; *Bergamot, Cajeput, Coriander, Eucalyptus, Lemon-grass, Niaouli, Black-pepper, Chamomile, Jasmine, Lavender, Marjoram, Peppermint, Rosemary and Ginger.* In some cases Anti-depressant essential oil like; *Basil, Bergamot, Lemongrass, Clary Sage, Geranium, Jasmine, Lavender, Melissa, Orange Blossom, Patchouli, Rose, Sandalwood and Ylang Ylang.* Warming (Rubefacients) essential oils like; *Bergamot, Eucalyptus, Thyme, Black Pepper, Camphor, Juniper, Lavender, Peppermint, Pine and Ginger.* Auto-immune enhancers like; *Cinnamon leaf, Clove bud, Frankincense.*

Disease or Disorder	HEARTBURN (PYROSIS)
Description	This is a common symptom of gastric distress consisting of a burning sensation which extends up into the oesophagus from the base of the sternum and is quite often felt to rise into the throat and may be accompanied by a sour belch. Heartburn is usually caused by the reflux of gastric contents into the esophagus but may be caused by gastric hyper-acidity or peptic ulcer.
Possible Allopathic Treatment	Anti-acids relieve the symptoms but do not cure the heartburn
Possible Holistic Aromatherapy Treatment	After a medical doctor has diagnosed the problem you could attempt to help the recovery by using... Anti-inflammatory essential oils like; *Caraway, Teatree, Camphor, Chamomile, Fennel, Geranium, Jasmine, Peppermint, Benzoin, Frankincense, Myrrh and Patchouli.* Mixed with Pain-killing analgesic oils like; *Bergamot, Cajeput, Coriander, Eucalyptus, Lemon-grass, Niaouli, Black-pepper, Chamomile, Jasmine, Lavender, Marjoram, Peppermint, Rosemary and Ginger.* In some cases Anti-depressant essential oil like; *Basil, Bergamot, Lemongrass, Clary Sage, Geranium, Jasmine, Lavender, Melissa, Orange Blossom, Patchouli, Rose, Sandalwood and Ylang Ylang.* Warming (Rubefacients) essential oils like; *Bergamot, Eucalyptus, Thyme, Black Pepper, Camphor, Juniper, Lavender, Peppermint, Pine and Ginger.* Auto-immune enhancers like; *Cinnamon leaf, Clove bud, Frankincense.*

Disease or Disorder	HEPATITIS
Description	Hepatitis, or inflammation of the liver, characterized by jaundice, hepatomegaly, anorexia, abdominal and gastric discomfort, abnormal liver function, clay-coloured stools, and tea-coloured urine. Hepatitis is sometimes caused by alcohol or by certain drugs or chemicals, bacterial or viral infection, parasitic infestation, but in many instances it is the result of one kind of three viruses, known as type A, type B and non-A, non-B. That awkward designation for the third virus comes from the fact that the specific agents have yet to be identified, doctors only know that it isn't either A or B. Hepatitis 'C' (non-A, non-B) A type of hepatitis transmitted largely by blood.
Possible Allopathic Treatment	Regardless of type, viral hepatitis results in a common set of symptoms, which include fever, headache, sore throat, nausea, aching joints and muscles, loss of appetite, weakness, pain in the upper right abdomen, and jaundice. NOTE: Do not massage any person with a contagious disease. This disease can still be contracted after many years from the recovery date.
Possible Holistic Aromatherapy Treatment	Because of the number of incidents concerning misdiagnoses, Unless you are medically trained, or fully understand the Hepatitis family and its inherent problems. Do-not treat.

Disease or Disorder	HEPATITIS A
Description	Primarily a disease of young adults or children is spread through faecally contaminated food, water or contaminated objects. Although victims may feel miserable, the illness almost never has lasting consequences. A form of infectious viral hepatitis caused by the hepatitis "A" virus. Also called acute infective hepatitis. Prophylaxis with immune globulin is effective in household and sexual contacts.
Possible Allopathic Treatment	Regardless of type, viral hepatitis results in a common set of symptoms, which include fever, headache, sore throat, nausea, aching joints and muscles, loss of appetite, weakness, pain in the upper right abdomen, and jaundice. NOTE: Do not massage any person with a contagious disease. This disease can still be contracted after many years from the recovery date.
Possible Holistic Aromatherapy Treatment	Because of the number of incidents concerning misdiagnoses, Unless you are medically trained, or fully understand the Hepatitis family and its inherent problems. Do-not treat.

Disease or Disorder	HEPATITIS B
Description	A form of viral hepatitis caused by the hepatitis B virus. The virus is transmitted in contaminated serum in blood transfusion, sexual contact with an infected person, or by contaminated needles and instruments. The infection may be severe and result in prolonged illness, destruction of liver cells, cirrhosis, or death. On the other hand is caused by chronic liver inflammation in about 10% of all patients and can be serious for the elderly or those in poor health. Serum hepatitis, as this ailment used to be called, is transmitted through blood transfusions, injections with unsterile needles, or intimate contact (body fluids, saliva, semen or tears).
Possible Allopathic Treatment	Regardless of type, viral hepatitis results in a common set of symptoms, which include fever, headache, sore throat, nausea, aching joints and muscles, loss of appetite, weakness, pain in the upper right abdomen, and jaundice. NOTE: Do not massage any person with a contagious disease. This disease can still be contracted after many years from the recovery date.
Possible Holistic Aromatherapy Treatment	Because of the number of incidents concerning misdiagnoses, Unless you are medically trained, or fully understand the Hepatitis family and its inherent problems. Do-not treat.

Disease or Disorder	DIVERTICULITIS
Description	Inflammation of small pouches, called "diverticula" on the colon. If faecal matter penetrates through the thin wall of the diverticula it will cause inflammation and possible abscess formation in the tissues surrounding the colon. During this period the lumen of the colon often narrows and may become obstructed. The patient will experience crampy pain, particularly over the area of the sigmoid colon, fever, and leucocytosis are also present.
Possible Allopathic Treatment	Barium enemas and proctoscopy are performed to rule out carcinoma of the colon, (which exhibits many of the same symptoms). Non-invasive treatment may include, bed rest, intravenous fluids, antibiotics and nothing taken by mouth. In acute cases, bowel resection of the affected part greatly reduces mortality and morbidity.
Possible Holistic Aromatherapy Treatment	Anti-spasmodic essential oils like; *Aniseed, Basil, Bergamot, Black Pepper, Cajeput, Chamomile, Clary-Sage, Coriander, Cypress, Fennel, Ginger, Hyssop, Jasmine, Juniper, Lavender, Marjoram, Melissa, Orange, Peppermint, Patchouli, Pettitgrain, Rosemary, Thyme.* Anti-inflammatory essential oils like; *Caraway, Teatree, Camphor, Chamomile, Fennel, Geranium, Jasmine, Peppermint, Benzoin, Frankincense, Myrrh and Patchouli.* Mixed with Pain-killing analgesic oils like; *Bergamot, Cajeput, Coriander, Eucalyptus, Lemon-grass, Niaouli, Black-pepper, Chamomile, Jasmine, Lavender, Marjoram, Peppermint, Rosemary and Ginger.* In some cases Anti-depressant essential oil like; *Basil, Bergamot, Lemongrass, Clary Sage, Geranium, Jasmine, Lavender, Melissa, Orange Blossom, Patchouli, Rose, Sandalwood and Ylang Ylang.* Warming (Rubefacients) essential oils like; *Bergamot, Eucalyptus, Thyme, Black Pepper, Camphor, Juniper, Lavender, Peppermint, Pine and Ginger.* Auto-immune enhancers like; *Cinnamon leaf, Clove bud, Frankincense.*

Disease or Disorder	DUODENAL ULCER
Description	More commonly referred to as peptic ulcer. Ulceration of the stomach or first part of the duodenum from excessive acid in the stomach or inadequate resistance to acids of the mucosal lining. Ulcers may be acute or chronic. Acute lesions are almost always multiple and superficial. Chronic ulcers are deep, single, persistent and symptomatic. The muscular coating of the stomach wall does not regenerate; during healing a scar will form permanently marking the site. Ulcers are caused by a variety of poorly understood or misunderstood factors, that include, excessive secretion of gastric acid, inadequate protection of the mucus membrane, stress, heredity, and the taking of certain drugs including corticosteroids, anti-hypertensive and anti-inflammatory medication.
Possible Allopathic Treatment	Short term symptomatic relief is provided with antacids and frequent, small, simple meals. Haemorrhage may be caused by perforation of the muscle and blood vessels and often requires surgical resection of the damaged area. The diagnosis and evaluation of peptic ulcers involve serial X-rays using a contrast medium and endoscopy.
Possible Holistic Aromatherapy Treatment	Anti-spasmodic essential oils like; *Aniseed, Basil, Bergamot, Black Pepper, Cajeput, Chamomile, Clary-Sage, Coriander, Cypress, Fennel, Ginger, Hyssop, Jasmine, Juniper, Lavender, Marjoram, Melissa, Orange, Peppermint, Patchouli, Pettitgrain, Rosemary, Thyme.* Anti-inflammatory essential oils like; *Caraway, Teatree, Camphor, Chamomile, Fennel, Geranium, Jasmine, Peppermint, Benzoin, Frankincense, Myrrh and Patchouli.* Mixed with Pain-killing analgesic oils like; *Bergamot, Cajeput, Coriander, Eucalyptus, Lemon-grass, Niaouli, Black-pepper, Chamomile, Jasmine, Lavender, Marjoram, Peppermint, Rosemary and Ginger.* In some cases Anti-depressant essential oil like; *Basil, Bergamot, Lemongrass, Clary Sage, Geranium, Jasmine, Lavender, Melissa, Orange Blossom, Patchouli, Rose, Sandalwood and Ylang Ylang.* Warming (Rubefacients) essential oils like; *Bergamot, Eucalyptus, Thyme, Black Pepper, Camphor, Juniper, Lavender, Peppermint, Pine and Ginger.* Auto-immune enhancers like; *Cinnamon leaf, Clove bud, Frankincense.*

Disease or Disorder	GASTRITIS
Description	Acute inflammation of the stomach that may be due to chemical irritation or infection that occurs in two forms; acute and chronic. Acute gastritis, may be caused by severe burns, major surgery, aspirin or other anti-inflammatory agents, corticosteroids, drugs, food allergens, viral, bacterial, or chemical toxins. The symptoms of anorexia, nausea, vomiting and discomfort after eating, usually abate after the causative agent has been removed. Chronic gastritis may occur if the irritation is continued for a long period, and is usually a sign of an underlying disease, such as peptic ulcer, stomach cancer, severe peptic ulceration (zollinger-Ellison syndrome), or pernicious anaemia. Differential diagnosis is by endoscopy with biopsy.
Possible Allopathic Treatment	If torrential bleeding occurs the reported mortality rate is 60%. Surgical intervention with low recovery effects. Anti-secretory ulcer drugs, vasoconstrictors and coagulation medication have proven useful. Acute onset is a happier picture, prevention and/or early treatment before bleeding is a problem will increase the probability of recovery.
Possible Holistic Aromatherapy Treatment	Only treat after conventional medicine has been exhausted or during recovery, oils that may prove useful are... Anti-spasmodic essential oils like; *Aniseed, Basil, Bergamot, Black Pepper, Cajeput, Chamomile, Clary-Sage, Coriander, Cypress, Fennel, Ginger, Hyssop, Jasmine, Juniper, Lavender, Marjoram, Melissa, Orange, Peppermint, Patchouli, Pettitgrain, Rosemary, Thyme.* Anti-inflammatory essential oils like; *Caraway, Teatree, Camphor, Chamomile, Fennel, Geranium, Jasmine, Peppermint, Benzoin, Frankincense, Myrrh and Patchouli.* Mixed with Pain-killing analgesic oils like; *Bergamot, Cajeput, Coriander, Eucalyptus, Lemon-grass, Niaouli, Black-pepper, Chamomile, Jasmine, Lavender, Marjoram, Peppermint, Rosemary and Ginger.* In some cases Anti-depressant essential oil like; *Basil, Bergamot, Lemongrass, Clary Sage, Geranium, Jasmine, Lavender, Melissa, Orange Blossom, Patchouli, Rose, Sandalwood and Ylang Ylang.* Warming (Rubefacients) essential oils like; *Bergamot, Eucalyptus, Thyme, Black Pepper, Camphor, Juniper, Lavender, Peppermint, Pine and Ginger.* Auto-immune enhancers like; *Cinnamon leaf, Clove bud, Frankincense.*

Disease or Disorder	HAEMORRHOIDS
Description	Venous distension in the anal area causing dilation of the blood vessels and swelling of the mucosa overlying them. Internal haemorrhoids originate above the internal sphincter of the anus. If they become large enough to protrude from the anus, they may become constricted and painful. Small internal haemorrhoids often bleed with defecation. External haemorrhoids appear outside the anal sphincter. They are usually not painful, and bleeding does not occur unless a haemorrhoidal vein ruptures or thromboses.
Possible Allopathic Treatment	Treatment includes local applications of a topical medication to lubricate, anaesthetize, and shrink the haemorrhoids, sitz baths and cold or hot compresses are also soothing. As a last resort surgery may be necessary.
Possible Holistic Aromatherapy Treatment	Vasoconstrictors like, camomile, cypress and rose. Anti-inflammatory essential oils like; *Caraway, Teatree, Camphor, Chamomile, Fennel, Geranium, Jasmine, Peppermint, Benzoin, Frankincense, Myrrh and Patchouli.* Mixed with Pain-killing analgesic oils like; *Bergamot, Cajeput, Coriander, Eucalyptus, Lemon-grass, Niaouli, Black-pepper, Chamomile, Jasmine, Lavender, Marjoram, Peppermint, Rosemary and Ginger.* In some cases Anti-depressant essential oil like; *Basil, Bergamot, Lemongrass, Clary Sage, Geranium, Jasmine, Lavender, Melissa, Orange Blossom, Patchouli, Rose, Sandalwood and Ylang Ylang.*

Disease or Disorder	MUMPS
Description	Virus infection of the salivary glands that may also involve the pancreas. Swelling of the parotid glands caused by paramyxovirus. Normally it effects children between 5-15 years of age. Adults that are infected react severely. The mumps paramyxovisus lives in the saliva of the effected individuals and is transmitted in droplets or by direct contact. The virus is present in the saliva from 6 days before to 9 days after the onset of the swelling of the parotid glands. The disease sometimes involves complications, such as arthritis, pancreatitis, myocarditis, oophoritis, and nephritis. About one half of the men with mumps suffer some atrophy of the testicles, sterility rarely results. Symptoms include, anorexia, headache, malaise, low grade fever, earache, parotid gland swelling and a temperature of 101 - 104 degrees F.
Possible Allopathic Treatment	Respiratory isolation and analgesics, antipyretics and plenty of fluids
Possible Holistic Aromatherapy Treatment	Anti-inflammatory essential oils like; *Caraway, Teatree, Camphor, Chamomile, Fennel, Geranium, Jasmine, Peppermint, Benzoin, Frankincense, Myrrh and Patchouli.* Auto-immune enhancers like; Cinnamon leaf, Clove bud, Frankincense. Mixed with Pain-killing Analgesic oils like; *Bergamot, Cajeput, Coriander, Eucalyptus, Lemongrass, Niaouli, Black-pepper, Chamomile, Jasmine, Lavender, Marjoram, Peppermint, Rosemary and Ginger.* In some cases Anti-depressant essential oil like; *Basil, Bergamot, Lemongrass, Clary Sage, Geranium, Jasmine, Lavender, Melissa, Orange Blossom, Patchouli, Rose, Sandalwood and Ylang Ylang.*

Disease or Disorder	ULCERATIVE COLITIS
Description	Colitis is an inflammatory condition of the large intestine, with symptoms of diarrhea, bleeding and ulceration of the mucosa of the intestine, weight loss and pain. Ulcerative colitis is a chronic episode of colitis with increased symptomology.
Possible Allopathic Treatment	Diagnosis is based on clinical signs, barium X-Ray of the colon and colonoscopy with biopsy. Steroids, fluids, electrolytes, antibiotics are used with colitis and chronic ulcerative colitis may be treated with corticosteroids and anti-inflammatory agents. Surgery may be an option if drug therapy is ineffective
Possible Holistic Aromatherapy Treatment	Anti-spasmodic essential oils like; *Aniseed, Basil, Bergamot, Black Pepper, Cajeput, Chamomile, Clary-Sage, Coriander, Cypress, Fennel, Ginger, Hyssop, Jasmine, Juniper, Lavender, Marjoram, Melissa, Orange, Peppermint, Patchouli, Pettitgrain, Rosemary, Thyme.* Anti-inflammatory essential oils like; *Caraway, Teatree, Camphor, Chamomile, Fennel, Geranium, Jasmine, Peppermint, Benzoin, Frankincense, Myrrh and Patchouli.* Auto-immune enhancers like; *Cinnamon leaf, Clove bud, Frankincense.* Mixed with Pain-killing Analgesic oils like; *Bergamot, Cajeput, Coriander, Eucalyptus, Lemon-grass, Niaouli, Black-pepper, Chamomile, Jasmine, Lavender, Marjoram, Peppermint, Rosemary and Ginger.* In some cases Anti-depressant essential oil like; *Basil, Bergamot, Lemongrass, Clary Sage, Geranium, Jasmine, Lavender, Melissa, Orange Blossom, Patchouli, Rose, Sandalwood and Ylang Ylang.* Warming (Rubefacients) essential oils like; *Bergamot, Eucalyptus, Thyme, Black Pepper, Camphor, Juniper, Lavender, Peppermint, Pine and Ginger.*

Essential Oils

CARAWAY

Latin name: *carum carvi*   Botanical family: *Umbelliferae*

Three main areas where this oil can help:

1. Digestive tonic
2. Respiratory disorders
3. Bruising

Properties	Uses
Digestive *(to promote or aid digestion)*	Flatulence, gastric spasms, stomach disorders, appetite stimulant, diarrhea
Expectorant *(helps promote the removal of mucous from the respiratory system)*	Bronchitis, pleurisy, bronchial asthma
Stimulant *(helps promote the removal of mucous from the respiratory system)*	Lethargy, circulatory stimulant, fatigue, mental fatigue

Place of Origin
Caraway *(carum carvi)* grows to a height of about two feet with fern-like leaves. It develops small, curved brown fruits with tufted pink/white flowers. Caraway originates in Holland, Russia and N. Europe, though it is now a native of Asia.

Method of Extraction
The essential oil is distilled from the seeds and sometimes the dried fruit of the herb. Its colourless with a strong, sweet spicy odour. The main constituents are carvone, limonene, and aldehydes.

Traditional Uses
An old spice dating back as far as the Stone Age, it is believed the name comes from the Arabic term *"Karawya"*, which is still used in the East. Caraway is used in bread making as an aromatic ingredient as well as for its carminative properties.

Herbal Medicine
A powerful antiseptic commonly used for the relief of toothaches. It is valued digestive remedy. It will help soothe stomach and digestive problems such as flatulence, indigestion, stomach spasms and nervous dyspepsia.

Aromatherapy

Stomach problems respond well with the use of caraway. It will soothe the stomach and aid digestion, while helping such complaints as gastric spasms, diarrhea, pain, and flatulence. It is known to stimulate the appetite, potentially finding use for those suffering from anorexia nervosa.

The expectorant properties make this oil useful with bronchitis, bronchial asthma, coughs, laryngitis or other respiratory disorders that require an antispasmodic effect in relation to breathing difficulties. It is used in cases of vertigo due to its ability to help balance the inner ear.

Warning: *This oil may irritate sensitive skin. Use with caution.*

CLOVE

Latin name: *eugenia caryophyllata*   Botanical family: *Myrtacae*

Three main area where this oil can help:

1.   Gum infections or toothache
2.   Digestive problems
3.   Cancer treatment

Properties   Uses

Digestive *(to promote or aid digestion)*	Diarrhea, intestinal spasms, dyspepsia, flatulence
Analgesic *(to deaden pain)*	Toothache, rheumatism, arthritis, headaches, gum infections
Expectorant *(helps promote the removal of mucous from the respiratory system)*	Asthma, bronchitis, pleurisy, tuberculosis
Antimicrobial/antiviral	Scabies, intestinal worms, measles
Stimulant *(an agent which quickens the physiological functions of the body)*	Mental fatigue, loss of concentration, impotence, frigidity

Place of Origin
Essential oil of clove *"eugenia caryophyllata"* is a small evergreen tree with grey leaves and a smooth bark. It grows in the Moluccas, Reunion, the Antilles, and Madagascar.

Method of Extraction
The essential oil of clove is obtained from the buds or leaves of the tree. After being dried naturally, they are then steam distilled. The scent is a sweet but spicy warming fragrance. The principal known constituents are eugenol, acteugenol, methyl alcohol, methyl salicylate, furfurol, pinene, vanillin, and caryophyllene.

Traditional Uses
Historically, clove was the most expensive of all the spices. In ancient Chinese medical writing, cloves are one of the earliest medicinal spices mentioned. It has a history of use during the Plague and during the times other infectious illnesses. Its antiseptic properties have been used in the prevention of contagious diseases and epidemics.

Herbal Medicine

Clove is said to contain one of the most powerful germicidal agents in the herb kingdom. It increases blood circulation and promotes digestion. This herb is used for relieving toothache, especially pain from infection and nerve exposure.

Aromatherapy

Antibacterial and antiviral in nature, clove prevents contagion which explains its extensive historical usage to combat plagues. It is good for respiratory problems such as colds, asthma bronchitis and pleurisy. It has been proven effective against tuberculosis. Very valuable to utilize *(in a vapourizer)* as a germicide or bactericide and prevent the spreading of disease

The use of cloves proves beneficial to digestive problems. It also eases nausea and combats bad breath-especially that which is due to gastric fermentation. Essential oil of clove is effective against vomiting, flatulence, intestinal spasms, diarrhea and parasites.

Considered a stimulant, clove will help dispel mental fatigue or help improve concentration. It has an uplifting effect especially when one is feeling tired and lethargic

For aromatherapy purposes, only clove bud oil should be used

Warning: *Contraindicated during pregnancy. Possible skin irritant.*

PEPPERMINT

Latin name: *mentha piperita*   Botanical family: *Labiatae*

Three main areas where this oil can help:

      1.   Upset stomachs and diarrhea
      2.   Migraines and headaches
      3.   Influenza

Properties	Uses
Stomachic *(digestive aid and tonic, improving appetite)*	Colic, diarrhea, dyspepsia, gall stones, gastralgia, halitosis, nausea, vomiting, constipation, food poisoning, travel sickness, sluggish digestion, indigestion
Expectorant *(helps promote the removal of mucous from the respiratory system)*	Bronchitis, asthma, colds, influenza, sinusitis, pneumonia, dry coughs, sinusitis, allergies
Stimulant *(an agent which quickens the physiological functions of the body)*	Fainting, mental fatigue, shock, dizziness
Analgesic *(an agent which quickens the physiological functions of the body)*	Headaches, migraines, aches and pains, rheumatism
Nervin *(strengthening and toning to the nerves and the nervous system)*	Neuralgia, nervous disorders, paralysis, palpitations, vertigo, hysteria, depression

Place of Origin
A native of the Mediterranean, peppermint is cultivated in many parts of the world including Italy, USA, Japan, and Great Britain, The USA produces more oil than any other country in the world, but the European oils are regarded as being superior in quality to any other oil. This is due to the fact that the plant prefers a damp climate.

Method of Extraction
Mentha piperita, or peppermint essential oil is steam distilled from the leaves and the flowering tops. The plant grows to approximately 3 feet in height and has serrated leaves with purple flowers. The active ingredients of peppermint oil include menthol, mentone, limonene, menthene and phellandrene.

Traditional Uses
Greek mythology tells a tale of Mint who was once the nymph called Mentha, whom Pluto found extremely attractive. Persephone, his jealous wife, pursued Mentha and trod her into the ground. Pluto then changed Mentha into a delightful herb.

A popular tonic for the past few thousand years, peppermint has been used in the East. Derived from the Latin term of *"menthe"* meaning thought, the Romans considered it a tonic for the brain.

Herbal Medicine
Popularly used for many different types of stomach complaints, due to its strengthening abilities, peppermint is said to help with nausea, vomiting, nausea and flatulence. It is anti-spasmodic in nature which will assist in relieving pains in the alimentary canal.

Aromatherapy
As with herbal medicine, the use of peppermint is beneficial in the treatment of digestive and stomach disorders. This essential oil has the ability to relax the muscles of the digestive tract and stimulate bile flow. It proves useful for a variety of complaints including indigestion, nausea *(all types ie: travel sickness, morning sickness, etc.)*, vomiting, colic, flatulence and diarrhea.

It helps to break up gallstones, has a detoxifying effect on the liver and may also be good for kidney stones. Remember to use it well diluted on the abdomen and massage it in a clockwise direction only.

Due to its high amount of menthol, it is cooling and serves as an analgesic. Colds and flu respond well with the treatment of peppermint essential oil. It offers a cooling effect especially in feverish conditions. Simultaneously, peppermint induces sweating which in turns helps alleviate fevers in a natural way.

Respiratory disorders such as asthma, bronchitis, sinusitis and coughs show improvement either through the use of steam inhalation or topical applications in the chest and/or sinus areas. Steaming can also assist with problems like acne, by decongesting the skin and through the antiseptic effect, help control bacteria found on the skin. *(Only use a single drop when steaming due to the strength of this essential oil.)*

Headaches and migraines respond well to peppermint. The cephalic properties will stimulate the brain and clear thinking. It is excellent for the treatment of mental fatigue, shock, nervousness and fainting.

External application on the breast will relieve the problem of curdled or congested milk and prevent infection.

Rats and mice, ants and cockroaches show a strong dislike to the odour of peppermint. This makes a pleasant and safe alternative to poisons, posing no risk what-so-ever to either pets or young children.

Warning:
1)   *The use of peppermint may antidote homeopathic remedies.*
2)   *Do not use peppermint in the evening as it is a stimulant and can cause alertness. It is unwise to use over long periods, as it may cause disturbance of a normal sleep pattern.*

PETITGRAIN

Latin name: *citrus vulgaris*   Botanical name: *Rutacae*

Three main areas where this oil can help

    1.   Anti-spasmodic within the digestive system
    2.   Antidepressant
    3.   Skin problems

Properties	Uses
Antidepressant *(helps alleviate depression)*	Depression, sadness, grief
Sedative *(reduces functional activity, calming)*	Anxiety, insomnia, tachycardia
Antispasmodic *(to prevent or ease muscle spasm or convulsions)*	Muscle spasms, digestive complaints, flatulence, gastric problems
Deodorant *(corrects, masks or removes unpleasant odours)*	Acne, skin care, eczema, dermatitis, pimples

Place of Origin
Essential oil of petitgrain is obtained from the bitter orange tree *(citrus bigaradia)* which also gives us neroli. There is similarities between the two essential oils. The best petitgrain comes from the Mediterranean region, like other citrus oils. A cheaper grade is imported from Paraguay. A good petitgrain oil has a fresh, flowery if somewhat earthy or woodsy aroma.

Method of Extraction
Petitgrain essential oil is steam distilled from the leaves and young twigs, but in the earlier centuries the oil was extracted from the small unripe oranges, picked when they were still green and very small. *(No bigger than a cherry)*. Hence, came the name *"petit grains"* meaning small grains.   Uneconomical to produce, while also creating a shortage of the mature fruit, the old name was gradually transferred to the oil from the leaves and the twigs. Chemically it shares many of the constituents of neroli but contains higher portions of linalol and linalyl acetate.

Herbal Use
There is no herbal use associated with petitgrain other than as herbal tea.

Aromatherapy

A safe, non-toxic essential oil, petitgrain is very similar to neroli, but has a gentler response to problems and at a fraction of the price.

A tonic to the nervous system, it calms anxiety, especially that which is accompanied by rapid heart beat. Insomnia responds well. Apply a drop to the pillow at night to ease tension and help obtain a good nights sleep.

Calming on both the mind and body, relief is found during periods of sadness, anger, disappointment and depression.

Its antispasmodic properties will aid gastric problems like flatulence, dyspepsia, and digestive problems by calming the stomach muscles.

Petitgrain possesses deodorant properties making it popular in the bath to help refresh the body. As a skin tonic it shows promise in the treatment of pimples, acne and eczema and dermatitis.

Question and Answer Sheets

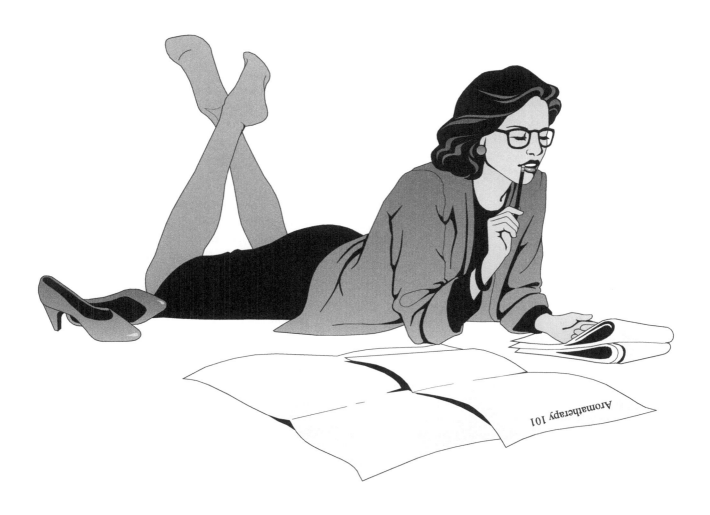

Please keep the questions for review.
Circle the correct answer/s on the Answer Sheets at the back of the book and
<u>return these sheets only</u> to your instructor.

Questions - Lesson #3

1. Essential oils break down into what chemical constituents?
a. Terpenes
b. Alcohols
c. Crystals
d. Phenols
e. Aldeloids
f. Aldehydes
g. Acids
h. Esteroxides
I. Esters
j. Oxides
k. Alcoterpines
l. Lactones

2. What three main industries use essential oils other than aromatherapists?
a. Food industries
b. Pharmaceutical industries
c. Agriculture industries
d. Perfume industries
e. Clothing industries

3. All essential oils are?
a. Anti-fungal
b. Anti-bacterial
c. Anti-septic
d. Anti-spasmodic

4. What does biotic mean?
a. Strengthens the neurological system whilst killing bacteria
b. Strengthens living tissue whilst killing bacteria
c. Strengthens living tissue whilst killing diseases
d. Strengthens living tissue whilst killing insects

5. There are two essential oils that are of animal origin?
a. Deer
b. Musk
c. Amber
d. Ambergris
e. Camel
f. Clove

6. Name the common properties of essential oil?
a. are volatile and evaporate quickly
b. Soluble in alcohol
c. Partially soluble in water

d. Soluble in carrier oils
e. Unsuitable for soaps
f. All of the above

7. Top notes are?
a. Light fragrant oils that are often used for acute problems and evaporate quickly
b. Are calming and stimulating, balancing
c. Heavy, strong smelling oils that are used for chronic problems and evaporate slowly

8. Middle notes are?
a. Light fragrant oils that are often used for acute problems and evaporate quickly
b. Are calming and stimulating, balancing
c. Heavy, strong smelling oils that are used for chronic problems and evaporate slowly

9. Base notes are?
a. Light fragrant oils that are often used for acute problems and evaporate quickly
b. Are calming and stimulating, balancing
c. Heavy, strong smelling oils that are used for chronic problems and evaporate slowly

10. Name two absolutes?
a. Jasmine
b. Orange
c. Rosemary
d. Rose
e. Frankincense
f. Myrrh

11. Name two resinoids?
a. Jasmine
b. Orange
c. Rosemary
d. Rose
e. Frankincense
f. Myrrh

12. Name three methods of obtaining essential oils?
a. Steam
b. Mulching
c. Pressing
d. Enfleurage
e. Centrifugal extraction
f. Microwave extraction
g. Soft earth and clay method

13 What part of the plant is used to obtain essential oil of caraway?
a. the flowering tops
b. the seeds and dried fruit
c. the leaves and buds
d. the roots

14. What three main areas will caraway help most?
a. bruises
b. menstrual problems
c. digestive tonic
d. headaches
e. respiratory disorders

15. What do you have to be careful of when using caraway?
a. during pregnancy
b. people want to drink it
c. skin and mucous membrane irritant
d. sensitive skin irritant

16. What three main areas will clove help most?
a. bruises
b. menstrual problems
c. digestive tonic
d. gum infections or tooth-ache
e. cancer treatment

17. What two things do you have to be careful of when using clove?
a. during pregnancy
b. people want to drink it
c. skin and mucous membrane irritant
d. sensitive skin irritant

18. What part of the plant is used to obtain essential oil of clove?
a. the flowering tops
b. the rind of the fruit
c. the leaves and buds
d. the wood

19. What three main areas will peppermint help most?
a. bruises
b. menstrual problems
c. upset stomach and diarrhoea
d. headaches and migraine
e. respiratory disorders and influenza

20. What do you have to be careful of when using peppermint?
a. will antidote homeopathic remedies

b. people want to drink it
c. causes wakefulness and disturbed sleep patterns
d. sensitive skin irritant

21. What part of the plant is used to obtain essential oil of peppermint?
a. the leaves & flowering tops
b. the rind of the fruit
c. the leaves and young twigs
d. the wood

22. What three main areas will petitgrain help most?
a. anti-spasmodic for digestive system
b. headaches
c. skin healing
d. depression and anxiety
e. tonic to the body

23. What do you have to be careful of when using petitgrain?
a. people want to drink it
b. skin irritant
c. during pregnancy
d. no contra-indications noted

24. Describe in your own words the purpose of the digestive system?

25. How long does it take for a meal to be converted from solids to semi-solids in the stomach?
a. 2 - 4 hours
b. 3 - 6 hours
c. 5 - 7 hours
d. 4 - 6 hours

26. Which organ of digestion controls the rate at which the stomach moves food along?
a. a sphincter
b. the duodenum
c. the esophagus

27. When the stomach is full, which hormone is released to speed up digestion?
a. pepsin
b. bromelin
c. gastrin

28. Associated with the digestive system are five other related organs, they are?
a. the liver
b. the tongue
c. the large intestine
d. the teeth
e. the salivary glands
f. the appendix
g. the pancreas

29. What are the four functions of the mouth?
a. to break up food by chewing
b. to assist in breathing
c. to lubricate food with saliva
d. to communicate
e. to assist in regulating body temperature
f. to consciously initiate swallowing

30. The upper surface of the tongue is covered with papillae, of which there are three forms, they are?
a. filiform
b. folioform
c. fungiform
d. vallate
e. valioform

31. There are believed to be only four primary tastes, they are:
a. hot
b. sweet
c. sour
d. cold
e. bitter
f. salty

32. How many teeth are there in the average adult?
a. 24
b. 36
c. 30
d. 32

33. There are three pairs of salivary glands, they are:
a. carotid glands
b. parotid glands
c. sublingual glands
d. bicuspid glands
e. submandibular glands

34. The pharynx is muscular tube with 7 openings, they are?
a. the mouth

b. two at the back of the nose
c. the sacrum
d. the larynx
e. the two eustachian tubes
f. the oesophagus
g. the ilium

35. From the pharynx food passes into which organs of digestion?
a. the stomach
b. the duodenum
c. the oesophagus

36. The stomach is divided into three parts, they are?
a. the body
b. the serous
c. the cardiac
d. the hiatus
e. the pyloric

37. The stomach has three coats or coverings, they are?
a. the outer coat of serous membrane
b. the inner tripe membrane
c. the inner mucous membrane
d. the middle muscular coat
e. the middle acid coat

38. Which type of acid is secreted into the stomach?
a. sulphuric acid
b. hydrochloric acid
c. mephanimic acid

39. What keeps the stomach from digesting itself?
a. the liquid we take in with food
b. the constant intake of liquids and solids
c. the mucous lining, which is alkaline, coats the gastric lining

40. The duodenum is located where and is what shape?
a. at the base of the stomach and is a "C" shape
b. at the top of the stomach and is round
c. at the top of the stomach and is a "C" shape

41. The gallbladder secretes what?
a. gall
b. bile
c. digestive enzymes

42. The pancreas secretes what?
a. alkaline juices
b. hormones
c. mucus

43. The liver produces what?
a. vitamins A,B,E, and K
b. bile
c. fatty acids

44. What are villi?
a. part of the digestive system
b. a type of mucous membranes
c. finger-like projections in the small intestine

45. What is the function of "Peyers Patches"?
a. to fight infection
b. to break down proteins and sugars
c. to control movement of the small intestine

46. Name the four flexure points on the large intestine?
a. ilium flexure
b. appendix flexure
c. ascending flexure
d. ileo-caecal flexure
e. ascending flexure
f. hepatic flexure
g. duodenum flexure
h. transverse flexure
i. splenic flexure
j. descending flexure
k. descending flexure
l. sigmoid flexure
m. rectum flexure

47. Describe the liver.

48. Which vitamins are stored in the liver?
a. Vit A
b. Vit B
c. Vit D
d. Vit E
e. Vit C
f. Vit K

49. The liver removes a yellow pigment called?
a. bilirubin
b. jaundice
c. bile
d. beta carotene

50. If the liver is unable to remove the yellow pigment, what is the resulting illness called?
a. bilirubin
b. jaundice
c. bilious
d. carotenism

51. Describe the pancreas.

52. What do the islets of langerhans do?
a. manufactures peptones and polypeptides
b. manufactures amino acids
c. manufactures insulin
d. manufactures enzymes and hormones

53. What is diabetes mellitus?
a. excess blood sugar, too little insulin
b. excess insulin, too little blood sugar
c. excess blood pressure, too little insulin
d. excess insulin, insufficient growth hormone

54. What are proteins converted into?
a. red blood cells
b. peptones and polypeptides
c. energy
d. disaccharides

55. What is peristalsis?
a. the process of digestion in the large intestine
b. the movement of food through the small intestine
c. the wave like movements along the digestive tract
d. the process of converting sugar into glucose

56. Where would you find the pyloric valve?
a. at the top of the stomach where it merges with the small intestine
b. at the bottom of the stomach where it merges with the small intestine
c. at the joining of the small intestine to the large intestine
d. at the end of the digestive tract

57. Describe in your own words the meaning of the word "appendicitis".

58. What is the cause of cirrhosis of the liver?
a. a malfunction of the liver due to over exposure to toxic substances including alcohol
b. a malfunction of the liver due to over exposure to alcohol
c. a malfunction of the liver due to genetic misinformation
d. a breakdown of the liver due to over exposure to toxic substances including alcohol

59. What is jaundice?
a.   yellowed skin due to an excess of bile pigments in the circulatory system
b.   yellowed skin due to excess of carotenes in the circulatory system
c.   yellowed skin due to excess of melanin pigments in the circulatory system
d.   a very biased point of view

60. What is your understanding of the disorder called "hepatitis"?

61. What does enterogastrone do?
a.   slow down the gastric action
b.   speeds up the gastric action
c.   signals the stomach to release food
d.   signals that the stomach is full

62. What is the purpose of the ileo-caecal valve?
a.   it allows food to pass into the duodenum but not return to the stomach
b.   it allows chyme to pass into the ileum but not return to the duodenum
c.   it allows chyme to pass into the caecum but not return to the ileum
d.   it allows chyme to exit the body but not return to the rectum

63. What does insulin do?
a.   controls the glucose level in the blood stream
b.   controls the rate that sugar in converted into glucose
c.   controls the amount of gastric enzymes
d.   controls the conversion of peptones into amino acids

64. What is diverticulitis?
a.   inflammation of the branches of the digestive tract
b.   inflammation of small pouches on the colon
c.   inflammation of the lining of the stomach
d.   inflammation of the lining of the bowel

65. What is gastritis?
a.   acute inflammation of the branches of the digestive tract
b.   acute inflammation of small pouches on the colon
c.   acute inflammation of the lining of the stomach
d.   acute inflammation of the lining of the bowel

66. Label the diagram of the digestive tract.
(SEE ANSWER SHEET FOR DIAGRAM)

Answer Sheet - Lesson #3

(Keep the questions for review. Circle the correct answer/s and return these sheets only to your instructor.)

1. A   B   C   D   E   F   G   H   I   J   K   L

2. A   B   C   D   E

3. A   B   C   D

4. A   B   C   D

5. A   B   C   D   E   F

6. A   B   C   D   E   F

7. A   B   C

8. A   B   C

9. A   B   C

10. A   B   C   D   E   F

11. A   B   C   D   E   F

12. A   B   C   D   E   F   G

13. A   B   C   D

14. A   B   C   D   E

15. A   B   C   D

16. A   B   C   D   E

17. A   B   C   D

18. A   B   C   D

19. A   B   C   D   E

20. A   B   C   D

21. A   B   C   D

22. A   B   C   D   E

23. A   B   C   D

24. _____

_____

_____

25. A   B   C   D

26. A   B   C

27. A   B   C

28. A   B   C   D   E   F   G

29. A   B   C   D   E   F

30. A   B   C   D   E

31. A   B   C   D   E   F

32. A   B   C   D

33. A   B   C   D   E

34. A   B   C   D   E   F   G

35. A   B   C

36. A   B   C   D   E

37. A   B   C   D   E

38. A   B   C

39. A   B   C

40. A   B   C

41. A   B   C

42. A   B   C

43. A   B   C

44. A   B   C

45. A   B   C

46. A   B   C   D   E   F   G   H   I   J   K   L   M

47. _____

_____

48.   A   B   C   D   E   F

49.   A   B   C   D

50.   A   B   C   D

51.   _____

      _____

      _____

      _____

52.   A   B   C   D

53.   A   B   C   D

54.   A   B   C   D

55.   A   B   C   D

56.   A   B   C   D

57.   _____

      _____

      _____

      _____

58.   A   B   C   D

59.   A   B   C   D

60.   _____

      _____

      _____

      _____

61.   A   B   C   D

62.   A   B   C   D

63.   A   B   C   D

64.   A   B   C   D

65.   A   B   C   D

66.   Label the diagram of the digestive tract

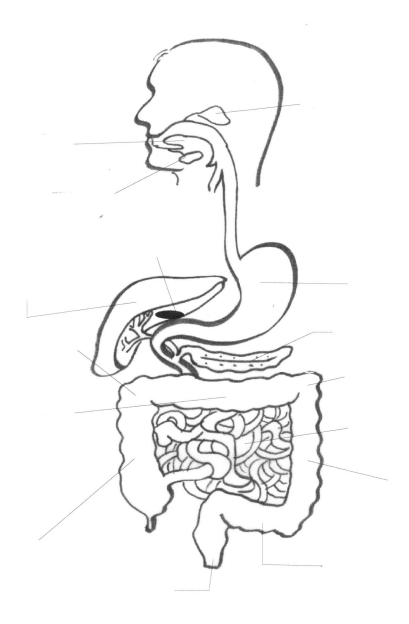

LESSON FOUR

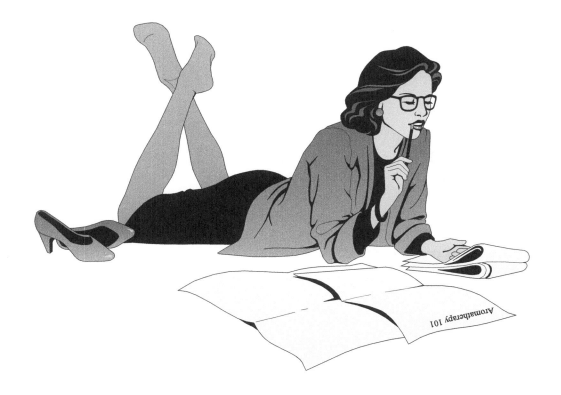

Lesson #4

Table of Contents

Aromatherapy Client Record Sheet

Therapist	Date	Case Number
Your name goes in here	Day of the first visit	Numerically expressed

Client's Name

The clients full name is entered here

Client's Address

The clients full postal address is entered here

D.O.B. Place the clients date of birth here	Tel: telephone number here, inc. area code

All month dates should be entered as a three letter word, ie. Jan, Feb, Mar, etc.

Occupation Job title   State if their job causes them to be active (mobile) or inactive

Medical History	Medication
Enter all medical information here, regarding hospitalization and ask if they have consulted a doctor about their problem.	Enter all medication taken here Enter all vitamins or diet supplements taken as well as allergies etc.

Medical History: Enter here all relevant information regarding the medical history that the client wishes to share with you. This information will also help you to build up the overall picture of the clients health problems. Ask questions eg: When was the last time you were in hospital? What was it for? What was the result? And does it effect you now? Repeat these questions again until you have exhausted the hospital history. Also ask, when was the last time you visited your doctor? What was it for? What was the result? And does it effect you now? Repeat these questions again until you have exhausted the visits that are relevant to their personal medical history with their doctor.

Medication: List all medication and at some later time refer to your books on prescribed drugs to learn about the side effects if any. All too often people come complaining about a health problem and the source could be the side effects experienced with new drugs. Also the information on the drugs as described will also give you a clearer picture into the health problems experienced by the client.

Ask the following questions:

Headaches		Sleep	
Bowel		Digestive	4 main food groups Yes or No
Reproductive		General Health	Energy level high or low

Headaches: Do you suffer from headaches?

If yes, how often, how severe? What makes them come and what makes them go? Would you consider them mild, moderate or severe?

Sleep: How do you sleep? Do you have interrupted sleep? What causes the interruption? Do you wake up tired? Do you have trouble getting off to sleep?

Bowel: Are you regular? Are you more prone to going too often or not enough?

Digestive: Are you eating the four main food groups? Are you drinking enough water? Do you have problems digesting fats? Do you have any food allergies? Do you suffer from any gas, bloating or stomach pain?

Reproductive: Are you pregnant? Is there any possibility that you might be pregnant? Are there any problems with your reproductive system that you know of?

General Health: How would you describe your general health today? Do you feel that your energy level is high or low?

Contra-indications: Have you suffered or do you suffer from any of the following; TB, HIV, epilepsy, hepatitis, dermatitis, high or low blood pressure, or any thing else that you would like to tell me? If they answer "Yes" ask them if they would like to disclose any information?

The remainder of the chart is completed by observation and body analysis, during the practical examination and assessment of the client.

Assessment

Headaches		Cellulite	High Med Low
Sleep		Lymph	Axillaries. Inguinal.
Bowel		Circulation	Feet Hand Legs
Digestive	4 main groups YES or NO	Respiratory	Thoracic / Abdominal / Deep or Shallow
Reproductive	Pregnant Y or No	Glands	neck Throat
General Health	High energy - Low energy	Eyes	Clear or Congested
Contra-Indications	Epilepsy Hepatitis HIV Dermatitis TB High/Low blood Cancer Other	Three Levels & Spine and posture	Shoulder Scapular Hips
Spine	C# T# L#	Sinus	Clear or Congested
Posture	Good or Poor	Arms	abnormalities
Test Lines	C T L	Skin	Norm-Oil Norm-Dry
Kidneys	L R		
Legs		Stress Level	High Medium Low

This area or block is designed to give you the therapist the standard fault-finding questions and observations to assist you in understanding your clients obvious and not-so obvious health care problems.

Posture: This is to ascertain if the discomfort they are experiencing is related to posture. A good description in this box will be of tremendous value as time goes on.

Spine: Checking the spine while standing allows us to assess the condition of the spine under normal daily stress. Note in this space if there appears to be any problem areas or abnormalities as far as you can discern.
C = cervical, T = thoracic, L = lumbar, # = to indicate the vertebrae involved.
Checking the spine while prone allows us to assess the condition of the spine while relaxed. Note in this space if there appears to be any problem areas or abnormalities as far as you can discern.

3 Levels: Checking the levels of the shoulders, scapula and pelvis we are able to determine much about the body by using the law of comparison.

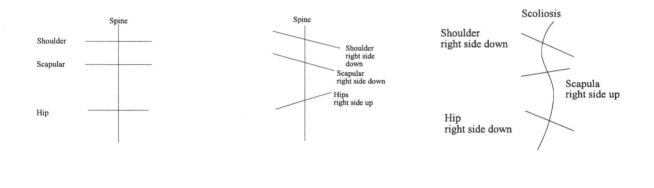

In perfect shape   Right sided problems   A mess

The above diagrams are a few suggested ways of expressing the rear view of the spine in relation to the three areas of postural concern, ie. Shoulders, scapula and hips.

Test Lines: Using the side of the nail on both thumbs, draw them firmly but gently down both sides of the spine without actually touching the spine itself. The resulting red-lines displayed will indicate the amount of free or congested areas on the back. This subject is covered more thoroughly during the practical part of the course.
C=cervical, T=thoracic, L=lumbar.

Kidneys: Check kidney area for tenderness by palpating

Legs: Check for bruises, thread-veins, muscle tone, skin condition, feet condition, mobility in knee and ankle joints.

Cellulite: Only required for ladies. Measure to your own standards, ie. high, medium or low.

Circulation: Test hands and feet. Cold feet do not indicate poor circulation, it may be that they have deep circulation which will cause the surface skin to be cool most of the time. The easiest way to check this is to apply pressure to the nails and observe the change of colour, if it changes colour quickly and returns to normal then it is safe to assume that the circulation is relatively good in that area. If it seems to take its time returning to normal then you should suspect a problem. Other reasons may include endocrine.

Eyes: Look for stress lines and anaemia. The eyes are the windows to the soul. In timeyou will learn a lot about the person just by looking into the eyes.

Skin: There are very few people with perfect skin. Normal to oily or normal to dry would be a good description.

Arms: Check the arms as you would the legs. People with respiratory problems, hay fever, asthma and emphysema normally have a marked roughness on the skin of the outer upper arm.

Lymph: Check the inguinal and axillary lymph nodes for congestion. If they are congested they will feel lumpy.

Sinus: Palpate the sinus area to assess any congestion.

Glands: Palpate the glands around the neck and throat to assess if they are swollen.

Respiratory: Observe respiration without making it obvious that this is what you are doing. Should the client realize that you are checking the rate of respiration they could change their normal breathing. Th= thoracic, Abdom= abdominal. Just circle two on the chart, ie. are they breathing deep or shallow, from the thoracic area or abdominal area.

Stress Level: The stress levels should be determined by the therapist. Theoretically you should not ask the client what these levels are. This should be assessed by you via observation of: muscle tone, lines in the face, eye condition, sleep patterns, bowel regularity, etc.

Spare Box: This should be used by you for any observation or complaint not covered.

Having assessed your client, you must decide which problems you are going to help, in order of priority. Stress is always treated as the main condition. You will need to choose the secondary and third condition in which to treat your client for.

List the oils in order of: TOP, MIDDLE AND BASE NOTES. Cross reference them and pick three oils to blend. Add this to the carrier of your choice. *(This is explained later and is taught in the video or during the practical portion of the course).*

Aromatherapy Student Client Record Sheet

Therapist	Date	Case Number
Client's Name in full		
Client's Address		
D.O.B.	Tel:	
Occupation:		Active or Inactive

Last visit/s to Doctor	Allergies	
Hospitalization	Vitamins	
Medical History	Medication	

Headaches	Cellulite	High	Med	Low
Sleep	Lymph	Axil.	Ing.	
Bowel	Circulation	Feet	Hands	
Digest (4 main groups Y or No)	Respiratory	Thor / Abdom - Deep /Shallow		
Reproductive (Pregnant Y or No)	Glands	Sub-mandib / Sub-clave		
General Health (Energy Level High or Low)	Eyes	Clear or Congested		
Contra-indications (Epilepsy, Hepatitis, Aids, Dermatitis, T.B., H/L blood, Cancer, Other)	Posture & Three levels of Spine	Shoulder, Scapular, Hips		
Spine (C# T# L#)	Sinus	Clear or Congested		
Test lines (C# T# L#)	Arms	Skin		
Kidneys (L R)	Skin	Normal-Oil, Normal-Dry		
Legs	Stress level	High, Medium, Low		

Main Condition | Secondary Condition | Third Condition
STRESS

TOP	MID	BASE	TOP	MID	BASE	TOP	MID	BASE
Bas	Cham	Ben						
Ber	Ger	C/w						
C/S	Hys	Frank						
Lem	Jun	Imm						
Mand	Lav	Jas						
Orang	Marj	Lind						
Pet	Mel	Myr						
Thym	Pep	Ner						
Yar	Pine	Pat						
	R/M	Rose						
	R/W	S/W						
		Vet						
		Y Y						

Please indicate.......... Acute Blend   Chronic Blend   Synergistic Blend

Essential Oils Chosen

Carrier Oil Added	Drops #	Drops #	Drops #
Grapeseed _____ ml	5% of		

Home Treatment Remarks

1. This is to acknowledge that I have been informed about the Aromatherapy treatment being offered and I fully understand and accept that this treatment is being performed by a student Aromatherapist.

2. I also agree to this information being stored and used as part of the mandatory case studies required by the above student and consent to the treatment offered.

3. I do not wish to have this personal information given to any other person or business and I understand that I may be contacted at some time from the school to verify that I did in fact receive a treatment from the above named Aromatherapy student therapist.

4. I also understand that the Aromatherapist performing this treatment is not a medical doctor, nor is he/she diagnosing, prescribing or replacing my family doctor.

5. I do not wish to have this personal information given to any other person or business and I understand that I may be contacted at some time from the school to verify that I did in fact receive a treatment from the above named student.

signed:_____   date:_____

Introduction to the Vascular System

This system which is sometimes called the circulatory system, consists of the heart, blood vessels, blood, lymphatic vessels and lymph.

The centre of the circulatory system, is the heart, which is a muscular organ that rhythmically contracts, forcing the blood through a system of vessels. The heart itself weighs approximately nine ounces (225 grammes) in a fully grown adult and lies one-third to the right and two-thirds to the left of the thoracic cavity. At birth it beats about 130 times a minute, at six years about 100 times a minute, reducing in adult life to between 65-80 beats a minute, giving an average of about 74.

During the 24 hour period, an adult human heart will pump about 9,000 litres of blood through approximately 12,000 miles of blood vessels.

THE HEART

The heart is encapsulated in a fibrous pericardium containing the serous pericardial sac, holding a small amount of fluid that allows frictionless movement.

The heart is divided into four chambers. These are the right and left atrium (*or auricles*). In the upper part of the heart, and the right and left ventricles in the lower part of the heart. The right side of the heart is divided vertically by a solid wall or septum, which prevents the venous blood in the right side from coming into contact or mixing with the arterial blood in the left side of the heart. The right side pumps deoxygenated blood through to the lungs, and the left side pumps oxygenated blood from the lungs. This is known as the systemic circulation (pulmonary circulation).

To keep the heart beating the *Sino-Atrial Node* located in the right atrium sends impulses through the two atria, causing atrial systole. It then stimulates the atrio-ventricular node to pass rapidly down a muscle called "The Bundle of His", to cause *ventricular systole*.

Circulation is divided into two principle systems, the general or systemic circulation and the pulmonary circulation. The systemic system has two particular branches - the portal and the coronary circulation - but for the purposes of this text we will confine ourselves to the two principle systems: the systemic and the pulmonary.

DIAGRAM OF THE HEART

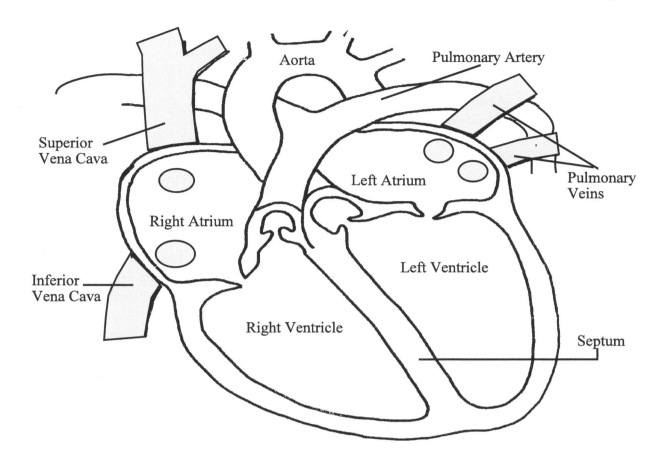

Blood vessels which proceed from the heart are known as arteries. These are hollow, elastic tubes which start off fairly large and gradually decrease in diameter as they spread throughout the body until they become known as arterioles and finally very fine hairlike blood vessels known as capillaries. The blood vessels which proceed towards the heart are known as veins. These are elastic tubes which have one way valves to prevent a backwards flow of the blood. The veins empty their contents through the inferior and superior venacava into the right hand side of the heart, first of all into the right atrium, from there it passes into the right ventricle. Then on through to the pulmonary artery into the lungs where it is re-oxygenated and then returned to the heart via the pulmonary veins into the left atrium and then into the left ventricle until finally, into the body, through the ascending and descending aortas.

The descending aorta divides into two iliacs. When the iliac reaches the groin it then becomes the femoral, passing underneath the knee when it becomes the popliteal. It further sub-divides into the anterior tibial and the posterior tibial, then to the dorsalis pedis and the plantar arches. The ascending aorta divides into two subclavian which then pass underneath the arm. In the armpit it becomes the axillary then the brachial for the length of the upper arm when it divides into the radial and ulna culminating in the palmer arches. When it reaches the subclavian junction another branch goes upwards through the common carotid (neck region) to the facial, temporal and occipital branches.

BLOOD

Blood is alkaline in pH. Its quantity amounts to something like six litres in the average adult. It is very complex in nature but has four principle constituent parts:

1.   Plasma
2.   Erythrocytes *(red blood cells)*
3.   Leucocytes *(white blood cells)*. Corpuscles is Latin for little bodies.
4.   Platelets

Plasma provides the liquid basis of the blood, this is a clear straw coloured liquid which holds various substances in solution. These include:
water, glucose, amino acids, mineral salts and enzymes, etc.

Erythrocytes are inert biconcave discs, that are made in the red bone marrow. They get their colour from haemoglobin which has the ability to absorb oxygen *(when it becomes oxy-haemoglobin, which is bright red in colour)* and carbon dioxide *(when it becomes carboxi-haemoglobin which becomes very dark red, bordering on a muddy brown colour)*. Their function is to carry oxygen from the lungs to the tissues and carbon dioxide from the tissues to the lungs during respiration. The average life span of an erythrocyte is 120 days. As they age, they lose their elasticity and are trapped in the small blood vessels, spleen and other organs. Their eventual disintegration takes place in the spleen, being finally completed in the liver.

DIAGRAM OF THE CIRCULATION SYSTEM

The arteries

Direction of circulation

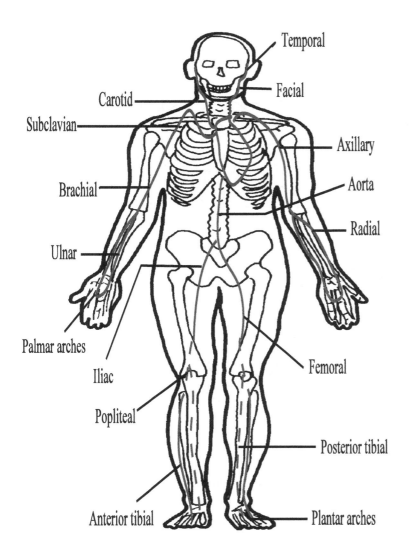

Temporal

Facial

Carotid

Subclavian

Axillary

Brachial

Aorta

Radial

Ulnar

Palmar arches

Iliac

Femoral

Popliteal

Posterior tibial

Anterior tibial

Plantar arches

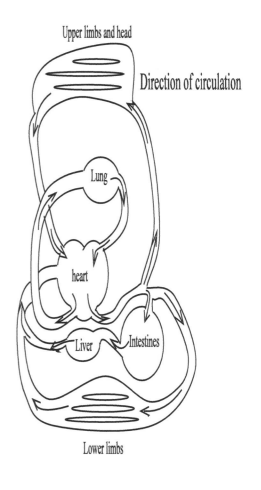

Upper limbs and head

Direction of circulation

Lung

heart

Liver   Intestines

Lower limbs

The following diagram shows the circulation of blood through the heart. This diagram is not drawn accurately. But this method of drawing makes it easier to understand.

THE CIRCULATION OF BLOOD THROUGH THE HEART

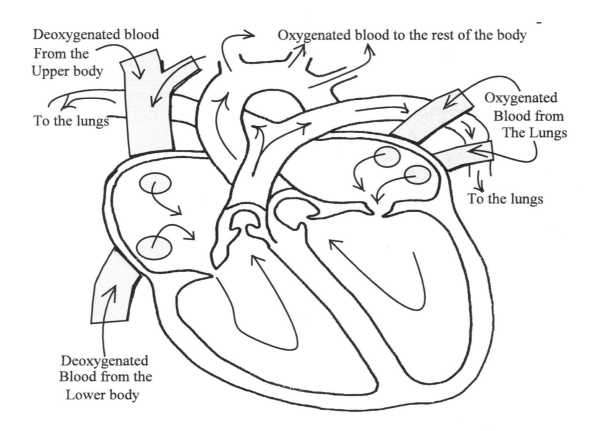

Deoxygenated blood From the Upper body

To the lungs

Oxygenated blood to the rest of the body

Oxygenated Blood from The Lungs

To the lungs

Deoxygenated Blood from the Lower body

In health, the erythrocytes total about five million per cubic millimetre of blood, which gives a total of somewhere in the region of 25 billion in a human adult. If these cells were placed end to end they would form a ribbon sufficiently long enough to encircle the world more than four times. These cells are the body's transporters, they carry food and oxygen to all parts of the body and on their return journey pick up waste products, primarily carbon-dioxide.

Leucocytes (phagocytes) or white corpuscles are larger than erythrocytes, have an irregular shape and a nucleus. They are produced in the bone marrow and, in health, they total about eight thousand per cubic millimetre. They act as the protectors or soldiers of the body. Their chief role being to protect the body against infection by their power of ingesting bacteria: A process which is known as phagocytosis.

When the body is subject to serious infection the leucocytes increase rapidly by a process of division known as mitosis.

Then we have platelets or thrombocytes. These average 250 thousand per cubic millimetre of blood, they are derived from large multinucleated cells in the bone marrow and are essential to the blood for coagulation, (clotting).

DIAGRAM OF VEIN VALVES

This diagram shows the open and
closed vein valves:

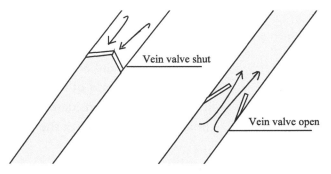

Veins convey blood to the heart

Vein valve shut

Vein valve open

BLOOD TYPES

The existence of human blood types was established by Karl Landsteiner in 1902, when he began a study to determine why fatalities occurred following some blood transfusions. He discovered that the cause was incompatibility between the blood of the donor and the blood of the recipient. Arising from this work came the Landsteiner classification of blood groups which classified blood into the four main blood types: "A;", "B", "AB", and "O".

Type "O" is sometimes called the universal donor because it may give blood to all blood types, but it can only receive from type "O".

On the other hand, type "AB" is sometimes called the universal recipient because it can receive from any group but can only give to the "AB" group.

Type "A" can give to both "A" and "AB" and receive only from blood types "A" and "O".
Type "B" can give to type "B" and "AB" and receive only from blood types "B" or "O".

In 1940 Landsteiner and A.S. Weiner, recognized the "Rh" (Rhesus) factor, a substance found in red blood cells. This was discovered during their experiments with Rhesus monkeys, hence the name Rhesus or an abbreviation for Rhesus (Rh). It is estimated that 85% of white people have a Rh positive factor and the other 15% are Rh negative. The presence or absence of antigen makes the individual either Rhesus positive or Rhesus negative. Antibodies are not found in Rhesus negative people.

Terminology

Angiology: The science of dealing with blood and lymph vessels.

Cholesterol: A major fat found in the blood and a constituent in animal fats and oils. There are different types of cholestrol found in the body. LDL (low density lipo-proteins) is considered a bad cholestrol and is present in many foods such as fast food and other modern day products. They increase the chances of hypertension and other cardio-vascular conditions. HDL (high density lipo-proteins) is considered s good choloestrol as it helps remove excess cholestrol off the sides of the arteries.

Coronary: Usually relating to the blood.

Diastolic pressure: Is the pressure measured during the relaxing phase of the cardiac cycle.

Haemorrhoids (piles):   Are dilated veins in the rectum and anus either internal or external.

Hypertension: A term relating to high blood pressure.

Hypotension: A term relating to low blood pressure.

Phlebitis: An inflammation of the vein walls, mostly found in the legs, which may lead to thrombo-phlebitis, which is a complication caused by an obstructing blood clot.

Systolic pressure: The pressure measured during the contraction phase of the cardiac cycle.

Thrombus: A clot of blood found within the heart or blood vessels.

Endocarditis: Inflammation of the heart lining, usually the valves.

Pericarditis: Inflammation of the pericardium.

Atrial fibrillation: Irregular, rapid heart beat due to disorder of the Sino-Atrial Node.

Common Diseases and Disorders

Disease or Disorder	SIMPLE ANAEMIA
Description	This is probably the most common blood complaint. Anaemia means, loss of normal balance between the productive and destructive blood processes. This can be due to a drop in the blood volume after a haemorrhage, or the drop in the number of red blood cells, or in the amount of haemoglobin, or a combination of any two or more of these factors. There are many forms of anaemia, but we are primarily concerned with two categories: 1. simple anaemia. 2. pernicious anaemia. In simple anaemia there are two direct causative factors, the first is a marked nutritional deficiency of iron, frequently seen with pregnant women, and premature infants, as well as in growing children. The second causative factor is through chronic blood loss, during menstruation or because of an accident. One of the characteristics of pernicious anaemia is the presence of giant red cells (macrocytes), each cell appearing to be overloaded with haemoglobin, while the total red cell count is decreased. As recently as 1925 this disease was invariably fatal, today the life expectancy of the properly treated patient is no different from that of the general population. Pernicious anaemia results from failure of the red blood cells to develop and mature normally. While a decreased number of red blood cells is indicative of anaemia, a continuously increasing number of white blood cells can be indicative of leukaemia. Reference has already been made to the fact that white blood cells increase in number by mitosis, in the presence of necessary stimuli such as an infection and the normal eight thousand per cubic millimetre of blood can increase to as many as sixty thousand, in a case of severe pneumonia. However, when the condition is cured, the mitosing effect ceases and the white blood count returns to normal. In leukaemia the leucocytes and/or lymphocytes do not remain at the normal number, but gradually increase.
Possible Allopathic Treatment	The therapeutic response to anaemia depends on the cause. Moderate to severe anaemia may require a blood transfusion. If the condition is acute, a supplement of the deficient component will be administered.
Possible Holistic Aromatherapy Treatment	No aromatherapy treatment will help with an anaemia problem. However, aromatherapy will greatly assist recovery and maintain immune levels during or/and after treatment.

Disease or Disorder	BRUISES
Description	A bruise could be described as a discolouration in or below the skin tissue, when tiny blood vessels or capillaries are ruptured. Blood seeps into tissues and the red cells break. Discolouration disappears as the red cells degenerate and are reabsorbed, a bruise disappears usually in about 14 days. A blue bruise appears if the overlying tissue is pink. Haemoglobin the principle pigment in red cells turns blue when oxygen is removed. Tissues quickly use up oxygen and it is not resupplied because the blood vessels are broken. A yellow bruise occurs due to the breakdown products of haemoglobin. The pigment is eventually removed by white blood cells. One of the reasons for the yellow colour is due to an iron deficiency. With certain blood disorders that affect the platelets there can be unusual bruising which can be caused with only very slight pressure on the skin.
Possible Allopathic Treatment	In the case of trauma to the head, (contusions) the patient should be closely observed for changes in neurological signs, including mental status, vital signs, pupillary findings, focalization or lateralizations of signs and seizures.
Possible Holistic Aromatherapy Treatment	Arnica cream will help relieve and cause the bruising to come to the surface quicker. Fennel, hyssop and lavender are effective in a ice-compress. Later when the bruise is developed and changes colour, add rosemary to the blend using a light local massage to increase circulation. Often chamomile, black pepper and lavender together in a solution of St. Johns Wort or borage will prove useful.

Disease or Disorder	VARICOSE VEINS
Description	A network of veins serves to drain the capillary beds and body tissue of "used" blood, and returns this blood to the heart. Venous flow is assisted in its return to the heart by the rhythmic suction action of breathing, the muscular contraction in the extremities and the valves located in the veins. Gravity assists the venous blood from the neck and head to return to the heart, but venous flow from the legs is against the pull of gravity, and for most of the day has to run up hill. The valves in the veins prevent back flow and when some of these valves become impaired or cease to function, the veins become permanently dilated. There are many causes of varicosity but these include; 1. congenital factors; heredity 2. environmental factors: people whose work necessitates Those who stand still for long periods of time are at particular risk. Varicose veins are also quite often, a complication of pregnancy.
Possible Allopathic Treatment	The saphenous veins of the legs are most often affected. Elevation of the legs and the use of elastic stocking are often advised. Surgery (ligation & stripping) may be required. Injection of sclerosing solutions help prevent or treat postphlebitic syndrome.
Possible Holistic Aromatherapy Treatment	Aromatherapy treatment needs to be aimed chiefly at improving the general tone of the veins and should be combined with dietary and other advice. One of the most important oils for strengthening the veins is cypress, which should be used as a bath oil, and applied, very gently, over the area of the affected veins. Massage can be used above the affected area (ie. On that part of the leg that is close to the heart) but must never be used below the varicosity as this will only increase pressure in the vein. Garlic capsules will strengthen the circulation, as will vitamin E & C. Gentle exercise and elevate legs for 20-30 minutes a day. As the treatment progresses lavender, juniper and rosemary may also be used. Application must be daily to have any effect. Note: massaging varicose areas is strictly prohibited...

Disease or Disorder	HAEMOPHILIA
Description	This is the best known of the bleeding diseases. It is an hereditary disease where the victim almost always is male, the disease being passed on by the mother, who is the carrier. It is a disease in which there is a deficiency in the clotting of the blood.
Possible Allopathic Treatment	The primary objective is to prevent bleeding and to make the environment as safe as possible.
Possible Holistic Aromatherapy Treatment	The primary objective is to prevent bleeding and to make the environment as safe as possible. There is no possible holistic aromatherapy treatment that would reverse or help this disorder other than to use uplifting oils like, *Basil, Bergamot, Clary Sage, Geranium, Jasmine, Grapefruit, Lavender, Lemongrass, Mandarin, Melissa, Neroli, Orange Blossom, Patchouli, Petitgrain, Rose, Sandalwood and Ylang Ylang.*

Disease or Disorder	ARTERIOSCLEROSIS AND ATHEROSCLEROSIS	
Description	Arteriosclerosis:	Arteriosclerosis is a general term used to describe different conditions relating to hardening of the arteries. Some hardening will occur as we age. It can be caused by atherosclerosis.
	Atherosclerosis:	This is where a build up of fats, plaque (fibrous tissue, cholestrol and calcium) on the inside of the artery reducing the size of the wall.
Possible Allopathic Treatment	Diet and lifestyle changes including exercise are recommended. Vasodilators and exercise may relieve symptoms, but there is no specific treatment for the disorder. Surgery may be an option with chronic severe cases.	
Possible Holistic Aromatherapy Treatment	Preventative measures include therapy of predisposing diseases, adequate rest and exercise, and avoidance of stress. Gentle application with Analgesic Pain-killing oils like; *Bergamot, Cajeput, Coriander, Eucalyptus, Lemon-grass, Niaouli, Black-pepper, Chamomile, Jasmine, Lavender, Marjoram, Peppermint, Rosemary and Ginger.* Anti-depressant essential oil like; *Basil, Bergamot, Clary Sage, Geranium, Jasmine, Grapefruit, Lavender, Lemongrass, Mandarin, Melissa, Neroli, Orange Blossom, Patchouli, Petitgrain, Rose, Sandalwood and Ylang Ylang.* Anti-inflammatory essential oils like; *Caraway, Teatree, Camphor, Chamomile, Fennel, Geranium, Jasmine, Peppermint, Benzoin, Frankincense, Myrrh and Patchouli.* Warming (Rubefacient) essential oils like; *Bergamot, Eucalyptus, Thyme, Black Pepper, Camphor, Juniper, Lavender, Peppermint, Pine and Ginger.*	

Essential Oils

CYPRESS

Latin name: *cupressus sempervirens*   Family: *Cupresacae*

Three main areas where this oil can help:

  1.   Respiratory problems
  2.   Regulation of the menstrual cycle
  3.   Cancer retarding action (no scientific proof)

Properties   Uses

Vasoconstrictor	Varicose veins, skin care, haemorrhoids, haemorrhages, hot flashes
Uterine	Dysmenorrhea, enuresis, menopause
Hepatic	Liver disorders
Antispasmodic	Asthma, diarrhea, spasmodic cough, whooping cough, bronchitis, hay fever

Place of Origin
The cypress tree is tall and conical shaped. Its small flowers are succeeded by round cones, or nuts as they are call which are coloured greyish-brown. Cypress trees are coniferae *(Perennial)* and originated in the East.

Method of Extraction
The essential oil of cypress is distilled from the leaves and the cones. The chemical constituents include d-pinene, d-camphene, d-sylvestrene, cymene, sabinol, terpenic alcohol and camphor of cypress.

Traditional Uses
Commonly found in gardens and cemeteries, this began years back from the Egyptian and Roman tradition of dedicating the tree to the gods of death and the underworld. The cypress was given its name from the island of Cyprus, where it used to be worshipped. The Latin name of "sempervirens" comes from *"ever-living"* which may possible refer to the evergreen nature of the leaves.
Historically the wood was used for building ships and homes as well as sarcophagi.

Herbal Medicine
Best known as an astringent and a styptic today, although in the past it was a well-known ingredient for whooping cough.

Aromatherapy

One of the strongest vasoconstrictors in the aromatherapy field, combined with its astringent action, makes the essential oil of cypress valuable in the treatment of varicose veins and haemorrhoids. *(Apply locally to the varicosed area and very gently apply oils with light strokes towards the heart. Never massage directly over varicose veins.)*

The antispasmodic properties, especially when dealing with the bronchi makes it ideal for asthma, bronchitis, or whooping cough. Diffusing this oil would be a good idea as far as taking preventative measures

Cypress is considered a tonic to the uterus and is or importance to use when dealing with its related disorders. Abnormalities such as painful periods (dysmenorrhoea), heavy flow, prolonged bleeding or other menstrual problems improve with the use of this oil. It helps balance the female hormonal system and gynecological problems due to it ability to stimulate estrogen.

Deodorant and astringent in nature, it controls excessive discharges including water loss. Excessive sweating (cypress will reduce the amount of perspiration as well as the unpleasant odour that often accompanies this problem), excessive urination and most forms of haemorrhage will benefit with this essential oil.

It has been suggested that cypress might help in some forms of cancer. However, there is no definite proof on this subject. There is now an investigation into this potential ability of Cypress taking place in England.

Cypress is an effective insect repellant. Most dogs will tolerate the smell of this essence to allow you to apply it in the form of a spritzer to help keep them free of fleas. Combined with the deodorant properties, it will reduce the *"dog smell"* so commonly found during summer.

Warning: *Do not use this essential oil during pregnancy.*

Hyssop

Latin name: *hyssopus officinalis*   Botanical family: *Labiatae*

Three main areas where this oil can help

1. Chest infections
2. Treatment of bruises
3. Sore throats

Properties | Uses

Expectorant	Colds, bronchitis, whooping cough, catarrh, asthma, sore throats, tuberculosis
Digestive/Antispasmodic	Loss of appetite, flatulence, constipation, colic
Cicatrisant	Skin care, eczema, dermatitis, wounds, scars
Sedative	Anxiety, hysteria

Place of Origin
Hyssop is a member of the labiatae family and is a native of the Mediterranean. It grows between two to three feet in height with spikes of flowers that may be blue, white, pink or mauve.

Method of Extraction
Steam distillation of the flowering tops produce the essential oil. The active ingredients include a high proportion of pinocamphene with pinene and traces of geraniol, borneol, thujone and phellandrene. Because of the high ketone content, this oil is considered borderline in the terms of toxicity.

Traditional Uses
Hyssop was regarded by both the Greeks and the Hebrews as a sacred herb and is mentioned several times in the old testament. It was used to clean out temples and sacred places, quite literally by using bundles of the herb as a broom. Later, it was a popular strewing herb and these uses might lead us to consider burning or vaporising hyssop to disinfect a room as a preventative measure against infection.

Herbal Medicine
Mainly used in herbal medicine as an expectorant for coughs, asthma and shortness of breath. It has also been found useful during fevers. An infusion is taken to induce perspiration. Hyssop is a circulatory stimulant and will reduce blood pressure in hypertensives. An infusion of the dried herb one ounce to one pint of boiling water taken in doses of two fluid ounces three or four times a day. It can also be combined in equal parts with other cough remedies such as horehound and coltsfoot.

Aromatherapy

Caution should be exercised when dealing with this essential oil. Two circumstances to avoid the oil altogether are:

1)   Epilepsy - Hyssop must never be used on a client suffering from epilepsy as it may trigger an attack

1)   Pregnancy - This oil may not be used during pregnancy because of its high toxicity and   action on the nervous system as well as it astringent characteristics. It may harm the developing baby or interfere with the mothers symbiotic relationship with the baby.

Hyssop has some therapeutic applications, so with caution in mind, it may be considered in some of the following:

- ▸ Hyssop has an affinity for the respiratory system due to its expectorant properties. Where ever there is thick mucous present, such as coughs, chest infections, or catarrh, hyssop is indicated for use. It possesses a stimulating and tonic effect on the respiratory system by clearing the chest and easing the constriction that is commonly found in respiratory complaints.
- ▸ Antispasmodic in nature, as well as a digestive aid, use of this essence shows improvement in cases of flatulence, constipation, colic and even loss of appetite.
- ▸ Another use is to help dispel bruising. Used with a cold compress as soon as possible after the bruising has occurred. Compresses with hyssop may prove valuable in the treatment of arthritis and rheumatism.
- ▸ Essential oil of hyssop is cephalic. It leads to mental clarity that will result in a feeling of alertness. It helps to calm emotions especially in cases of anxiety and hysteria.

Warning: *USE WITH CAUTION*

THYME

Latin name: *thymus vulgaris*   Botanical family: *Labiatae*

Three main areas where this oil can help:

1.   Stimulates the auto-immune system
2.   Raises low blood pressure
3.   Strong anti-septic

Properties   Uses

Expectorant	Asthma, coughs, colds, chest infections, respiratory infections, bronchitis
Nervine	Stimulates central nervous system, exhaustion, debility, poor memory
Immunostimulant	Stimulates immune system, stimulates white blood cells, HIV, viruses, infections
Stimulant	Circulatory system, low blood pressure, anaemia, arthritis, rheumatism
Antiseptic	Dysentery, gastro-enteritis, lice, worms

Place of Origin
Common thyme *(thymus vulgaris)* is a member of the labiatae. Native to the Mediterranean area, it is cultivated in France among other places. There are several vanities of thyme, but the common thyme is the one normally used in aromatherapy.

Method of Extraction
The pink flowered variety of common thyme is considered to yield an essential oil superior to the white flowered variety. The oil is steam distilled twice from the leaves and flowering tops, to remove irritant substances present in the plant. The active constituents of the oil include thymol and carvacrol, together making us about 60% of the volume, with terpinene, cymene, borneo and linalol.

Traditional Uses
This plants medicinal reputation grew over the centuries. It was used to help battle plagues that occurred throughout Europe. As recently as World War 1, the essential oil served as a battle field antiseptic.

The origin of the word thyme comes from the Greek *"thymos"* which means to *"perfume"*. Today, two of the active constituents, carvacrol and thymol are frequently isolated and used in perfumery.

Herbal Medicine
This herb has readily been used in cooking and is a digestive remedy for stomach disorders including colic, gastritis and loss of appetite. An antiseptic expectorant, it will strengthen the lungs in cases of bronchial infection, whooping cough and asthma. An infusion is made of adding one ounce of dried herb to one pint of boiling water and drink two fluid ounces two to three times per day. You can gargle with this for sore throats and the infusion also improves the appetite.

Aromatherapy

Thyme is a powerful essential oil, but must be used in low doses because it can be an irritant, especially on mucous membranes. A strong antiseptic oil, it is valuable for treatment in gastric infections and can help expel intestinal worms of many varieties including tapeworms, threadworms, and roundworms.

Respiratory conditions such as infections, colds, asthma, bronchitis, and coughs as well as mouth and throat infections will benefit from the expectorant properties. As little as 0.1% of essential oil of thyme in a toothpaste is effective against the bacteria that causes mouth and gum infections.

Thyme is a circulatory stimulant. It will raise low blood pressure. Also an immune stimulant, thyme will increase the production of white blood cells thereby increasing immunity. It is said to be one of the main essential oils to be used in the treatment of HIV- related diseases.

It is particularly effective when dealing with debility, exhaustion, fatigue or lethargy. Thyme stimulates the appetite which is generally poor after an illness.

It aids in strengthening the mind and body. Through stimulating the central nervous system, thyme activates the brain cells improving both the memory and concentration abilities. It balances the adrenal cortex when there e is an overproduction of adrenaline hormones or acetylcholine, which would help aid kidney malfunction and other digestive problems.

Thyme is sometimes used in hot compresses to relieve rheumatic pain. A good first aid treatment of insect bites and stings is the crushed fresh herb. Do not use neat essential oil for this as it will sting. Remember to pre-dissolve the essential oils if using them in the bath.

YLANG YLANG

Latin name: *cananga odorata*   Botanical family: *Anonaceae*

Three main areas where this oil can help:

1.   High blood pressure and rapid heart beat
2.   Stress, anxiety, pms and depression
3.   Aphrodisiac

Properties	Uses
Antidepressant	Depression, sadness, grief, apathy, lack of confidence
Aphrodisiac	Frigidity, impotence
Hypotensive	High blood pressure, hyperpnoea *(rapid breathing)*, tachycardia, hyperventilation
Sedative	Insomnia, anxiety, nervous tension, palpitations, anger, tension
Hormone Balancer	PMS, menopause, tonic to the womb

Place of Origin
The essential oil of ylang ylang is obtained from the flowers of a small tropical tree which grows in the Philippines, Java, Sumatra and Madagascar. The tree grows to a height of sixty feet and there are pink, mauve, and yellow flowered varieties. The name Ylang ylang means *"flower of flowers"*.

Method of Extraction
The finest essential oil is extracted from the yellow flowered varieties and is obtained by steam distillation. The first part of the oil which is of the best quality and it is this which is sold under the name of ylang ylang. The remainder of the oil obtained during the latter part of the process, *(known as "tail of the distillate)* is of poorer quality and is usually sold under the name Canaga.
The oil varies in colour from almost colourless to pale yellow and the aroma is very sweet and exotic. The oil contains eugenol, geraniol, linalol, safrol, ylangol, terpenes, pinene, benzoic, formic salicylic and valeric acids.

Herbal Medicine
There is no herbal remedy associated with this beautiful plant other than as a herbal tea.

Aromatherapy

Ylang ylang works on a physical level by relaxing the central nervous system *(although with prolonged use it may have the opposite effect)*. High blood pressure, rapid breathing, tachycardia and hyperventilation seen to ease with the use of this essential oil. It has a profound effect on the cardiovascular system and deals well with emotions like shock, anger, fear and others that stem from an emotional cause.

Well known for its aphrodisiac properties, Ylang helps dispel problems such as frigidity and impotence. It can be used to ease anxiety about sexual inadequacy and through its sedative qualities release pent up nervous tension, lack of confidence and help with anxiety in general as well as insomnia.

Depression, sadness, grief and apathy show improvement with Ylang ylang. A hormonal balancer, ylang is responsive in the treatment of problems that are associated with the reproductive system. PMS, and menopause are specifically helped with the use of this oil. It is also reported that in order to keep the breast tissue firm, a topical preparation of ylang is needed.

A balance of sebaceous secretions *(sebum)*, ylang ylang can be used in skin care on both oily and dry skin conditions as well as a scalp stimulant.

Warning: *Excessive use could cause headaches*

Question and Answer Sheets

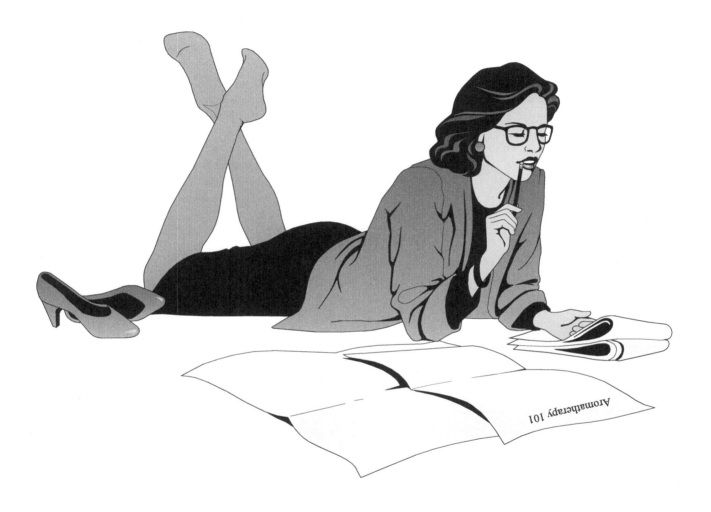

Please keep the questions for review.
Circle the correct answer/s on the Answer Sheets at the back of the book and
<u>return these sheets only</u> to your instructor.

Questions - Lesson #4

1. Under medical history what information is required?
a. hospital treatments
b. last visit to the vet
c. consultations with a doctor
d. consultations with a dentist

2. What question(s) should you ask regarding headaches?
a. how severe & how often
b. what makes them come and what makes them go
c. how frequently do you take medication for it
d. is it related to a sinus disorder

3. What question(s) should you ask regarding sleep?
a. do you have interrupted sleep
b. what causes the interruption
c. do you wake-up tired
d. do you have trouble getting off to sleep

4. What question(s) should you ask regarding reproduction?
a. are there any problems with your reproductive system
b. is there any possibility you might be pregnant
c. are you pregnant
d. is the world already over populated

5. Why do you check posture?
a. to encourage them to work-out more
b. to understand body mechanics better
c. to ascertain if their discomfort is related to poor posture.
d. to ascertain if their discomfort is related to poor muscle failure

6. Does cold feet always indicate poor circulation?
a. yes
b. no
c. I don't know
d. yes and no

7. Should you ask the client to indicate their own stress levels?
a. yes
b. no
c. I don't know
d. only if you didn't know what you were doing

8. What encapsulates the heart?
a. fibrous pericardium
b. fibrous myocardium
c. pericardium systole
d. pericardia system

9. The heart is divided into four chambers, they are?
a. the right atriale   e. the right pulmonary
b. the right atrium   f. the right ventricle
c. the left atriale   g. the left pulmonary
d. the left atrium   h. the left ventricle

10. What is the wall called that divides the left side of the heart from the right side and what is its purpose?
a.   the septum and it keeps the venous blood from coming in contact with the arterial blood
b.   the cardiac wall and it keeps the venous blood from coming in contact with the arterial blood
c.   the septum and it keeps the heart beat regular
d.   the cardiac wall and it keeps the blood flowing

11. Which side of the heart pumps deoxygenated blood to the lungs?
a. the left side
b. the right side
c. they both do

12. Complete the missing words that describe what keeps the heart beating,
The sino-atrial node located in the right_____
sends impulses through the two atria, causing
_____. It then stimulates the atrio-ventricular node to pass rapidly down the _____ to cause ventricular systole.

13. The circulation is divided into two principal systems, they are?
a. systemic circulation   b. pulmonary circulation
c. venous circulation   d. arterial circulation

14. Blood vessels which proceed from the heart are known as?
a. veins   b. arteries
c. arterioles   d. capillaries

15. These hollow elastic tubes which start off fairly large gradually decrease in diameter to become known as?
a. veins   b. arteries
c. arterioles   d. capillaries

16. Finally they decrease into fine hairlike blood vessels known as?

a. veins   b. arteries

c. arterioles   d. capillaries

17.   Blood vessels that proceed towards the heart are known as?

a. veins   b. arteries

c. arterioles   d. capillaries

18. What prevents the backflow of blood in veins?

a. gravity

b. one way valves

c. blood only gets pumped one way

d. compression of the vessels by the muscles

19. Which vessels return blood directly into the heart and on which side of the heart does this occur?

a. the inferior and superior venacava into the right side of the heart

b. the inferior and superior venacava into the left side of the heart

c. the inferior and superior pulmonary artery into the right side

d. the inferior and superior pulmonary artery into the left side

20. Which blood vessel leaves the heart to take the blood to the lungs?

a. the pulmonary vein   b. the pulmonary artery

c. the ascending aorta   d. the descending aorta

21. After reoxygenated blood leaves the lungs, which blood vessel returns the blood to the heart?

a. the pulmonary vein   b. the pulmonary artery

c. the ascending aorta   d. the descending aorta

22. Which chamber of the heart receives oxygenated blood first?

a. the right atrium   b. the left atrium

c. the right ventricle   d. the left ventricle

23. Which blood vessel(s) dispatch oxygenated blood from the heart to the body in the first instance?

a. the pulmonary vein   b. the pulmonary artery

c. the ascending aorta   d. the descending aorta

24. The descending aorta divides into two vessel, what are they called?

a. the iliacs   b. the femorals

c. the popliteals   d. the brachials

25. When this artery reaches the groin it divides to traverse down the upper legs, what is it now called?

a. the iliac   b. the femoral

c. the popliteal   d. the brachial

26. Having passed underneath the knee it then becomes the?

a. the iliac   b. the femoral

c. the popliteal   d. the brachial

27. What is the artery in the lower legs called?

a. the popliteal

b. the anterior tibial and the posterior tibial

c. the dorsalis pedis and the plantar arches

d. the axillary and the brachial

28. Name the two arteries in the feet.

a. the popliteal and the femoral

b. the anterior tibial and the posterior tibial

c. the dorsalis pedis and the plantar arches

d. the axillary and the brachial

29. Name the artery that subdivides from the ascending aorta.

a. the subclavian   b. the submandibular

c. the axillary   d. the brachial

30. Name the artery in the armpit.

a. the submandibular   b. the axillary

c. the brachial   d. the palmar arch

31. Name the artery in the upper arm.

a. the axillary   b. the brachial

c. the radial   d. the palmar arch

32. Name the two arteries in the lower arm.

a. the axillary and the brachial

b. the radial and the ulna

c. the palmar and the plantar arches

d. the temporal and occipital

33. Name the artery in the hand.

a. the common carotid   b. the radial

c. the palmar arch   d. the temporal

34. Name the artery in the neck.

a. the common carotid   b. the temporal

c. the palmar arch   d. the occipital

35. Name the two facial arteries.
a. the axillary and the brachial
b. the temporal and the facial
c. the occipital and the femoral
d. the iliac and the subclavian

36. What type of substance is blood?
a. acidic   b. alkaline
c. combination   d. liquid

37. Name the four principle constituent parts of blood.
a. plasma   b. erythrocytes
c. water   d. leucocytes
e. platelets   f. oxygen
g. carbon dioxide

38. The main substances held in solution in plasma are?
a. glucose   b. insulin
c. amino acids   d. mineral salts.
e. water   f. enzymes
g. oxygen

39. Erythrocytes or red corpuscles get their colour from?
a. iron
b. oxygenated haemoglobin
c. carbon dioxide
d. protein

40. What is oxy-haemoglobin?
a. oxygen rich erythrocytes
b. carbon dioxide rich erythrocytes
c. oxygen rich lymphocytes
d. oxygen lacking lymphocytes

41. What is carboxi-haemoglobin?
a. oxygen rich erythrocytes
b. carbon dioxide rich erythrocytes
c. oxygen rich lymphocytes
d. carbon dioxide rich lymphocytes

42. What is the average life span of an erythrocyte?
a. 20 days   b. 60 days
c. 120 days   d. 100 days

43. Where are erythrocytes formed?
a. the red bone marrow   b. the spleen
c. the liver   d. the kidneys

44. The eventual disintegration of erythrocytes takes place in what organs?
a. the spleen   b. the liver
c. the kidneys   d. the stomach

45. White corpuscles are also known as?
a. white cells   b. leucocytes
c. lymphocytes   d. thrombocytes

46. What is the chief role of the white corpuscles?
a. protectors or soldiers   b. cleaners
c. feeders   d. clotters

47. The white corpuscles ability to digest bacteria is called?
a. phagomitosis   b. phagocytosis
c. mitosis   d. thrombosis

48. Leucocytes increase by a process of division called?
a. phagomitosis   b. phagocytosis
c. mitosis   d. thrombosis

49. What is the purpose of the platelets or thrombocytes?
a. blood clotting   b. blood cleaning
c. blood health   d. blood clearing

50. Which action do you think would assist in the venous return of blood to the heart?
a. walking or movement of the legs
b. breathing and the muscular contraction in extremities
c. the involuntary contraction of the muscles
d. the signals from the medulla oblongata

51. What are the three causes of varicose veins?
a. congenital factors   b. poor eating habits
c. environmental factors   d. pregnancy
e. lack of exercise

52. What is haemophilia?
a. deficiency of clotting factor of the blood
b. deficiency of haemoglobin
c. deficiency of proper lymphocytes
d. deficiency of proper red cells

53. Which sex is more prone to haemophilia, and how do they contract it?
a. females via heterosexual intercourse with infected males
b. males via genetics from the mother
c. males via genetics from the father
d. females via genetics from the mother

54. What does the term angiology mean?
a. the disease affecting the heart valves
b. the science dealing with the circulatory system
c. the diseases affecting the heart and its immediate arteries
d. the science dealing with blood and lymph vessels

55. What is cholesterol?
a. a type of fat found in blood & animal fats
b. a constituent of all animal fats and oils
c. a constituent of any type of oils that creates problems when ingested in very large quantities
d. animal fats and oils

56. What is phlebitis?
a. inflammation of the pericardium
b. inflammation of the heart lining
c. inflammation of the vein walls, usually in the legs
d. inflammation of the lining of the colon

57. What is thrombus?
a. inflammation of the heart lining
b. a clot of blood found within the heart or blood vessels
c. narrowing of the vessels, leading to blockage
d. irregular, rapid heart beat due to a malfunction of valves

58. What is endocarditis?
a. inflammation of the pericardium
b. inflammation of the heart lining
c. inflammation of the vein walls
d. inflammation of the abdominal cavity

59. What is pericarditis?
a. inflammation of the pericardium
b. inflammation of the heart lining
c. inflammation of the vein walls
d. inflammation of the abdominal cavity

60. What is atrial fibrillation?
a. irregular, rapid heart beat due to a malfunction of valves
b. irregular, rapid heart beat due to excess stomach acid
c. irregular, rapid heart beat due over exertion
d. irregular, rapid heart beat due to a disorder of the sino-atrial node

61. Label the diagram of the heart.
(SEE ANSWER SHEET FOR DIAGRAM)

62. Label the diagram of the arteries.
(SEE ANSWER SHEET FOR DIAGRAM)

63. What part of the plant is used to obtain essentia oil of cypress?
a. the seeds of the plant
b. the flowering tops
c. the leaves and cones
d. the roots
e. the fruit or berries of the plant
f. the wood

64. What three main areas will cypress help most?
a. calming on the respiratory system
b. calming on the genito-urinary system
c. regulating menstrual cycle
d. stimulating to the circulatory system
e. helpful in cancer
f. balancing of the nervous system

65. What should you be careful of when using cypress.
a. people who suffer from asthma
b. skin sensitivity
c. not to be used during pregnancy
d. liver disorders

66. What part of the plant is used to obtain essential oil of hyssop?
a. the seeds of the plant
b. the leaves
c. the flowering tops
d. the roots
e. the fruit or berries of the plant
f. the wood

67. What three main areas will hyssop help most?
a. respiratory system stimulant
b. healing on skin injuries
c. treatment of muscles spasms and sinus problems
d. chest infections
e. sore throats

68. What two main areas should be avoided when using hyssop?
a. low blood pressure   b. high blood pressure
c. epilepsy   d. diabetes
e. pregnancy   f. geriatrics

69. Name three things that essential oil of thyme can help?
a. stimulates the auto-immune system
b. raises low blood pressure
c. stimulates mitosis
d. helps with thrombosis
e. anti-septic

70. How is essential oil of thyme produced?
a. steam distillation of the flowers
b. steam distillation of the roots
c. solvent extraction of the flowers
d. cold pressing the plant

71. What do you have to be careful of when using essential oil of thyme?

a. high blood pressure

b. should not be used on people trying to lose weight

c. Should not be used during pregnancy

d. none of the above

72. Name three things that essential oil of ylang ylang can help?

a. stimulates the auto-immune system

b. high blood pressure and rapid heart beat

c. stress, anxiety, pms and depression

d. helps with thrombosis

e. strong aphrodisiac

73. How is essential oil of ylang ylang produced?

a. steam distillation of the flowers

b. steam distillation of the roots

c. solvent extraction of the flowers

d. cold pressing the plant

Answer Sheet - Lesson #4

(Keep the questions for review. Circle the correct answer/s and return these sheets only to your instructor.)

1.   A   B   C   D

2.   A   B   C   D

3.   A   B   C   D

4.   A   B   C   D

5.   A   B   C   D

6.   A   B   C   D

7.   A   B   C   D

8.   A   B   C   D

9.   A   B   C   D   E   F   G   H

10. A   B   C   D

11. A   B   C

12.   To keep the heart beating the Sino-Atrial Node located in the right_____sends impulses through the

two atria, causing _____. It then stimulates the atrio-ventricular node to pass rapidly down

the _____ to cause ventricular systole.

13. A   B   C   D

14. A   B   C   D

15. A   B   C   D

16. A   B   C   D

17. A   B   C   D

18. A   B   C   D

19. A   B   C   D

20. A   B   C   D

21. A   B   C   D

22. A   B   C   D

23. A   B   C   D

24. A   B   C   D

25. A   B   C   D

26. A   B   C   D

27. A   B   C   D

28. A   B   C   D

29. A   B   C   D

30. A   B   C   D

31. A   B   C   D

32. A   B   C   D

33. A   B   C   D

34. A   B   C   D

35. A   B   C   D

36. A   B   C   D

37. A   B   C   D   E   F   G

38. A   B   C   D   E   F   G

39. A   B   C   D

40. A   B   C   D

41. A   B   C   D

42. A   B   C   D

43. A   B   C   D

44. A   B   C   D

45. A   B   C   D

46. A   B   C   D

47. A   B   C   D

48. A   B   C   D

49. A   B   C   D

50. A   B   C   D

51. A   B   C   D   E

52. A   B   C   D

53. A   B   C   D

54. A   B   C   D

55. A   B   C   D

56. A   B   C   D

57. A   B   C   D

58. A   B   C   D

59. A   B   C   D

60. A   B   C   D

61. Label the diagram of the heart

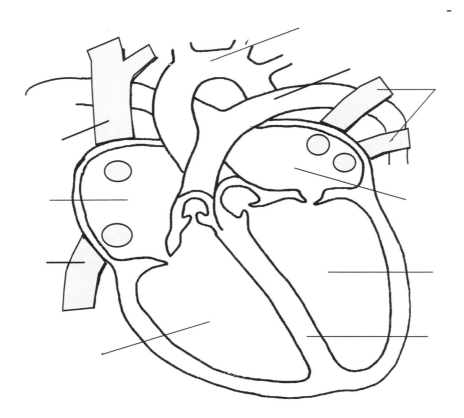

62. Label the diagram of the arteries.

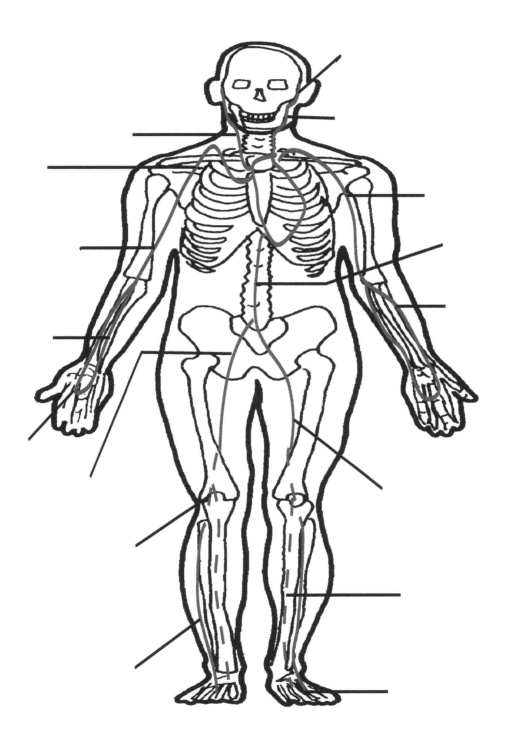

63. A   B   C   D   E   F

64. A   B   C   D   E   F

65. A   B   C   D

66. A   B   C   D   E   F

67. A   B   C   D   E

68. A   B   C   D   E   F

69. A   B   C   D   E

70. A   B   C   D

71. A   B   C   D

72. A   B   C   D   E

73. A   B   C   D

LESSON
FIVE

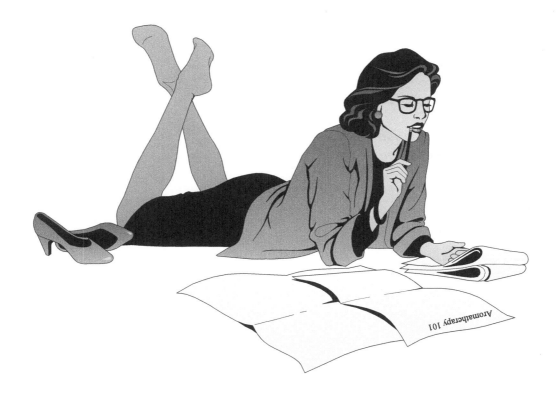

Lesson #5

Table of Contents

How to Use the Cross Reference Chart

Before we decide which oils to use we must first decide which pathology we are going to treat. The holistic way is to complete an assessment as described in the last lesson and attempt to look after three disorders at the same time. Stress is the number one disorder. Stress is responsible for 98% of all disorders *(unless, hereditary, traumatic, congenital or environmental)*, so it makes sense to treat stress first. We also know that stress makes an illness worse and will lower the immune system.

The next pathology to be treated should be the most troublesome to the patient, ie. migraine, diarrhoea, constipation, low back pain etc.

The third disorder should be something that contributes to the first and second disorder, ie. Headaches could be an offshoot of constipation.

Having decided which disorders you will be treating, you must then refer to the Cross Reference Chart and locate the offending disorder found in the reference chart *(or a close cousin)* and write the top notes in the top note column, the middle notes in the middle note column and the base notes in the base note column. To help squeeze them in, only use the first three or four letters of the oils, ie. lavender = lav, eucalyptus = euc, and so on. Double-barrelled names like clary sage become = C/S and ylang ylang becomes = Y/Y, one more for luck? Rosemary = R/M.

The next process in cross referencing is to cross match the essential oils. This is done by looking down the top note column in the first (stress column) disorder and comparing the oils listed with those in the first column of the second and third disorders. If you find oils that are repeated in those (second & third) columns write a "2" next to the oil in the top note column if it is repeated in the second condition, and a "3" if it appears in the third condition top note column, ie

FIRST CONDITION			SECOND CONDITION			THIRD CONDITION		
TOP	MIDDLE	BASE	TOP	MIDDLE	BASE	TOP	MIDDLE	BASE
BAS 23	B/P 3	C/W	BAS	CYP	CLOV	BAS	B/P	CYP
EUC 23	CYP 2	JAS	LEM	CHAM	Y/Y	T/T	FEN	IRIG
PET	CHAM 23	MYRR	EUC	FEN	ROSE	EUC	R/M	N/M
BERG	FEN 23	PAT 23	CORI	MEL	PAT	G/F	CHAM	PAT

Above you can see that in the top note column of the first condition, bas *(basil)* and euc *(eucalyptus)* shows a "2" *(mentioned in the second condition)* and a "3" *(mentioned in the third condition)*. This also is repeated for cham *(chamomile)* and fen *(fennel)* in the middle notes and pat *(patchouli)* in the base note section. Whereas cyp *(cypress)* is only repeated once in the second condition, and B/P *(blackpepper)* is only repeated once in the third condition.

Basil, eucalyptus, chamomile, fennel and patchouli, are oils that are useful for all three conditions. The only thing we have to do now is to decide which oils to use. To help us we have rules of selection.

RULE 1

▸ Only use three oils, per blend, per treatment.
▸ Only use one base note, per blend, per treatment.
▸ Only use indicated oils. *(These are oils that are indicated by a "2" and a "3" next to them).*
▸ If there are not enough indicated oils to choose from, use the second condition *("2")* as a priority before using the third condition oil.

RULE 2

▸ To make an ACUTE blend: Use two middle notes, and one top note
▸ To make a CHRONIC blend: Use two middle notes and one base note
▸ To make a SYNERGISTIC blend: Use one top note, one middle note and one base note

RULE 3

▸ Acute blends treat acute disorders
▸ Chronic blends treat chronic disorders
▸ Synergistic blends treat disorders that conflict or are unknown

RULE 4

▸ Use 4 drops of each top note essential oil to create your blend
▸ Use 3 drops of each middle note essential oil to create your blend
▸ Use 1 drop of each base note essential oil to create your blend
This means that;
an acute blend will measure 10 drops in total
a chronic blend will measure 7 drops in total
a synergistic blend will measure 8 drops in total

In a perfect world this is the results, unfortunately this is not always possible, therefore;
three top notes will measure out to be 12 drops in total
three middle notes will measure out to be 9 drops in total
and three base notes are improper and should not be used

RULE 5

▸ Only use high quality essential oils.
▸ Other schools and essential oils will claim purity and quality. But the bottom line is this; why do they suggest more drops in a blend if their oils are as therapeutically strong as the oils used by this school. More does not mean better, the results will speak for themselves.

Try the following test, by completing the cross reference chart on the following page and comparing it with the answer sheet.

Which blend of essential oils would you use for the following condition:

Main Condition	Secondary Condition	Third Condition
1. STRESS	2. BRONCHITIS	3. ECZEMA

TOP	MIDDLE	BASE	TOP	MIDDLE	BASE	TOP	MIDDLE	BASE

ESSENTIAL OILS CHOSEN FOR AN ACUTE PROBLEM (show amount of drops)

1	2	3

ESSENTIAL OILS CHOSEN FOR A CHRONIC PROBLEM (show amount of drops)

1	2	3

ESSENTIAL OILS CHOSEN SHOWING A SYNERGISTIC BLEND (show amount of drops)

1	2	3

_____

_____

_____

Which blends of essential oils you would use for the following condition: *example*

Main Condition   Secondary Condition   Third Condition

1. STRESS			2. BRONCHITIS			3. ECZEMA		
TOP	MIDDLE	BASE	TOP	MIDDLE	BASE	TOP	MIDDLE	BASE
BAS 23	CHAM 3	BEN 23	BAS	ANI	BEN	BAS	CHAM	BEN
BERG 23	GER 3	C/W 23	BERG	B/P	C/W	BERG	GER	C/W
C/S	HYS 23	FRANK 23	CAJ	CAMP	CLO	CAJ	HYS	FRANK
LEM 2	JUN 23	IMM 23	CARA	CYP	FRANK	EUC	JUN	IMM
MAND	LAV 23	JAS	EUC	HYS	GIN	NIAO	LAV	MYRR
ORANG 2	MARJ 2	L/B	LEM	JUN	IMM	THY	MEL	PAT
PET	MEL 3	MYRR 23	NIAO	LAV	MYRR	YAR		ROSE
THY 23	PEP 2	NERO	ORANG	MARJ	ORIG	SAG		S/W
YAR 23	PIN 2	PAT 3	THY	PEP	S/W			
	R/M 2	ROSE 3	T/T	PIN				
		S/W 23	YAR	R/M				
		VET	SAG					
		Y/Y						

The oils that are *"indicated"* are;
* basil, bergamot, and thyme from the top notes.
* hyssop, juniper, and lavender from the middle notes.
* benzoin, cedarwood, frankincense, and myrrh from the base notes.
        (acute blends require two middle notes, one top)

ESSENTIAL OILS CHOSEN FOR AN **ACUTE PROBLEM** *(show amount of drops)*

1. Bergamot (4 drops)	2. Juniper (3 drops)	3.Lavender (3 drops)

        (chronic blends require two middle notes, one base)
ESSENTIAL OILS CHOSEN FOR AN **CHRONIC PROBLEM** (show amount of drops)

1. Cedarwood (1 drop)	2. Juniper (3 drops)	3. Lavender (3 drops)

        (synergistic blends require one top, one middle, one base)
ESSENTIAL OILS CHOSEN SHOWING A **SYNERGISTIC BLEND** (show amount of drops)

1. Bergamot (4 drops)	2. Juniper (3 drops)	3. Cedarwood (1 drop)

As long as you have used indicated oils from the selection above * you will be correct. As time goes by you will become more knowledgeable about the properties of the essential oils and this knowledge will improve your choices.

Therapeutic Cross Reference Chart

TOP NOTES	MIDDLE NOTES	BASE NOTES
Basil	Aniseed	Benzoin
Bergamot	**Black Pepper**	Cedarwood
Cajuput	Camphor	Clove
Caraway	**Chamomile**	**Frankincense**
Clary Sage	Cypress	Ginger
Coriander	**Fennel**	Immortelle
Eucalyptus	Geranium	**Jasmine**
Grapefruit	Hyssop	Linden Blossom
Lemon	**Juniper**	**Myrrh**
Lemongrass	**Lavender**	Neroli
Mandarin	**Marjoram**	Nutmeg
Niaouli	Melissa	Origanum
Orange	**Peppermint**	Patchouli
Petitgrain	**Pine**	**Rose**
Sage	**Rosemary**	Sandalwood
Thyme		Vetivert
Tea tree		**Ylang Ylang**
Yarrow		

* Bold print indicates oils most used.

DIGESTIVE DISORDERS

PROBLEM	TOP NOTES	MIDDLE NOTES	BASE NOTES
COLIC	Bergamot Yarrow	Black Pepper Fennel Hyssop Juniper Lavender Peppermint	Cinnamon Sandalwood
CONSTIPATION	Basil Coriander Mandarin Orange	Black Pepper Chamomile Camphor Fennel Hyssop Juniper Marjoram Rosemary	Ginger
DIARRHOEA	Caraway Eucalyptus Lemon Orange Yarrow	Chamomile Cypress Geranium Juniper Lavender Marjoram Peppermint Rosemary	Clove Cinnamon Ginger Linden Blossom Myrrh Neroli Nutmeg Sandalwood
FLATULENCE (Gas)	Basil Bergamot Caraway Coriander Sage Yarrow	Aniseed Camphor Fennel Hyssop Juniper Lavender Peppermint Rosemary	Cinnamon Ginger Myrrh
GASTRO-ENTERITIS	Basil Cajuput Niaouli Thyme Tea tree	Chamomile Juniper Peppermint	
HAEMORRHOID	Bergamot Cajuput Clary Sage Niaouli Tea tree Yarrow	Cypress Geranium	Myrrh Neroli Patchouli Sandalwood

PROBLEM	TOP NOTES	MIDDLE NOTES	BASE NOTES
INDIGESTION	Basil	Aniseed	Clove
	Bergamot	Black Pepper	Ginger
	Grapefruit	Chamomile	Immortelle
	Lemongrass	Juniper	Linden Blossom
	Sage	Lavender	
	Thyme	Pine	
		Peppermint	
LIVER PROBLEMS	Grapefruit	Chamomile	Immortelle
	Lemon	Cypress	Linden Blossom
	Sage	Geranium	Myrrh
		Juniper	Rose
		Peppermint	
		Rosemary	
LOSS OF APPETITE	Bergamot	Black Pepper	Ginger
	Caraway	Chamomile	Origanum
	Coriander	Fennel	
	Mandarin	Hyssop	
	Lemongrass	Juniper	
NAUSEA	Basil	Black Pepper	Ginger
	Caraway	Fennel	Rose
	Mandarin	Lavender	Sandalwood
		Melissa	
		Peppermint	
SLUGGISH DIGESTION	Coriander	Black Pepper	Ginger
	Orange	Fennel	Nutmeg
	Yarrow		Origanum
STOMACH ACHE	Bergamot	Chamomile	
		Fennel	
		Lavender	
		Peppermint	
		Rosemary	
VOMITING	Basil	Black Pepper	Ginger
	Lemon	Chamomile	Rose
		Melissa	
		Peppermint	
		Fennel	

HEAD AND NECK DISORDERS

PROBLEM	TOP NOTES	MIDDLE NOTES	BASE NOTES
COLDS (see also Respiratory)	Basil Eucalyptus Lemon Niaouli Tea Tree Thyme Yarrow	Black Pepper Cypress Geranium Juniper Lavender Marjoram Peppermint Pine Rosemary	Benzoin Cedarwood Frankincense
SINUS PROBLEMS (see also Respiratory)	Basil Cajuput Eucalyptus Lemon Niaouli Thyme Tea Tree	Lavender Peppermint Pine	Clove Frankincense
SORE THROAT	Bergamot Cajuput Clary Sage Eucalyptus Lemon Niaouli Sage Thyme Tea Tree	Geranium Lavender Peppermint	Cedarwood Ginger Myrrh Sandalwood
MIGRAINE HEADACHES	Basil Eucalyptus Grapefruit Lemon Yarrow	Aniseed Chamomile Lavender Marjoram Peppermint Rosemary	Immortelle Linden Blossom Rose
HEADACHES	Eucalyptus Grapefruit Lemon	Chamomile Lavender Marjoram Melissa Peppermint Rosemary	Immortelle Linden Blossom

Neck Pain - see Muscular & Joint Disorders

MENSTRUAL DISORDERS

PROBLEM	TOP NOTES	MIDDLE NOTES	BASE NOTES
HEAVY PERIODS	Yarrow Sage	Chamomile Cypress Geranium Juniper	Frankincense Rose
IRREGULAR OR SPOTTY PERIODS (ADD 5-10% CALENDULA CARRIER OIL).	Clary-Sage Basil Thyme	Chamomile Fennel Hyssop Lavender Peppermint	Rose
PAINFUL PERIODS (ADD 5-10% CALENDULA CARRIER OIL).	Basil Cajuput Sage Yarrow	Aniseed Chamomile Cypress Juniper Marjoram Melissa Peppermint	Frankincense Jasmine
P.M.S.	Clary Sage Grapefruit Yarrow	Chamomile Geranium Lavender Melissa	Jasmine Neroli Rose

MUSCULAR & JOINT DISORDERS

PROBLEM	TOP NOTES	MIDDLE NOTES	BASE NOTES
ABDOMINAL CRAMPS	Basil	Aniseed	Clove
	Bergamot	Black Pepper	Immortelle
	Caraway	Fennel	Neroli
	Clary Sage	Marjoram	Nutmeg
	Orange	Melissa	
	Yarrow	Peppermint	
ACHES & PAINS	Basil	Black Pepper	Benzoin
	Cajuput	Camphor	Clove
	Caraway	Chamomile	Ginger
	Coriander	Geranium	Immortelle
	Eucalyptus	Juniper	Nutmeg
	Sage	Lavender	Origanum
	Thyme	Marjoram	
		Melissa	
		Peppermint	
		Rosemary	
ARTHRITIS	Bergamot	Black Pepper	Benzoin
	Cajuput	Camphor	Cedarwood
	Caraway	Chamomile	Clove
	Coriander	Cypress	Frankincense
	Eucalyptus	Fennel	Ginger
	Grapefruit	Geranium	Myrrh
	Lemon	Juniper	Nutmeg
	Niaouli	Lavender	Origanum
	Sage	Marjoram	Vetivert
	Thyme	Pine	
	Yarrow	Rosemary	
RHEUMATISM	Basil	Aniseed	Benzoin
	Cajuput	Chamomile	Ginger
	Coriander	Cypress	Immortelle
	Eucalyptus	Fennel	Nutmeg
	Lemon	Hyssop	Origanum
	Niaouli	Lavender	
	Sage	Marjoram	
	Thyme	Rosemary	
	Yarrow	Juniper	

MUSCULAR & JOINT DISORDERS *continued...*

PROBLEM	TOP NOTES	MIDDLE NOTES	BASE NOTES
MUSCLE SPASM OR MUSCLE CRAMP	Basil	Black Pepper	Ginger
	Bergamot	Camphor	Immortelle
	Cajuput	Chamomile	Jasmine
	Caraway	Cypress	Linden Blossom
	Clary Sage	Fennel	Neroli
	Coriander	Hyssop	Nutmeg
	Eucalyptus	Juniper	Origanum
	Mandarin	Lavender	Rose
	Orange	Marjoram	
		Peppermint	
		Rosemary	
SPRAINS/STRAINS	Eucalyptus	Black Pepper	Clove
	Thyme	Camphor	Ginger
		Chamomile	Immortelle
		Hyssop	Rose
		Lavender	Vetivert
		Marjoram	
		Peppermint	
		Rosemary	
IMPROVE MUSCLE TONE	Grapefruit	Black Pepper	Ginger
	Lemongrass	Lavender	
		Marjoram	
		Pine	
		Rosemary	

NERVOUS OR MENTAL DISORDERS

PROBLEM	TOP NOTES	MIDDLE NOTES	BASE NOTES
STRESS (Anxiety)	Basil	Chamomile	Benzoin
	Bergamot	Geranium	Cedarwood
	Clary Sage	Hyssop	Frankincense
	Lemon	Juniper	Immortelle
	Mandarin	Lavender	Jasmine
	Orange	Marjoram	Linden Blossom
	Petitgrain	Melissa	Myrrh
	Thyme	Peppermint	Neroli
	Yarrow	Pine	Patchouli
		Rosemary	Rose
			Sandalwood
			Vetivert
			Ylang Ylang
DEPRESSION	Basil	Chamomile	Cinnamon
	Bergamot	Camphor	Frankincense
	Grapefruit	Cypress	Immortelle
	Niaouli	Geranium	Neroli
	Orange	Lavender	Patchouli
	Petitgrain	Hyssop	Rose
	Ti-Tree	Juniper	Sandalwood
	Thyme	Marjoram	Vetivert
	Clary Sage	Pine	Ylang Ylang
		Rosemary	Jasmine
		Melissa	
EMOTIONAL STRESS	Basil	Juniper	Benzoin
	Clary Sage	Lavender	Jasmine
		Marjoram	
HYSTERIA	Basil	Camphor	Cedarwood
	Orange	Chamomile	Frankincense
	Petitgrain	Lavender	Immortelle
		Marjoram	Neroli
		Melissa	Ylang Ylang
		Peppermint	

NERVOUS OR MENTAL DISORDERS *continued...*

PROBLEM	TOP NOTES	MIDDLE NOTES	BASE NOTES
INSOMNIA	Basil	Camphor	Linden Blossom
	Orange	Chamomile	Neroli
	Mandarin	Juniper	Rose
	Petitgrain	Lavender	Sandalwood
	Thyme	Marjoram	Ylang Ylang
	Yarrow	Melissa	
IRRITABILITY	Bergamot	Chamomile	Jasmine
	Clary Sage	Cypress	Linden Blossom
	Grapefruit	Lavender	Neroli
	Orange	Marjoram	Rose
		Melissa	Ylang Ylang
SUDDEN STRESS	Basil	Juniper	Benzoin
		Lavender	Neroli
		Marjoram	Rose
		Peppermint	

CIRCULATION DISORDERS

PROBLEM	TOP NOTES	MIDDLE NOTES	BASE NOTES
HIGH BLOOD PRESSURE	Basil	Juniper	Immortelle
	Clary sage	Lavender	Ylang Ylang
	Lemon	Marjoram	Linden Blossom
	Mandarin	Melissa	
	Yarrow	Hyssop	
LOW BLOOD PRESSURE	Eucalyptus	Black Pepper	Benzoin
	Thyme	Camphor	Ginger
	Lemon	Chamomile	Immortelle
	Niaouli	Hyssop	
	Sage	Rosemary	
FLUID RETENTION	Eucalyptus	Cypress	Benzoin
	Grapefruit	Fennel	Cedar Wood
	Lemon	Geranium	Linden Blossom
	Petigrain	Hyssop	Patchouli
	Sage	Juniper	
	Yarrow	Lavender	
		Rosemary	

CIRCULATION DISORDERS *continued...*

PROBLEM	TOP NOTES	MIDDLE NOTES	BASE NOTES
KIDNEY COMPLAINTS	Eucalyptus	Fennel	Cedarwood
	Grapefruit	Geranium	Linden Blossom
	Lemon	Juniper	Sandalwood
	Sage	Lavender	
	Thyme	Pine	
INFLAMED KIDNEYS	Coriander	Fennel	Clove
	Eucalyptus	Geranium	Myrrh
	Lemon	Hyssop	Sandalwood
	Sage	Juniper	Cedarwood
	Thyme	Pine	
		Lavender	
CYSTITIS	Basil	Chamomile	Clove
	Cajuput	Hyssop	Sandalwood
	Coriander	Juniper	
	Eucalyptus	Peppermint	
	Niaouli		
	Thyme		
CONGESTED LYMPH	Lemon	Black Pepper	Benzoin
	Grapefruit	Camphor	Ginger
	Niaouli	Chamomile	Frankincense
	Tea Tree	Juniper	Immortelle
	Yarrow	Rosemary	Linden Blossom
	Sage	Cypress	Rose
		Geranium	
		Melissa	
		Lavender	
VARICOSE VEINS (*****Do not massage*****)	Lemon	Cypress Peppermint	Neroli
THREAD VEINS	Lemon	Chamomile	Frankincense
	Orange	Cypress	Neroli
	Yarrow	Lavender	Patchouli
		Peppermint	Rose

RESPIRATORY DISORDERS

PROBLEM	TOP NOTES	MIDDLE NOTES	BASE NOTES
ALLERGIES	Basil	Chamomile	Benzoin
	Eucalyptus	Geranium	Frankincense
	Lemon	Hyssop	Immortelle
	Thyme	Melissa	
ASTHMA	Basil	Aniseed	Benzoin
	Bergamot	Black Pepper	Clove
	Cajuput	Chamomile	Frankincense
	Eucalyptus	Cypress	Neroli
	Lemon	Hyssop	Origanum
	Mandarin	Lavender	Immortelle
	Niaouli	Marjoram	Rose
	Thyme	Melissa	
	Sage	Peppermint	
		Pine	
		Rosemary	
BRONCHITIS	Basil	Aniseed	Benzoin
	Bergamot	Black Pepper	Cedarwood
	Cajuput	Camphor	Clove
	Caraway	Cypress	Frankincense
	Eucalyptus	Hyssop	Ginger
	Lemon	Juniper	Immortelle
	Niaouli	Lavender	Myrrh
	Orange	Marjoram	Origanum
	Thyme	Peppermint	Sandalwood
	Tea Tree	Pine	
	Yarrow	Rosemary	
	Sage		
CATARRH	Basil	Black Pepper	Cedarwood
	Cajuput	Hyssop	Frankincense
	Eucalyptus	Lavender	Ginger
	Lemon	Marjoram	Myrrh
	Niaouli	Peppermint	Sandalwood
	Thyme		
	Tea Tree		

PROBLEM	TOP NOTES	MIDDLE NOTES	BASE NOTES
COUGH	Basil	Aniseed	Benzoin
	Cajuput	Black Pepper	Cedarwood
	Eucalyptus	Camphor	Cinnamon
	Thyme	Hyssop	Ginger
	Tea Tree	Melissa	Immortelle
		Peppermint	Jasmine
		Pine	Myrrh
			Origanum
FLU	Basil	Cypress	Cinnamon
	Cajuput	Hyssop	Clove
	Coriander	Peppermint	Frankincense
	Eucalyptus	Pine	Ginger
	Lemon	Rosemary	Immortelle
	Niaouli		Linden Blossom
	Thyme		Myrrh
	Tea Tree		
	Yarrow		
	Sage		
PLEURISY	Caraway	Lavender	Clove
	Yarrow	Camphor	
WHOOPING COUGH	Basil	Fennel	Immortelle
	Naouli	Cypress	
	Thyme	Lavender	
	Tea Tree	Rosemary	

SKIN DISORDERS

For all skin disorders german chamomile is helpful because of the high azuline content. A 5% solution of calendula or oil of evening primrose is beneficial as well.

PROBLEM	TOP NOTES	MIDDLE NOTES	BASE NOTES
ABSCESSES/BOILS (Congested Skin)	Basil Bergamot Cajuput Lemon Niaouli Thyme Tea Tree	Chamomile Geranium Juniper Lavender Peppermint Rosemary	Clove Immortelle Myrrh Sandalwood
ACNE	Bergamot Cajuput Grapefruit Lemon Lemongrass Niaouli Orange Petitgrain Thyme Tea Tree Yarrow	Camphor Chamomile Geranium Juniper Lavender Rosemary	Benzoin Cedarwood Clove Frankincense Immortelle Patchouli Rose Sandalwood Vetivert
ALLERGIES **(Skin)**	Eucalyptus	Chamomile Hyssop Lavender Melissa	Immortelle Patchouli
ANTI-AGEING	Bergamot Clary Sage Orange	Geranium Lavender Marjoram	Frankincense Immortelle Linden Blossom Neroli Patchouli Rose Vetivert Ylang Ylang Sandalwood
ATHLETE'S FOOT	Lemongrass Tea Tree	Lavender Peppermint Pine	Cedarwood Frankincense Immortelle Myrrh Patchouli

PROBLEM	TOP NOTES	MIDDLE NOTES	BASE NOTES
ECZEMA	Basil	Chamomile	Benzoin
	Bergamot	Geranium	Cedarwood
	Cajuput	Hyssop	Frankincense
	Eucalyptus	Juniper	Immortelle
	Niaouli	Lavender	Myrrh
	Thyme	Melissa	Patchouli
	Yarrow		Rose
	Sage		Sandalwood
			Clove
ALLERGY PRONE OR SENSITIVE SKIN		Chamomile	Immortelle
		Lavender	Jasmine
			Neroli
			Rose
INFLAMED SKIN OR SUNBURNED	Clary Sage	Chamomile	Frankincense
	Tea Tree	Camphor	Sandalwood
	Yarrow	Geranium	Myrrh
		Lavender	Rose
		Peppermint	Benzoin
			Immortelle
			Patchouli
BROKEN CAPILLARIES	Lemon	Chamomile	Neroli
	Bergamot	Cypress	Rose
	Yarrow	Lavender	
		Peppermint	
BRUISES	Sage	Black Pepper	Myrrh
	Caraway	Camphor	Clove
		Chamomile	Ginger
		Fennel	
		Hyssop	
		Marjoram	
		Rosemary	
		Lavender	
BURNS	Sage	Chamomile	Benzoin
	Eucalyptus	Geranium	Linden Blossom
	Niaouli	Lavender	
	Tea Tree	Camphor	
	Yarrow		

SKIN DISORDERS *continued...*

PROBLEM	TOP NOTES	MIDDLE NOTES	BASE NOTES
CANDIDA	Tea Tree	Savory	Cinnamon
	Bergamot	Rosemary	Immortelle
	Eucalyptus		Myrrh
	Sage		Rose (Otto)
	Thyme		
CELLULITE	Lemongrass	Cypress	Cedarwood
	Sage	Juniper	Origanum
	Grapefruit	Fennel	Patchouli
		Geranium	Sandalwood
		Lavender	
		Rosemary	
DERMATITIS	Sage	Geranium	Benzoin
(Careful !)	Bergamot	Chamomile	Patchouli
	Cajuput	Hyssop	Cedarwood
	Eucalyptus	Juniper	Immortelle
	Thyme	Lavender	Rose (Otto)
		Peppermint	
DRY & CRACKED	Petigrain	Chamomile	Jasmine
SKIN	Yarrow	Geranium	Neroli
		Lavender	Sandalwood
			Rose
OEDEMA	Petitgrain	Fennel	Cedarwood
WATER RETENTION	Eucalyptus	Geranium	Benzoin
	Sage	Juniper	Patchouli
		Cypress	
		Lavender	
		Rosemary	
PSORIASIS	Bergamot	Lavender	Benzoin
	Cajuput	Geranium	Cedarwood
	Niaouli	Chamomile	Immortelle
CHICKENPOX	Bergamot	Chamomile	Immortelle
	Eucalyptus	Lavender	Sandalwood
	Tea Tree		
	Niaouli		

SKIN DISORDERS *continued...*			
PROBLEM	**TOP NOTES**	**MIDDLE NOTES**	**BASE NOTES**
SCABIES	Lemon	Lavender	Benzoin
	Bergamot	Peppermint	Clove
		Rosemary	Myrrh
			Neroli
FUNGAL SKIN INFECTIONS	Niaouli	Cypress	Patchouli
	Lemongrass	Geranium	Sandalwood
	Sage	Peppermint	Immortelle
	Tea Tree	Rosemary	
	Thyme	Pine	

DISEASES AND DISORDERS

PROBLEM	TOP NOTES	MIDDLE NOTES	BASE NOTES
DIABETES	Clary Sage Eucalyptus Lemon Thyme	Geranium Juniper Pine	Vetivert Ylang Ylang
EPILEPSY	Basil Cajuput Clary Sage Thyme	Lavender Marjoram Rosemary	
GOUT	Basil Lemon	Chamomile Fennel Juniper Pine Rosemary	
MENOPAUSE	Clary Sage Lemon Mandarin Sage	Aniseed Chamomile Cypress Fennel Geranium Lavender Melissa Peppermint Pine	Sandalwood Jasmine Ylang Ylang
OSTEOPOROSIS	Eucalyptus Lemon Sage	Lavender Rosemary	
TUBERCULOSIS	Cajuput Eucalyptus Niaouli Tea Tree		

The Lymphatic System

The lymphatic system is a type of **secondary circulation** inexplicably intertwined with the blood circulation. The basic material of the lymphatic system is the lymph which is **plasma** after it has exuded from the capillaries. It **gives nourishment** to the tissue cells and in return **takes away their waste** products. The liquid is drained off by tiny lymphatic vessels which join together to form larger lymph vessels and, as **these lymph vessels convey lymph towards the heart**, they are supplied with valves in much the same way as veins. Along their course towards the heart there are receiving or reservoir areas known as **lymph nodes**. They vary in size from pin head to a small almond.

The purpose of these lymph nodes is to filter the lymph and destroy foreign substances as it passes through and, in this way to help prevent infection passing into the blood stream and to produce and add lymphocytes to the lymph, and to produce antibodies.

Body cells live in tissue fluid, a liquid derived from the bloodstream. Water and dissolved substances, such as oxygen and nutrients, are constantly filtering through capillary walls into spaces between cells and as a result are adding volume to tissue fluids. Under normal conditions, fluid is also constantly removed so that it does not accumulate in the tissues. Part of this fluid simply returns (by diffusion) to the capillary bloodstream, taking with it some of the end products of cellular metabolism, including carbon dioxide and other substances. A second pathway for drainage of tissue fluid involves the lymphatic system. In addition to blood-carrying capillaries, there are microscopic vessels called lymphatic capillaries, which drain away excess tissue fluid that does not return to the blood capillaries. The relation between the circulatory system and the limbic system is shown below.

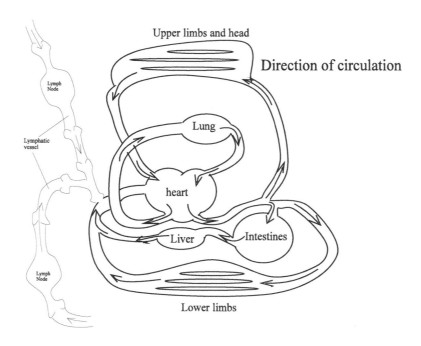

Another important function of the lymphatic system is to absorb protein from the tissue fluid and return it to the bloodstream. As soon as tissue fluids enters the lymphatic capillary, it is called "lymph". The lymphatic capillaries join to form the larger lymphatic vessels or ducts, and these vessels eventually empty into the veins. But, before the lymph reaches the veins, it flows through filters called "lymph nodes", this is where bacteria and other foreign particle are trapped and destroyed.

Lymphatic capillaries resemble blood capillaries in that they are made of one layer of flattened Squamous epithelial cells also called endothelium cells, which allows for easy passage of soluble material. Gaps between these endothelial cells allow the entrance of proteins and other relatively large suspended molecules. Unlike the blood stream the lymph seems to have no direction other than forwards and in the general direction of the heart.

The lymphatic vessels are thin walled and delicate and have a beaded appearance because of indentations where valves are located. These valves prevent back flow in the same way as veins by having a one-way valve positioned at intervals along the way.

Surface or **superficial lymph** is found within 2 cm below the skin surface, often near vein pathways. The deeper lymph vessels are larger and accompany the deep veins.

Lymph vessels are named according to location. For example, lymph found in the breast area is called *"mammary lymph"*, lymph vessels in the thigh are called *"femoral lymph vessels"*. All lymph vessels carry lymph to selected areas called **lymph nodes**. Lymphatic vessels carry lymph away from the regional nodes to eventually drain into one of two terminals. **The right lymphatic duct** or the **left thoracic duct**, to be emptied into the bloodstream.

Lymphoid tissue or specialized lymph glands are:
1. **Tonsils**
2. **Adenoids**
3. **Peyer's patches in the ileum.**

Eventually all lymph passes into two principal lymph vessels, the thoracic duct and the right lymphatic duct, which opens into the blood stream at the junctions of the right and left, **internal jugular** and **subclavian veins** where it becomes part of the general systemic circulation again. The right lymphatic duct is a short vessel about 1.25 cm long that receives lymph that comes from the upper right quadrant of the body *(right side of head, neck, arm and thorax)*. It empties into the **right subclavian vein** which is guarded by **two semilunar valves** to prevent blood from entering the duct. The rest of the body is drained by the **thoracic duct** which is much larger *(about 40 cm long)*. The duct begins in the posterior part of the abdomen, just below the diaphragm. The first part of the duct is enlarged to form a cistern or temporary storage pouch, called the **cisterna chyli**. The word *chyle comes from the milky fluid* formed by the combination of fat globules and lymph that comes from the intestinal lacteals.

The thoracic duct extends upwards through the diaphragm and along the back wall of the thorax up into the root of the neck of the left side. Here it receives the left jugular lymphatic vessels from the head and neck, the left subclavian vessels from the left upper extremity, and other lymphatic vessels from the thorax. All lymph from below the diaphragm empties into the cisterna chyli by way of the various lymph nodes.

There are approximately 600-1000 of these lymphatic nodes scattered throughout the body along the line of the lymphatic vessels.

The most common superficial ones being:

1. **Cervical nodes** or profundus on either side of the neck just below the ears, are divided into deep and superficial groups which drain certain parts of the head and neck. They often become enlarged during upper respiratory infections.

2. **Axillary glands** in the armpit. May become enlarged following infections of the upper extremities and breasts, cancer cells from the breasts often metastasize (spread) to the axillary nodes.

3. **Tracheobronchial nodes** are found near the trachea and around the larger bronchial tubes. People living in polluted areas, these nodes become filled with black carbon particle.

4. **Mesenteric nodes** are found between two layers of peritoneum that forms the mesentery (membrane around the intestines). There are about 100 - 150 of these nodes.

5. The **inguinals** in the groin. Receives lymph from the lower extremities and genital organs. When they are enlarged they are often referred to as buboes from which the bubonic plague got its name.

6. The ones in the **popliteal fossa** or depression behind the knee.

7. The **supratrochlea** or cubital nodes in the crutch of the elbow.

8. The **supraclavicular** glands.

9. The **submandibular nodes** underneath the mandible and the cervical, and occipital glands.

This is not a complete list of lymph nodes, but they are sometimes the most obvious of the superficial glands which swell when an infection is present in that part of the body.

DIAGRAM OF THE LYMPH NODES

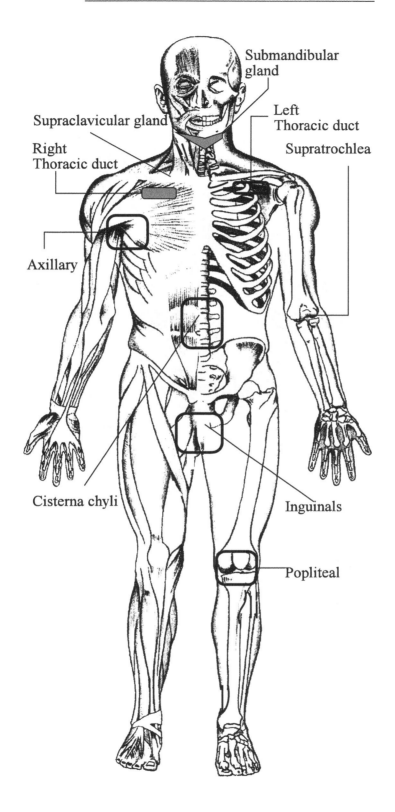

Submandibular gland

Supraclavicular gland

Left Thoracic duct

Right Thoracic duct

Supratrochlea

Axillary

Cisterna chyli

Inguinals

Popliteal

A lymph node consists of several points of entry and one point that exits, the points of entry are called afferent lymphatic angions and the exiting lymph angion is called efferent. There is an artery leading to the node and a vein leading out that supplies the lymph node with blood, the point of entry and exit into and out of the lymph node is called the helum. The node is split-up into areas called sinuses that are separated by walls called trabecula.

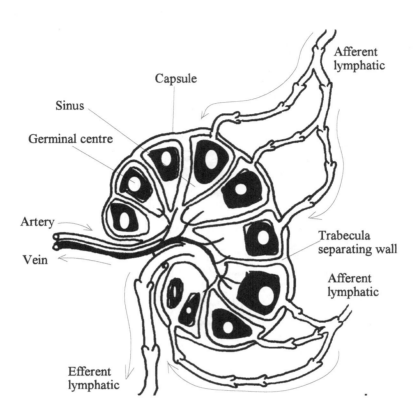

THE FUNCTION OF LYMPH

1. To filter out dust particles, and to remove, dyes, pathogens, waste and dead or dying cells.
2. The lymph nodes concentrate the lymph by removing 40 % of the fluid.
3. A lymph node can repair itself provided that there is a blood and nerve supply still intact.
4. To assist in immunity as one of the major sites of immune reactions..
5. Helps maintain blood fluid volume.
6. To circulate proteins around the body.
7. To transport fats, especially long chain cells and proteins.
8. To maintain connective tissue in a functional healthy state.
9. To remove excess water from the lymph via the veins.
10. To store or trap inorganic matter like dust particles.

Problems That Cause Restriction of Lymphatic Flow:
1. Chronic dehydration.
2. Elasticated clothing.
3. Cold will decrease lymph flow.
4. Heat above 104 degrees.
5. Night time or prolonged rest periods will shut the lymph system down.
6. Inflammation will close the lymph valves.
7. Paralysis.
8. Nerve lesions

The Effects of Lymphoedema:
1. Lowered lymph transport capacity.
2. Unable to break down proteins.
3. Swelling in subcutaneous tissue.
4. Excess protein build up.
5. Swelling gets worse as time goes on.
6. In time proteins break down.
7. Fibrosis is the final result.

What is Lymphoedema:
In long standing oedema the vascular action is increased and the body will lay down more connective tissue and fat cells. Gradually, the tissue becomes hard and lymph action ceases.
The appearance is normal, but the skin is taut. Pressing a finger causes a depression that remains after the finger is removed.

The Four Major Components of Lymph:
1. Water   2. Proteins   3. Fats   4. Cells

Three Minor Components of Lymph:
1. Dust   2. Dyes   3. Pathogens

Different Grades of Oedema:
Grade 1.   Is reversible, will recover with bed rest and appears soft and will pit with pressure
Grade 2.   Is irreversible, will not recover with bed rest and stronger pressure is required to cause pitting, fibrosis occurs, collagen and body connective tissue hardens.
Grade 3.   Severe and advanced oedema, sclerosis, elephantiasis, fibrosis around vessels and nerves causing damage, quite often lymphangiosarcoma forms.

LYMPHOSTATIC OEDEMA, is a high protein oedema that can be organic in origin, which means that there occurs a change in the pathway of the lymph at a body structure level. This change in the pathway often means that this type of oedema is often irreversible and cannot be cured. This type of oedema is called **ORGANIC OEDEMA**.

The other type of high protein lymphostatic oedema is called **FUNCTIONAL OEDEMA**. This type of oedema is treatable, and is caused by changes in the function of the body. Some of these changes are due to smooth muscle impairment, skeletal muscle paralysis, angion valve impairment or ruptured collagen filaments.

PRIMARY LYMPHOEDEMA is a branch of organic lymphoedema which normally manifests itself on one limb even though the problem exists in both limbs. It effects the lower extremities more than the upper limbs, and begins distally with a proximal spread. Lymph collector deficiency is the main cause, either congenital or hereditary. There are two types of Primary Lymphoedema, **Precox and Tarda**. Precox is more commonly found at an early age during puberty and adolescents. Tarda effects the remaining 17% after the age of 30 years, some of the effects are pale thin skin leading to hypokeratosis.

SECONDARY LYMPHOEDEMA is also a branch of organic lymphoedema. This type of oedema is caused by **outside intervention** like; Parasite (**nematode worm**) contracted by tropical mosquitoes that infect the blood and in time worms develop and live in the lymph giving rise to a disorder called filariasis disease. **Surgery** is also another major contributor of secondary oedema, where lymph nodes are removed or damaged. Cancers like, **lymphangiosarcoma** or Stewart-Treves Syndrome, or tumours, and lastly, **constricting clothing** like tight socks with elasticated tops, brasiers with wire or bone supports, underpants with elasticated or tight fitting legs seams. Any of these garments can cause inflammation in the area of constriction.

DYNAMIC OEDEMA unlike lymphostatic oedema is not a high protein oedema, but is in fact a low protein oedema that cannot be managed by manual lymphatic drainage treatment because it is caused by **congested heart failure**, varicose veins, kidney failure, right side heart failure (this causes blood in the veins to pool causing veins congestion).

LYMPHOSTATIC OEDEMA

HIGH PROTEIN OEDEMA

DYNAMIN OEDEMA

LOW PROTEIN OEDEMA
Contra-indicated for manual lymph therapies
congested heart failure
varicose veins
Kidney failure
Right side heart failure (causes venous blood
to pool causing venous congestion).

ORGANIC OEDEMA

MOSTLY IRREVERSIBLE
CHANGES IN PATHWAYS

FUNCTIONAL OEDEMA

REVERSIBLE
CHANGES IN FUNCTION

Smooth muscle impairment
Skeletal muscle paralysis
Angian valve impairment
Ruptured colagen filiments

PRIMARY OEDEMA

Congenital
Hereditary
difficiency of lymph vessels

SECONDARY OEDEMA

Paracite (Nematode worm causes filariasis disease transmitted
by tropical mosquitoes.
Surgery, or tumors.
Cancer (Lymphangiosarcoma) Stewart-Treves Sysdrome.
Constricting clothing causing inflammation.

PRECOX OEDEMA

At an early age
puberty and adolescence

TARDA OEDEMA

After age 30 yrs
Pale thin skin leading to
hypokeratosis

Although the lymphatic system appears primitive when compared to the other systems, it is in fact an amazing structure that works remarkably well. Every cell in the body must be supplied with nutrition, oxygen, hormones, water, essential minerals and protein. The metabolism requires not only the delivery of these substances but also the efficient removal of waste and other by-products, that's were the lymphatic system comes in.

The lymphatic system starts with tiny subcutaneous pre-lymphatic lymph vessels that cover the sub-surface of the entire body in zones and territories. These areas are defined and mapped out using watershed lines to show us the cut-off point for lymph travelling in a particular direction as seen below.

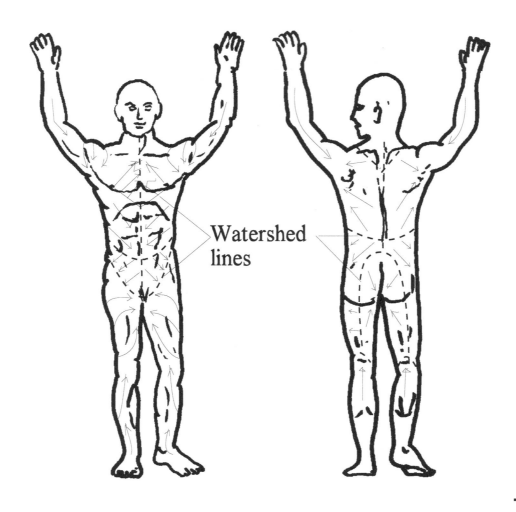

Watershed lines

The Spleen

The spleen is a mass of lymphoid tissue located in the upper left hypochondriac region of the abdomen and is normally protected by the lower part of the rib cage. It sits high under the dome of the diaphragm and is approximately the size of a fist
.

The spleen produces, monitors, stores and destroys blood cells. There is a white pulp and a red pulp area of the spleen. The white pulp is part of the immune system and produces lymphocytes that help the body fight against infections. The red pulp also contains white blood cells in the form of phagocytes. These are responsible for eating unwanted material in the blood like defective cells, bacteria, debris, etc. The red pulp will monitor the red blood cells and ultimately destroy those that are not functioning correctly whether due to age or defect.

The capsule of the spleen, as well as its structure is more elasticated than that of the lymph nodes. It contains involuntary or smooth muscle, which enables the spleen to contract or swell.

If the spleen is removed, the body's immune system will lose some of its capabilities to produce antibodies and remove bacteria from the blood. Hence, the body will be hard pressed to fight infection as it once used to.

MAJOR FUNCTIONS OF THE SPLEEN

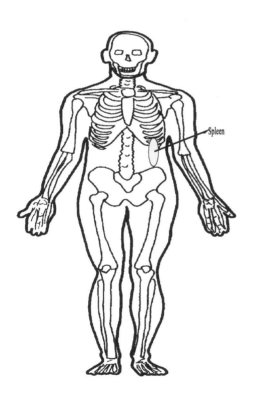

1. Cleaning the blood by filtration and phagocytosis.

2. Destroying old or worn-out red blood cells.

3. To produce red blood cells before birth.

4. To serve as a reservoir for blood, which can be returned to the bloodstream in case of haemorrhage or other emergencies.

Terminology

Analgesic   Pain-killing oils like; *Bergamot, Cajeput, Coriander, Eucalyptus, Lemon-grass, Niaouli, Black-pepper, Chamomile, Jasmine, Lavender, Marjoram, Peppermint, Rosemary and Ginger.*

Antibiotic   oils that combats infection within the body like, *Cajeput, Garlic, Manuka, Niaouli, Ravensara and Tea Tree.*

Anti-depressant   *Basil, Bergamot, Clary Sage, Geranium, Jasmine, Grapefruit, Lavender, Lemongrass, Mandarin, Melissa, Neroli, Orange Blossom, Patchouli, Petitgrain, Rose, Sandalwood and Ylang Ylang.*

Anti-inflammatory   *Caraway, Teatree, Camphor, Chamomile, Fennel, Geranium, Jasmine, Peppermint, Benzoin, Frankincense, Myrrh and Patchouli.*

Antispasmodics   prevent or relieves muscle spasm. *Chamomile, Cardamon, Clary-Sage, Ginger, Marjoram and Orange.*

Antiviral   oils kill or inhibit the growth of viruses, *Garlic, Bergamot, Eucalyptus, Lavender, Manuka, Ravensara and Tea Tree.*

Astringent   means to tighten the tissues and reduce fluid *loss. Cedarwood, Cypress, Frankincense, Juniper, Myrrh, Rose and Sandalwood.*

Bechic   (eases coughing), *Lavender, Sandalwood, and Thyme.*

Cephalic   oils clear the mind and stimulates mental activity. *Basil, Grapefruit, Rosemary and Thyme.*

Diuretic   aids in the production of urine and promotes urination - reduces swelling *Bergamot, Caraway, Eucalyptus, Lemon, Thyme, Black-pepper, Camphor, Cypress, Fennel, Geranium, Hyssop, Juniper, Lavender, Marjoram, Pine, Rosemary, Benzoin, Cedarwood, Frankincense, Patchouli and Sandalwood.*

Febrifuge   means to "reduce fever". *Bergamot, Chamomile, Eucalyptus, Melissa, Peppermint, Ravensara, Tea Tree.*

Fungicidal   oils will kill or inhibit the growth of yeasts and fungus. *Lavender, Myrrh, and Tea Tree.*

Hepatic   is to strengthen the liver. *Chamomile, Cypress, Lemon, Peppermint, Rosemary and Thyme.*

Immune enhancers   *Cinnamon leaf, Clove bud, Frankincense, Garlic, Lavender, Manuka, Ravensara, Rosewood and Tea Tree.*

Nervine or
Neurological stimulators   means to strengthen the nervous system. *Basil, Bergamot, Camphor wood, Chamomile (m), Cinnamon, Clary sage, Coriander, Cypress, Frankincense, Marjoram Sweet, Neroli, Nutmeg, Peppermint, Petigrain, Pine, Rose Otto and Rosemary.*

Rubefacient	means 'warming', *Black pepper, Eucalyptus, Juniper, Marjoram, Rosemary.*
Sedative	*Benzoin, Clary sage, Chamomile, Jasmine, Lavender, Marjoram, Melissa, Benzoin, Cedarwood, Frankincense, Myrrh, Neroli, Rose, Sandalwood and Ylang ylang.*
Vasoconstrictors	cause blood vessels to constrict. *Chamomile, Cypress, Rose.*
Vasodilators	cause the blood vessels to expand. *Marjoram.*
Vulnerary	helps wounds to heal. *Benzoin, Bergamot, Chamomile, Lavender, Myrrh and Tea Tree.*
Warming (Rubefacient)	*Bergamot, Eucalyptus, Thyme, Black Pepper, Camphor, Juniper, Lavender, Peppermint, Pine and Ginger.*

Common Diseases or Disorders

Disease or Disorder	ELEPHANTIASIS
Description	A great enlargement of an extremity resulting from blockage of lymphatic pathways. Usually this is the end stage of a lesion of filariasis, that has possibly lasted for years, it is characterized by tremendous swelling, usually of the external genitalia and legs. The overlying skin becomes dark, thick, and coarse.
Possible Allopathic Treatment	Not available at present. An option would be surgery and diuretics.
Possible Holistic Aromatherapy Treatment	****Only treat for pain and discomfort**** **Auto-immune enhancers** like; *Cinnamon leaf, Clove bud, Frankincense. Sedative oils like; Clary sage, Chamomile, Jasmine, Lavender, Marjoram, Benzoin, Cedarwood, Frankincense, Myrrh, Rose, Sandalwood and Ylang ylang.* **Anti-inflammatory** essential oils like; *Caraway, Teatree, Camphor, Chamomile, Fennel, Geranium, Jasmine, Peppermint, Benzoin, Frankincense, Myrrh and Patchouli.* **Analgesic** (Pain-killing)oils like; *Bergamot, Cajeput, Coriander, Eucalyptus, Lemon-grass, Niaouli, Black-pepper, Chamomile, Jasmine, Lavender, Marjoram, Peppermint, Rosemary and Ginger.* **Anti-depressant** essential oil like; *Basil, Bergamot, Lemongrass, Clary Sage, Geranium, Jasmine, Lavender, Melissa, Orange Blossom, Patchouli, Rose, Sandalwood and Ylang Ylang.*

Disease or Disorder	LYMPHADENITIS (LIM-FAD-EN-I-TIS)
Description	Inflammation of the lymph nodes, the nodes become enlarged and tender. Lymph node involvement may be generalized, with systemic infections or remain local. This condition reflects the body's attempt to combat an infection. Cervical lymphadenitis occurs during measles, scarlet fever, septic sore throat, diphtheria and frequently, the common cold. Chronic lymphadenitis may be due to the tubercle bacillus (TB). Infections of the upper extremities cause enlarged axillary nodes, as does cancer of the mammary glands. Infection of the external genitals or the lower extremities may cause enlargement of the inguinal lymph nodes.
Possible Allopathic Treatment	Treatment depends on underlying cause, hot, wet applications may help relieve pain. A lymph node biopsy will be necessary to determine the treatment.
Possible Holistic Aromatherapy Treatment	**Only treat for pain and discomfort** **Auto-immune enhancers** like; *Cinnamon leaf, Clove bud, Frankincense. Sedative oils like; Clary sage, Chamomile, Jasmine, Lavender, Marjoram, Benzoin, Cedarwood, Frankincense, Myrrh, Rose, Sandalwood and Ylang ylang.* **Anti-inflammatory** essential oils like; *Caraway, Teatree, Camphor, Chamomile, Fennel, Geranium, Jasmine, Peppermint, Benzoin, Frankincense, Myrrh and Patchouli.* **Analgesic** (Pain-killing) oils like; *Bergamot, Cajeput, Coriander, Eucalyptus, Lemon-grass, Niaouli, Black-pepper, Chamomile, Jasmine, Lavender, Marjoram, Peppermint, Rosemary and Ginger.* **Anti-depressant** essential oil like; *Basil, Bergamot, Lemongrass, Clary Sage, Geranium, Jasmine, Lavender, Melissa, Orange Blossom, Patchouli, Rose, Sandalwood and Ylang Ylang.*

Disease or Disorder	LYMPHADENOPATHY (LIMPH-ADEN-OPA-THEE)
Description	Lymphadenopathy is a term meaning "disease of the lymph nodes", Enlarged lymph nodes are common symptom in a number of infectious and cancerous diseases. An early sign of infection with HIV, the virus that causes AIDS, is a generalized lymphadenopathy. Infectious mononucleosis is an acute viral infection the hall mark of which is a marked enlargement of the cervical lymph nodes. Mononucleosis is fairly common among college students.
Possible Allopathic Treatment	Allopathic treatment would be too varied to specify here due to the onset of the disease, its progression and its cause. Treatment depends on underlying cause, but a hot, wet applications may help relieve pain. A lymph node biopsy will be necessary to determine the treatment.
Possible Holistic Aromatherapy Treatment	****Only treat for pain and discomfort**** **Auto-immune enhancers** like; *Cinnamon leaf, Clove bud, Frankincense. Sedative oils like; Clary sage, Chamomile, Jasmine, Lavender, Marjoram, Benzoin, Cedarwood, Frankincense, Myrrh, Rose, Sandalwood and Ylang ylang.* **Anti-inflammatory** essential oils like; *Caraway, Teatree, Camphor, Chamomile, Fennel, Geranium, Jasmine, Peppermint, Benzoin, Frankincense, Myrrh and Patchouli.* **Analgesic** (Pain-killing) oils like; *Bergamot, Cajeput, Coriander, Eucalyptus, Lemon-grass, Niaouli, Black-pepper, Chamomile, Jasmine, Lavender, Marjoram, Peppermint, Rosemary and Ginger.* **Anti-depressant** essential oil like; *Basil, Bergamot, Lemongrass, Clary Sage, Geranium, Jasmine, Lavender, Melissa, Orange Blossom, Patchouli, Rose, Sandalwood and Ylang Ylang.*

Disease or Disorder	SPLENOMEGALY
Description	An abnormal enlargement of the spleen, accompanies certain acute infectious diseases, including scarlet fever, typhus fever, typhoid fever and syphilis. Many tropical parasitic diseases cause splenomegaly. A certain blood fluke (flatworm) that is fairly common among workers in Japan and other parts of Asia causing marked splenic enlargement.
Possible Allopathic Treatment	Allopathic treatment would be too varied to specify here due to the onset of the disease, its progression and its cause. Treatment depends on underlying cause.
Possible Holistic Aromatherapy Treatment	****Only treat for pain and discomfort**** **Auto-immune enhancers** like; Cinnamon leaf, Clove bud, Frankincense. Sedative oils like; Clary sage, Chamomile, Jasmine, Lavender, Marjoram, Benzoin, Cedarwood, Frankincense, Myrrh, Rose, Sandalwood and Ylang ylang. **Anti-inflammatory** essential oils like; *Caraway, Teatree, Camphor, Chamomile, Fennel, Geranium, Jasmine, Peppermint, Benzoin, Frankincense, Myrrh and Patchouli.* **Analgesic** (Pain-killing) oils like; *Bergamot, Cajeput, Coriander, Eucalyptus, Lemon-grass, Niaouli, Black-pepper, Chamomile, Jasmine, Lavender, Marjoram, Peppermint, Rosemary and Ginger.* **Anti-depressant** essential oil like; *Basil, Bergamot, Lemongrass, Clary Sage, Geranium, Jasmine, Lavender, Melissa, Orange Blossom, Patchouli, Rose, Sandalwood and Ylang Ylang.*

Disease or Disorder	SPLENIC ANAEMIA
Description	Characterized by enlargement of the spleen, haemorrhages from the stomach, and accumulation of fluid in the abdomen.
Possible Allopathic Treatment	Allopathic treatment would be too varied to specify here due to the onset of the disease, its progression and its cause. Treatment depends on underlying cause, But in this disease and others of the same nature, splenectomy appears to constitute a cure.
Possible Holistic Aromatherapy Treatment	**Only treat for pain and discomfort** **Auto-immune enhancers** like; Cinnamon leaf, Clove bud, Frankincense. Sedative oils like; Clary sage, Chamomile, Jasmine, Lavender, Marjoram, Benzoin, Cedarwood, Frankincense, Myrrh, Rose, Sandalwood and Ylang ylang. **Anti-inflammatory** essential oils like; *Caraway, Teatree, Camphor, Chamomile, Fennel, Geranium, Jasmine, Peppermint, Benzoin, Frankincense, Myrrh and Patchouli.* **Analgesic** (Pain-killing) oils like; *Bergamot, Cajeput, Coriander, Eucalyptus, Lemon-grass, Niaouli, Black-pepper, Chamomile, Jasmine, Lavender, Marjoram, Peppermint, Rosemary and Ginger.* **Anti-depressant** essential oil like; *Basil, Bergamot, Lemongrass, Clary Sage, Geranium, Jasmine, Lavender, Melissa, Orange Blossom, Patchouli, Rose, Sandalwood and Ylang Ylang.*

Disease or Disorder	HODGKIN'S DISEASE
Description	Hodgkin's Disease is a chronic malignant disorder, most common in young men, characterized by painless enlarged lymph nodes. The nodes in the neck particularly, and often those in the armpit, thorax and groin. The spleen may become enlarged as well. The present of Reed-Sternberg cells, this is a large, abnormal multi nucleated reticuloendothelial cell found in the lymphatic system. Symptoms include anorexic type weight loss, generalized pruritus, low-grade fever, night sweats, anaemia and leucocytosis.
Possible Allopathic Treatment	Chemotherapy and radiation either separately or in combination, have been used with good results 50% of the time, affording patients many years of life.
Possible Holistic Aromatherapy Treatment	****Only treat for pain and discomfort**** **Auto-immune enhancers** like; Cinnamon leaf, Clove bud, Frankincense. Sedative oils like; Clary sage, Chamomile, Jasmine, Lavender, Marjoram, Benzoin, Cedarwood, Frankincense, Myrrh, Rose, Sandalwood and Ylang ylang. **Anti-inflammatory** essential oils like; *Caraway, Teatree, Camphor, Chamomile, Fennel, Geranium, Jasmine, Peppermint, Benzoin, Frankincense, Myrrh and Patchouli.* **Analgesic** (Pain-killing) oils like; *Bergamot, Cajeput, Coriander, Eucalyptus, Lemon-grass, Niaouli, Black-pepper, Chamomile, Jasmine, Lavender, Marjoram, Peppermint, Rosemary and Ginger.* **Anti-depressant** essential oil like; *Basil, Bergamot, Lemongrass, Clary Sage, Geranium, Jasmine, Lavender, Melissa, Orange Blossom, Patchouli, Rose, Sandalwood and Ylang Ylang.*

Disease or Disorder	**LYMPHOSARCOMA**
Description	Lymphosarcoma is a malignant tumour of the lymphoid tissue that is likely to be rapidly fatal. Fortunately, it is not a common disease. (Lymphoma, is any tumour, benign or malignant, that occurs in lymphoid tissue). Effects similar to Hodgkin's Disease.
Possible Allopathic Treatment	Early surgery in combination with appropriate radiotherapy offers the only possible cure at this time
Possible Holistic Aromatherapy Treatment	****Only treat for pain and discomfort**** **Auto-immune enhancers** like; Cinnamon leaf, Clove bud, Frankincense. Sedative oils like; Clary sage, Chamomile, Jasmine, Lavender, Marjoram, Benzoin, Cedarwood, Frankincense, Myrrh, Rose, Sandalwood and Ylang ylang. **Anti-inflammatory** essential oils like; *Caraway, Teatree, Camphor, Chamomile, Fennel, Geranium, Jasmine, Peppermint, Benzoin, Frankincense, Myrrh and Patchouli.* **Analgesic** (Pain-killing) oils like; *Bergamot, Cajeput, Coriander, Eucalyptus, Lemon-grass, Niaouli, Black-pepper, Chamomile, Jasmine, Lavender, Marjoram, Peppermint, Rosemary and Ginger.* **Anti-depressant** essential oil like; *Basil, Bergamot, Lemongrass, Clary Sage, Geranium, Jasmine, Lavender, Melissa, Orange Blossom, Patchouli, Rose, Sandalwood and Ylang Ylang.*

Essential Oils

CORIANDER

Latin name: *coriandrum sativum*   **Botanical family:** *umbelliferae*

The three main areas where this oil can help are:

1. Muscle relaxant
2. Detoxifier
3. Digestive problems

Properties	Uses
Antispasmodic	Colic, diarrhea, stomach cramps, flatulence, indigestion, nausea
Analgesic	Neuralgia, arthritis, rheumatism, headaches, aches and pains
Stimulant	Lymphatic stimulant, exhaustion, fatigue, hormonal stimulant, poor memory, loss of appetite *(anorexia)*
Antiseptic	Influenza, deodorant, body odour

Place of Origin
Coriander is an attractive plant which grows both wild and cultivated in the **Far East, Spain, North Africa, and Russia**. Some plants are found growing wild in parts of England. The seed has a very spicy and fresh aroma. It grows up to three 3 feet in height from a thin spindle shaped root with rounded leaves and tiny white to pink flowers.

Method Of Extraction
Essential oil of coriander is obtained through **steam distillation of the seeds of the ripe fruit and leaves.** The oil may be pale yellow or colourless. Its main chemical constituents include: coriandrol, pinene, geraniol and traces of phellandrene, dipentene, terpinene, cymene and borneol.

Traditional Uses
The fruits have been used since ancient times in both the culinary and medicinal fields. Used in cooking to delay the putrefaction process with meats, coriander is also known to help with digestive problems. After meals in the Victorian times, the seeds from the coriander plant were chewed to aid the digestion process as well as sweeten the breath. In the 17th Century it was used in liqueurs such as *Benedictine and Chartreuse.*

Herbal Uses
Drinking an infusion made from the coriander seed or chewing the seeds themselves will sooth an upset stomach or aid indigestion. To prepare the infusion, steep two tea spoons of dried seed in one cup of water on he next day you can drink it. Repeat daily until the problem goes away. Rheumatic pain responds well from a poultice made from the crushed seeds.

Aromatherapy

Essential oil of coriander is useful in the treatment of **digestive problems including colic, flatulence, indigestion and stomach cramps** due to its antispasmodic properties. It has been used in the treatment of anorexia nervosa because it has shown to increase the appetite.

A stimulant in general, **coriander will help remove wastes and detoxify the body by stimulating the spleen**. This can make it valuable to increase immunity and treat viral infections like flues and cold.

Fatigue, debility and exhaustion have improved with the use of this essential oil. An aid in battling infertility. At the same time it is a treatment for PMS and irregular menstrual cycles due to its ability to stimulate estrogen in females.

The oil has a **warming and analgesic effect** that can be utilized for arthritis, rheumatism, neuralgia, sprains and just general aches and pains. Combined with its known antispasmodic properties it will help relieve muscle spasms.

It is an effective antiseptic and deodorant essential oil. It will prevent body odour by way of killing the growth of bacteria and help mask the unpleasant smell that normally accompanies this problem. It si a wonderful addition to the bath or any bath products.

Warning: *This oil should be used in moderation as it can be stupefying in large doses.*

GRAPEFRUIT

Latin name: *citrus paradisi*   **Botanical family:**   *Rutaceae*

The three main areas where this oil can help are:

1. **Manic depression**
2. **Lymphatic stimulant**
3. **Drug addictions**

Properties	Uses
Stimulant	Lymphatic stimulant, cellulite, bile stimulant, fluid retention, appetite stimulant, fatigue, constipation
Antidepressant	Depression, grief, sadness, SAD *(seasonal affective disorder)*
Astringent	Acne, oily skin, stretch marks
Tonic	Liver, kidney, vascular system, gallstones

Place of Origin
Grapefruit is native to tropical **Asia and the West Indies**. However, the **USA is now the main producer** of the oil. This is a cultivated tree *(not grown wild)* that can grow to over 10 metres high. It has glossy leaves with white flowers and the familiar yellow fruits, which hang from the trees like large bunches of grapes flattened at the ends.

Method of Extraction
The essential oil is obtained through **expression of the peel** since the oil glands are embedded deep within the peel. This citrus contains much less oil than other citrus such as orange or lemon. Some oil is obtained through distillation, but this is an inferior quality oil and not to be used in aromatherapy. Active ingredients include mainly terpenes such as limonene, and alcohols such as geraiol and linalool.

Traditional Uses
It is not clearly known where grapefruit actually originated from. It was recorder in 1830, that it was finally accepted as a species and given the name citrus paradisi. It has been used in the food industry.

Herbal Uses
Other than use within the aromatherapy field, there is no herbal uses for grapefruit that the author is aware of.

Aromatherapy

An inexpensive, yet valuable oil to have in any aromatherapist repertoire, **grapefruit has a balancing effect on the central nervous system, making it useful in cases of manic-depression, depression, grief, nervous exhaustion or any instance where a light uplifting oil would benefit** the individual. When used in combination with other stimulating oils like peppermint, rosemary or other citrus oils, it can help revive a tired and weary body both physically and emotionally.

A **stimulant to both the spleen and the lymphatic system**, problems such as fluid retention, cellulite and weight gain show improvement by the action of removing any excess fluids and breaking down fats. Daily topical application of grapefruit is required to help disperse the cellulite. A combination of this oil and juniper have been found useful in the battle against cellulite. However, dietary changes need to be made, as well as regular exercise.

A tonic to the liver and kidney, essential oil of **grapefruit stimulates bile secretion and cleanses these organs and help dissolve kidney stones.** It may also be of assistance in dealing with those who are battling drug addiction.

A blood purifier and cleanser to the vascular system, problems like **gout, rheumatism or arthritis will benefit** from the application.

Astringent in nature, congested skin problems like acne, pimples or oily skin will benefit from the use of grapefruit essential oil. Combined with the uplifting attributes, this makes it valuable in the treatment of problem skin.

Remember most citrus oils are loved by the general population.

Warning: *As with any citrus oil, skin irritation could occur especially if exposed to ultraviolet radiation after application.*

LEMON

Latin Name: *citrus Limonium*   **Botanical name:** *Rutaceae*

The three main areas where this oil can help are:

1. **Circulatory problems**
2. **Immune stimulant**
3. **Wounds and cuts**

Properties	Uses
Tonic	Circulatory system, varicose veins, chilblains, broken capillaries, arteriosclerosis, digestive system
Anti-viral/ Immunostimulant	Influenza, respiratory infection, colds, catarrh, warts
Haemostatic	Cuts, nosebleeds, bleeding gums
Antiseptic	Infections, bronchitis, asthma, oily skin, pimples, acne

Place of Origin
The lemon tree is thought to have originated in India, and to have been introduced into Italy towards the end of the 5th Century. From **Italy,** cultivation spread throughout the **Mediterranean basin to Spain and Portugal**. **California** now rivals the traditional growing area in commercial terms.

Method of Extraction
The **essential oil of lemon is pressed from the outer rind of the lemons**. It takes as many as 3,000 of them to produce a kilo of essential oil. The oil is a pale yellow colour with a hint of green and obviously smells like the fresh clean scent of lemon. Its active constituents include pinene, limonene, phellandrene, camphene, linalol, acetates of linalol and geranyl, citral and citrinellal.

Traditional Uses
A plant dating back in history, it arrived in Europe during the Crusades. Long used for its antiseptic abilities, it has been used during infectious epidemics. The peel has known to be used to scent clothing as well as utilized as an insect repellant.
It was in the 17th Century that it was discovered to be valuable for its "medicinal" use *(due to the high Vitamin C content)* for infection and toxicity.

Herbal Uses
Lemon juice, especially first thing in the morning is an excellent digestive aid that will increase the digestive juices while cleansing and decongesting the liver. Also known for its cleansing abilities on the blood, it has been used as a styptic to help stop blood flow.

Aromatherapy

Similar to the herbal uses, lemon has a tonifying and stimulating action on many systems. Through the use of his essential oil, **the digestive system will find a reduction in gastric acidity. It can be used in cases of debility and loss of appetite.**

Lemon will stimulate both gastric and pancreatic secretions. *(It has been used in the treatment of diabetes).* The liver and kidneys will also benefit from the detoxifying and cleansing action of this essential oil.

Lemon possesses a unique ability to counteract acidity in the body even though the nature of lemon is acidic. However, the citric acid is neutralised during the digestion process. It will increase the carbonates and bi-carbonates of potassium and calcium and these in turn will help maintain the alkalinity of the system. Ulcers or cases where there is an imbalance in the acid/alkaline balance will find improvement. These disorders include problems where there is an excess of uric acid in the system such as **gout, rheumatism, arthritis**, etc. To further assist the elimination of internal uric acid, it would be wise to bath in 1 cup of dead sea salts, or epsom salts three times per week. The alkaline nature of these salts help disperse the acid build up found in the joints.

A powerful antiseptic, essential oil of lemon can be used for the treatment of colds, bronchitis, catarrh and in the prevention of infectious diseases. Lemon is a powerful bactericide which is another excellent reason to use it in the treatment of cuts. Dr. Jean Valnet cites research which has shown that essential oil will kill diphtheria bacilli in 20 minutes and even in a low dilution *(0.2%)*. It will render the tuberculosis bacilli completely inactive.
Furthermore **it is an immunostimulant** that increases the action of the white blood cells boosting the body's immune response to viruses and other immune disorders.

Haemostatic in nature, nosebleeds, minor cuts and wounds, and bleeding gums will benefit from its styptic properties. Bleeding gums, gingivitis or mouth ulcers will improve with the utilization of a mouthwash. For nosebleeds, soak a small piece of cotton into some lemon juice and insert it into the nostril.

Lemon has a tonic effect on the circulatory system and finds a use for varicose veins, arteriosclerosis, broken capillaries, high blood pressure and chilblains. Regular use improves sluggish circulation, by reducing blood viscosity and helps break down any hardened deposits.

Warning: Possible skin irritant. As with most citrus oils, lemon is photo toxic. UV lighting *(the sun or sun bed)* should be avoided after use of this essence.

YARROW

Latin name: *achillea millefolium*   **Botanical family:**   *Compositae*

The three main areas where this oil can help are:

1. **Immune system stimulant**
2. **Skin disorders**
3. **Digestive problems**

Properties	Uses
Tonic	Vascular system, menstrual problems, fluid retention
Stimulant	Digestive disorders, immune stimulant
Analgesic	Arthritis, aches and pains, rheumatism, headaches
Antispasmodic	Colic, diarrhea, flatulence
Anti-inflammatory	Arthritis, inflammation, skin problems, wounds, sores, acne

Place of Origin
A perennial herb found along country lanes, gardens and fields principally in **Europe, Western Asia and North America**. It grows to 3 feet and has fern-like feathery leaves with pink or white flowers, bonded in clusters on tough angular stems. The appearance is very similar to that of wild carrot, which is poisonous. However, the smell of the crushed leaves of yarrow is very bitter and unmistakable compared to wild carrot.

Method of Extraction
The most common method of obtaining this oil is through distillation of the dried leaves and flowering heads. The colour of this oil is tending to be more olive green with a blue tone, with a somewhat bitter smell.

The other method used is enfleurage (creating an absolute) *which produces a superior quality essential oil containing more azulene* making a dark blue with a fresher, less bitter smell. This oil seems less likely to cause skin irritation than the distilled oil.

Traditional Uses
Used throughout the centuries, yarrow was known for its healing potential in a wide variety of disorders. Today, it is listed in the British Herbal Pharmacopoeia for circulatory disorders such as hypertension and other thrombotic disorders.

Herbal Uses

Its ability to keep wound from becoming infected makes it a valuable herb that has been used for generations. An infusion of the dried herb combined with yarrow, elderflower and peppermint is on of the best remedies for the common cold and influenza. As a poultice is often used for piles and menstruation pain. Nose bleeds respond well when you crush the leaves and pack them up the nostrils.

Aromatherapy

As with german chamomile, yarrow has high azulene content. Because of this fatty substance, essential oil of **yarrow has anti-inflammatory and antispasmodic properties**. This makes it invaluable in relation to skin care problems such as acne, pimples, wounds, cuts, ulcers or lacerations.

Combined with its analgesic properties, inflammatory conditions like arthritis and rheumatism will find relief, as will other painful conditions such as headaches.

A stimulant to the digestive system, it will improve appetite by stimulating both the appetite and bile secretions. Helpful for **colic, flatulence and diarrhea**, yarrow will also improve problems that are associated with slow digestion. May also prove useful with cases of indigestion.

A tonic to the vascular system, yarrow is said to encourage blood renewal because it works directly on the bone marrow. **Varicose veins, arteriosclerosis, thrombosis, haemorrhoids and high blood pressure are circulatory conditions** where the use of this essential oil should show improvement.

Due to its balancing effect on the female hormonal system, this essence is a wonderful addition to assist with gynaecological problems. **Menstrual problems such as irregularity, heavy periods, fibroids, inflammation, pain and even fluid retention** are relieved with the use of the oil.

Yarrow has quite an affinity with the respiratory tract and its problems. It acts on braking up excess catarrh in the lungs and the nasal passages. It is one of the few oils that is of help in dealing with the problem of pleurisy. This oil promotes perspiration by opening the sweat glands encouraging a cleansing and cooling action needed when combatting infection.

Warning: *Prolonged use may cause headaches and possibly irritate sensitive skin. This is a potent oil and due to its affect on the female hormonal system, should be used with caution during pregnancy.*

FENNEL

Latin name: *Foeniculum vulgare*   **Botanical family**: *Umbelliferae*

The three main areas where this oil can help are:

1. **Anti-inflammatory**
2. **Digestive balancer, and diuretic**
3. **Detoxifier**

Properties	Uses
Diuretic	Water retention, kidney stones, cellulite, obesity
Splenetic	Alcoholism
Digestive	Constipation, indigestion, bloating, nausea, flatulence, colitis, vomiting, decrease appetite
Estrogenic	Menstrual irregularities, PMS, menopause, promotes lactation
Expectorant	Colds, catarrh, bronchitis, pulmonary infections

Place of Origin
Although found in many places throughout Europe, it is thought to be indigenous to the Mediterranean area. The plant grows to a height of up to five feet. It has strikingly bright golden yellow flowers. The name fennel is derived from the Latin of *"foenum"* meaning *"hay"*.

Method of Extraction
The essential oil of fennel is steam distilled from the crushed seeds. It contains the chemical constituents of anethole, fenchone, estragol, camphene and phellandrene. It has a pleasant flavour similar to aniseed, which unlike aniseed, which is fairly toxic, fennel is not.

Traditional Uses
A herb that has been used in the culinary arena as well as the medical field.
The Chinese and Hindus believed it was anti-venomous and very effective against poisonous bites or infections. It has been used as a sacred herb. It was believed to have warded off evil spirits.

Herbal Uses
Fennel tea will sooth the stomach and **is the main ingredient in *"Gripe Water"*** concocted to relieve infant from flatulence. Fennel tea can be made by pouring one half of a pint of boiling water onto the seeds and allowing them to infuse. This infusion can be gargled as a breath freshener, used as an eye wash and help to produce milk to nursing mothers. Chewing fennel seeds will stay the appetite and stop the stomach from becoming to acidic.

Aromatherapy

Essential oil of fennel possesses the ability to aid digestive problems like constipation, flatulence, bloating, nausea and more. Fennel tea has been popularly used as a digestive tonic. Fennel encourages the digestion process and will help dispel gas. It has been used to curb excessive eating by decreasing the appetite.

Fennel is **a strong diuretic that will assist with water retention** by increasing the removal of the fluid. It should be used when there is insufficient excretion of urine. It may prove useful with kidney stones by helping to dissolve them.

Cellulite and its related toxic build up in the adipose *(fat)* tissue will benefit from this diuretic property. Combined with its splenetic properties and the ability to cleanse the blood, liver, spleen and kidneys, it is a valuable oil. Occasionally used as a remedy for hangovers, it helps release the toxins from the liver.

Estrogenic in nature, due to it having a plant hormone similar to estrogen *(estragol)*, many menstrual irregularities or problems like **menopause, PMS, painful menstruation, irregular menstruation**, and others will show improvement. Remember that both sexes require estrogen in the body. It is responsible for maintaining muscle tone as well as the elasticity of the skin and the connective tissue.

Because of the plant hormone, fennel can be used to increase lactation for those who are breast feeding their infant.

Warning: *Contra-indicated in pregnancy*

Question and Answer Sheets

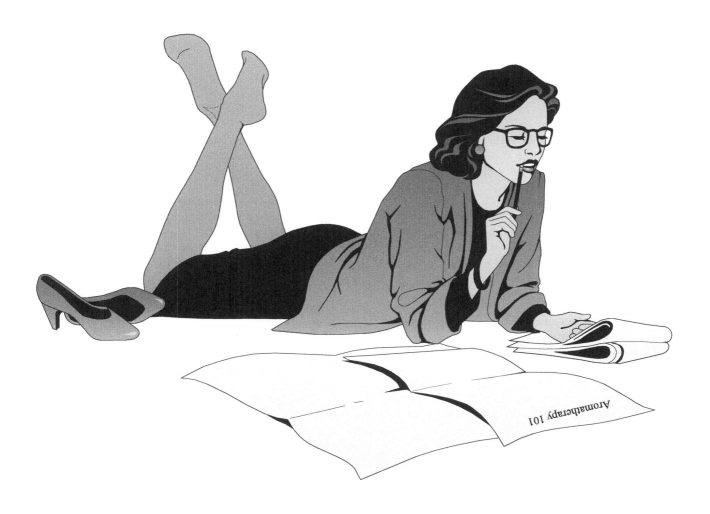

Please keep the questions for review.
Circle the correct answer/s on the Answer Sheets at the back of the book and
<u>**return these sheets only**</u> **to your instructor.**

Questions - Lesson #5

1. How many disorders do we treat for when using the cross reference sheet?
a. five
b. three
c. one
d. two

2. How do you decide which disorder takes precedent for treatment?
a. the one we have diagnosed
b. the one stated on their medic-alert bracelet
c. the most troublesome to the patient
d. anything their docotr told you to treat

3. How many essential oils are used in a blend?
a. one
b. two
c. three
d. four

4. An acute blend consists of the following oils.
a. 2 base notes and 1 top note
b. 1 base note, 1 middle note & 1 top note
c. 1 base note & 2 middle notes
d. 2 middle notes & 1 top note

5. A chronic blend consists of the following oils.
a. 2 base notes & 1 top note
b. 1 base note , 1 middle note & 1 top note
c. 1 base note, & 2 middle notes
d. 2 middle notes & 1 top note

6. A synergistic blend consists of the following oils.
a. 2 base notes & 1 top note
b. 1 base note, 1 middle note & 1 top note
c. 1 base note & 2 middle notes
d. 2 middle notes & 1 top note

7. How many drops are used when using a top note in blending?
a. three
b. four
c. one
d. two

8. How many drops are used when using a middle note in blending?
a. three
b. four
c. one
d. two

9. How many drops are used when using a base not in blending?
a. three
b. four
c. one
d. two

10. The lymphatic system contains reservoirs. These are called what?
a. lymph vessels
b. lymph nodes
c. lymphocytes
d. plasma stations

11. What is lymph and what does it do?
a. blood waste products, it keeps the cells clean
b. plasma, it nourishes and clears waste from the cells
c. white cells, it nourishes and clears waste from the cells
d. plasma, it destroys foreign cells

12. In which direction does all lymph travel?
a. around the circulatory system
b. through the brain and heart
c. towards the heart
d. towards the kidneys

13. What are lymph nodes and what is their purpose?
a. reservoir areas that filter lymph, destroy foreign substances and produce lymphocytes as needed
b. bumps under the skin that increase in size when an infection is present due to increased lymph
c. manufacturing areas that produce extra lymph in cases of trauma as needed
d. reservoir areas that filter and manufacture lymph in cases of trauma

14. Name three specialized lymph glands.
a. tonsils
b. lachrymals
c. peyer's patches
d. adenoids
e. salivaries

15. Eventually all lymph passes into which two principal lymph vessels?
a. peyer's patches duct
b. right lymphatic duct
c. lachrymal duct
d. thoracic duct

16. Name five of the common superficial lymph nodes.
a. axillary glands
b. salivary glands
c. inguinals
d. submandibular
e. supratrochlea
f. tonsils
g. femoral glands
h. in the popliteal fossa

17. Approximately how many lymph nodes are found in the body?
a. 600 - 1,000
b. 200 - 500
c. 1,000 - 1,500
d. unknown

18. State five functions of lymph.

19. **Which three of the following causes restriction of the lymphatic flow?**
a. elasticated clothing
b. nerve lesions
c. prolonged rest periods
d. warm baths
e. excessive exercise

20. **The four major components of lymph are?**
a. blood
b. water
c. red blood cells
d. proteins
e. fat
f. cells
g. dyes

21. **The three minor components of lymph are?**
a. dust, dyes & pathogens
b. dust, water & dyes
c. water, white blood cells & plasma
d. dyes, platelets & plasma

22. **If the spleen is removed, what will happen?**
a. the patient will die
b. the patient will require a transplant
c. antibiotics are necessary for life
d. the immune system will not function as well

23. **Name three major functions of the spleen.**

24. **Describe in your own words lymphadenitis.**

25. **What is Hodgkins disease?**
a. chronic malignant disorder, characterized by an enlarged spleen.
b. acute disorder, characterized by oedema
c. chronic malignant disorder characterized by painless enlarged lymph nodes
d. chronic malignant disorder characterized by tenderness within the liver.

26. **What is splenogomaly?**
a. enlargement of the spleen
b. viral infection of the spleen
c. cancer of the spleen

27. **What is elephantiasis?**
a. enlargement of an extremity due to circulatory problems.
b. inflammation of the lymph nodes
c. enlargement of an extremity resulting from blockage of the lymphatic pathways.
d. enlargement of an extremity due to trauma

28. **An analgesic oil ...**
a. reduces swelling
b. strengthens the nervous system
c. clears the mind and stimulates mental activity
d. is painkilling

29. **A cephalic oil ...**
a. reduces swelling
b. strengthens the nervous system
c. clears the mind and stimulates mental activity
d. is painkilling

30. **A nervine oil....**
a. reduces swelling
b. strengthens the nervous system
c. clears the mind and stimulates mental activity
d. is painkilling

31. **A diuretic oil.....**
a. reduces swelling
b. strengthens the nervous system
c. clears the mind and stimulate mental activity
d. is painkilling

32. **A hepatic oil...**
a. strengthens the liver
b. helps heal wounds
c. fights infection
d. reduces fever

33. **A vasoconstricting oil....**
a. reduces swelling
b. causes blood vessels to expand
c. causes blood vessels to constrict
d. tightens tissue

34. **In the white pulp of the spleen, what is produced?**
a. white cells
b. lymphocytes
c. phagocytes
d. leucocytes

35. **What does the red pulp contain?**
a. white cells
b. lymphocytes
c. phagocytes
d. leucocytes

36. **What is the purpose of the spleen?**
a. filtering the blood stream
b. regulates blood cells
c. an aid in the development of immunity
d. assists the diaphragm

37. **What part of the plant is used to obtain essential oil of coriander?**
a. the flowering tops
b. the rind of the fruit
c. seeds of the ripe fruit and the leaves
d. the wood

d. the wood

38. What three main areas will coriander help most?
a. urinary tract infection and mucous membranes
b. digestive problems
c. headaches
d. muscle relaxant
e. detoxifier

39. What do you have to be careful of when using coriander?
a. people want to drink
b. during pregnancy
c. stupefying in large doses
d. skin and mucous membranes

40. How is essential oil of grapefruit obtained?
a. distillation   b. extraction
c. maceration   d. enfleurage
e. pressing

41. What three main areas will grapefruit help most?
a. lymphatic stimulant   b. headaches
c. constipation   d. digestive problems
e. manic depression   f. drug addiction

42. What do you have to be careful of when using grapefruit?
a. people want to drink
b. during pregnancy
c. stupefying in large doses
d. skin irritant
e. photo toxic

43. What part of the plant is used to obtain essential oil of lemon?
a. the flowering tops
b. the rind of the fruit
c. the leaves
d. the wood

44. What three main areas will lemon help most?
a. balance acid levels
b. circulatory problems
c. immune stimulantcorpuscle production
d. respiratory tract infections and problems
e. wounds and cuts

45. What do you have to be careful of when using lemon?
a. people want to drink it.
b. skin irritant and photo toxicity
c. during pregnancy
d. people with high blood pressure

46. What part of the plant is used to obtain essential oil of fennel?
a. the seeds of the plant
b. the flowering tops
c. the leaves
d. the roots
e. the fruit or berries of the plant
f. the wood

47. How is fennel obtained?
a. distillation   b. extraction
c. maceration   d. enfleurage

48. What three main areas will fennel help most?
a. anti-inflammatory
b. digestive balancer
c. calming on headaches or migraines
d. detoxifying on the body
e. lowers blood pressure

49. What part of the plant is used to obtain essential oil of yarrow?
a. the seeds
b. dried leaves and flowering heads
c. the roots
d. the wood

50. What three main areas will yarrow help most?
a. headaches
b. stimulates the immune system
c. muscle relaxant
d. skin disorders
e. digestive problems

51. What do you have to be careful of when using yarrow?
a. skin irritant
b. prolonged use may cause headaches
c. use with care during pregnancy
d. all of the above

52. Label the diagram of the lymphatic system.
(SEE ANSWER SHEET FOR DIAGRAM)

Answer Sheet - Lesson #5

(Keep the questions for review. Circle the correct answer/s and return these sheets only to your instructor.)

1. A   B   C   D

2. A   B   C   D

3. A   B   C   D

4. A   B   C   D

5. A   B   C   D

6. A   B   C   D

7. A   B   C   D

8. A   B   C   D

9. A   B   C   D

10. A   B   C   D

11. A   B   C   D

12. A   B   C   D

13. A   B   C   D

14. A   B   C   D   E

15. A   B   C   D

16. A   B   C   D   E   F   G   H

17. A   B   C   D

18. Five functions of lymph are

    1)_____

    2)_____

    3)_____

    4)_____

    5)_____

19. A   B   C   D   E

20. A   B   C   D   E   F   G

21. A   B   C   D

22. A   B   C   D

23. Three major functions of the spleen include

     1)_____

     2) _____

     3) _____

24. Lymphadenitis is_____

_____

_____

_____

25. A   B   C   D

26. A   B   C

27. A   B   C   D

28. A   B   C   D

29. A   B   C   D

30. A   B   C   D

31. A   B   C   D

32. A   B   C   D

33. A   B   C   D

34. A   B   C   D

35. A   B   C   D

36. A   B   C   D

37. A   B   C   D

38. A   B   C   D   E

39. A   B   C   D

40. A   B   C   D   E

41. A   B   C   D   E   F

42. A   B   C   D   E

43. A   B   C   D

44. A   B   C   D   E

45. A   B   C   D

46. A   B   C   D   E   F

47. A   B   C   D

48. A   B   C   D   E

49. A   B   C   D

50. A   B   C   D   E

51. A   B   C   D

52. Label the following diagram of the lymphatic system.

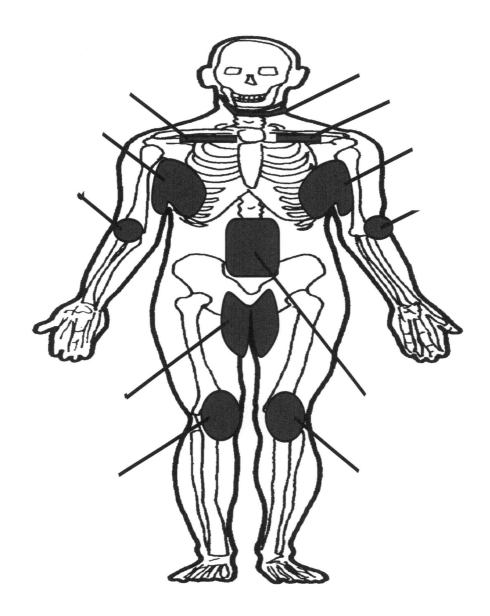

LESSON
SIX

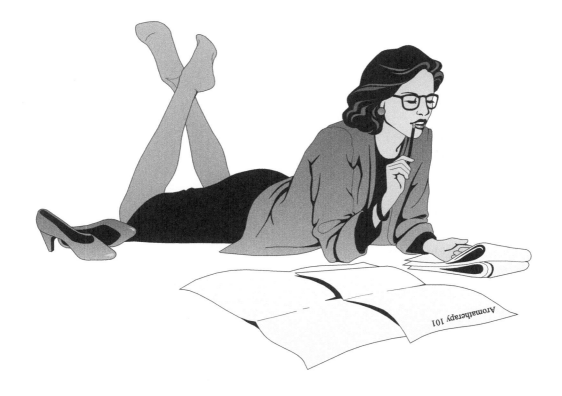

Lesson #6

Table of Contents

Chemistry and Essential Oils
(a brief overview)

The chemistry of essential oils was initially investigated in the early twentieth century. The chemical makeup and molecular structure were identified and then reproduced for commercial manufacturers. This started the boom of the synthetic and fragrant industry as well introducing the pharmacological approach to aromatherapy and essential oils.

Today there are active proponents in the aromatherapy industry who believe the most beneficial use of essential oils is through the method of "chemotyping". In other words, in order to determine the most effective use of specific oils, they will look to the chemical constituents of the essential oil and classify it according to the properties of the constituents. There is discrepancy in the ideology of chemotyping because of the varied content of the constituents due to;

1)   Varied environmental growing conditions from year to year, as well as the various countries that produce the same essential oil.

2)   It is strongly known that chemical components work in synergy with each other and the totality of the plants chemical make-up varies from the perceived make-up as analysed   through the chemical approach. In other words, *"The whole of an essential oil is greater than the sum of its parts."*

3)   Some plants can contain hundreds of chemical constituents. Many of these have not been identified as of yet.

Essential oils used in the perfumery and flavour industries are normally adulterated with other substances that are less expensive to produce. Aromatherapy essential oils can be adulterated as well. The adulteration of these oils involves taking a poor quality essence and in turn attempt to create a "saleable" product. Other known tricks in the industry will involve taking a good quality oil and "stretch" it by adding other substances to obtain greater profits due to the larger volume.

As a philosophy, it is best to remember that plants are very compatible with the human body. Historically we have relied on them for food and medicine and although modern technology is able to "copy" certain chemical compounds, it is important to know that these products are not the same as the natural plant. As such, it is wise to remember, the use of synthetic essential oils run a greater risk of unwanted side effects or reactions similarly as synthetic pharmacological drugs.

The constituents of essential oils are normally classified into either terpenes or oxygenated constituents and compounds which do not fall into either category.

Terpenes include:
1) monoterpenes (most commonly found terpene in essential oils)
2) sesquiterpenes
3) diterpenes

Oxygenated constituents include:

1)	Alcohols	5)	Caroxylic Acids
2)	Phenols	6)	Esters
3)	Aldehydes	7)	Lactones
4)	Ketones	8)	Ethers

Terpenes contain one carbon atom and one hydrogen atom. The number of isoprene units they contain will classify them into the appropriate terpene category. In other words, if a terpene has two isoprene units, it is called a monoterpene. Three isoprene units form sesquiterpenes and diterpenes are made from four isoprene units. When various oxygen-containing active groups are added to a monoterpene, other constituents are formed. These include the above list of oxygenated constituents.

ALCOHOLS

Alcohols are good anti-bacterial agents and posses little or no toxicity. Many essential oils that contain alcohols are favoured for skin-care application. Oils that are high in alcohols like geranium, bergamot and lavender have a natural deodorant effect. Alcohols are an ingredient most perfumers like to find in a product because of the agreeable fragrance, the up-lifting properties as well as the antiseptic properties.

Alcohols like monoterpenols, terpineol, geraniol, linalool and menthol, all end with, "ol" . These are strong bactericides, anti-infectious, antiviral, anti-fungal, stimulating, and warming constituents. Terpene alcohol molecules are mildly electropositive giving an enhanced antiseptic quality and a stronger bactericidal aspect to the oil.

Most alcohols are general nerve tonics or immune system balancers and hepatic with vasoconstrictive properties. There are few, if any hazards or contra-indications including skin irritation.

Alcohols like sesquiterpenols are normally good decongestants to the circulatory system (hypotensive), as well as stimulating to the heart and liver (hepatic). Similar to monoterpenols they are non-irritating, temperature reducing and considered a nerve tonic.
Sesquiterpenes alcohols are anti-allergic, anti-tumour or immune stimulant, glandular stimulant and anti-inflammative. Sesquiterpene alcohols are generally slightly less electropositive than monoterpene alcohols.

Alcohols like diterpenols, appear to have a balancing effect on the hormonal system because they are similar in nature to the human hormone

PHENOLS

Phenols also end with an "ol". This makes it important to distinguish the most common phenols. Phenols have strong antiseptic and antibacterial qualities, acting on the nervous and immune systems as a stimulant. Care should be exercised when using phenols as they tend to cause skin irritation if used incorrectly or in high dosages. They can be toxic to the liver and an irritant to the skin if they are used in high doses for an extended period of time.

Phenols are analgesic, anti-infectious, anti-spasmodic, antiviral, cicatrisant, digestive, diuretic, expectorant, mucolytic, sedative and a general tonic. Some examples of phenols include carvacol, eugenol, and thymol.

ALDEHYDES

Aldehydes and perfumery are as important to each other as cheese and crackers are to wine. Aldehydes often have strong aroma's. A few aldehydes are skin sensitizers and on people who have sensitive skin they can cause a reaction.

The citrus-like fragrance of lemonbalm is easily recognised. The aldehydes responsible for that fragrance is citral & citronella.

Aldehydes are anti-inflammatory, anti-infectious, anti-septic, anti-fungal, anti-viral, tonic, hypotensive, calming to the nervous system and they reduce temperatures. These effects are stronger if used in low concentrations. It is well known that citral and citronella exhibit their strongest sedative and antispasmodic effects when used in low dilutions and they have a reduced effect when using increased doses

Cinnamic aldehyde, when isolated from cinnamon bark oil and citral aldehyde just to name two, can be a skin sensitizer. When the whole oil is used, the problem of skin sensitivity really occurs.

Many of the known and unknown constituents act as a "quencher" to the individual problem chemicals. If this oil is stored incorrectly, it will not last too long because unwanted acids can form, destroying the therapeutic active ingredients.

KETONES

All ketone chemicals end with "one". A ketone which is not found in essential oils, but is recognised by most people is "acetone". It is not often that you find ketones in essential oils. They are neurotoxic. The toxic ketones most likely to be encountered in essential oils are thujones and pinocamphone

Essential oils that contain significant amounts of ketones are aniseed, caraway, hyssop and sage. Ketones like "pinocamphone" may provoke an epileptic fit and ketones like "thujone and pulegone" could cause a miscarriage, if they are used in large or frequent amounts.

The effects of ketones are, calming and sedative. They help break down mucus and fat and encourage the healing of wounds.

They are abortifacient, anti-coagulant, antifungal, anti-inflammatory, cicatrisant, digestive, lipolytic, mucolytic, and neurotoxic. Some ketones can also be digestive, analgesic, stimulant or expectorant.

ACIDS AND ESTERS

Acids and esters are anti-inflammatory by nature and seem to be free of contra-indications. Most acids found in essential oils are combined with esters and because of this there isn't a group dedicated to esters. An ester is the result of combining an organic acid with an alcohol. The last letters found in esters are "ate". They are usually very fruity and fragrant and because of this, they are used extensively in flavouring and edible fruit aromas.

Essential oils that have a large amount of esters are, lavender, clary sage, geranium, petitgrain and bergamot. Essential oils that have a lower amount of esters are juniper and roman chamomile. One of the important properties associated with esters is their anti-fungal and yeast retarding properties. Essential oil of geranium has a special importance in the treatment of candida. The anti-bacterial strength of geranium is not very high, but its anti-fungal properties are considerably potent.

Esters are gentle and free from hazards except for "methyl salicylate' found in wintergreen and birch pil. Esters are generally anti-inflammatory and anti-fungal and have an affinity for skin problems. They are good balancers to both the nervous (anti-spasmodic) and emotional (anti-depressant) systems.

OXIDES

Oxides are not commonly found in essential oils. Cineole, also known as eucalyptol, is found in a number of oils. Its major strength is its mucolytic property. This makes it a good expectorant for coughs and colds, as well as respiratory infections. Some skin irritation can occur if used in large quantity or over a prolonged period of time.

LACTONES

Lactones are easy to remember because they are more common in expressed oils or via solvent extraction. Lactones are good for reducing temperatures and relieving catarrh. The sesquiterpene lactone "helenalin", has been found to be one of the active ingredients of arnica. The antiphlogistics (anti-inflammatory) power of this compound was determined to be much higher than that of phenylbutazone, a common synthetic prescription antiphlogistic.

Lactones like coumarins are sedative and calming yet at the same time up-lifting and refreshing. They are also regarded for the anti-coagulating properties, which makes a good hypotensive. Sometimes photo toxic, but generally coumarins act as general tonics for most systems with emphasis on the nervous system.

Lactones like furocoumarins are closely related to coumarins. They are photosensitizers. Bergaptene, found in essential oil of bergamot, is a good example. Many are antiviral and antifungal.

The Neurological System

The neurological system is composed of nerve cells and supporting tissue. This control system has the ability to unify the body through various functions to maintain homeostasis. These functions are controlled by sending, receiving and carrying nerve impulses. The whole neurological system is based on chemical conductive materials related directly to the nerves and axons. The nerve cells are very sensitive and their fibres specialize in the transmission of impulses. This network runs throughout the body with a two-way connection.

The neurological system serves three main functions:

1) Sensory functions   It will sense changes within the body's internal and external environment.

2) Integrative functions   The body's ability to interpret these sensed changes.

3) Motor functions   The body's ability to respond to the interpreted changes and start the necessary action through either muscular contractions or glandular secretions.

The neurological system has two main divisions:
- ▶ Central (cerebrospinal) nervous system. (CNS)
- ▶ Peripheral nervous system. (PNS)

The Central Nervous System (CNS)

This is the control centre for the entire body. It consists of the brain and the spinal cord. The brain functions as the command centre while the spinal cord serves as an extension of the brain. The CNS uses both ascending and descending impulses to transfer the information it receives and gives to the peripheral nervous system. It serves as a source of motor commands for muscles and receives sensory input from the PNS.

The Peripheral Nervous System

This system is composed of a network of both cranial and spinal nerves (neuron processes) and ganglia (islands of neurons) that connect the central nervous system to other areas of the body. They are located outside of the CNS and include the Afferent (Sensory) System, the Efferent (Motor) System, the Somatic Nervous System, and the Autonomic Nervous System (which includes the Sympathetic and Parasympathetic systems.

Nerves of the peripheral nervous system generally have both fibres from the somatic system, which generates voluntary response and the autonomic system, which controls involuntary response. There are twelve pairs of cranial nerves and thirty one pairs of spinal nerves. These branches of spinal nerves are referred to as peripheral nerves. Their function is to relay sensations from the body to the brain and spinal cord and relay motor commands to all skeletal muscles.

CENTRAL NERVOUS SYSTEM

|

BRAIN & SPINAL CORD

|

CONTROLS MOTOR COMMANDS
AND SENSORY INPUT

PERIPHERAL NERVOUS SYSTEM

|

NETWORK OF NERVES
CONTROLS
AUTONOMIC NERVOUS FUNCTIONS

|

INCLUDES
SYMPATHETIC & PARASYMPATHETIC FUNCTIONS

HOW IS THIS INFO RELAYED?

The basis for the nervous system is the nerve cell or neuron. These pass the information to the central nervous system or peripheral nervous system. Neurons consist of a nerve cell body that has a receiving mechanism (dendrite) and a transmitting mechanism (axon).

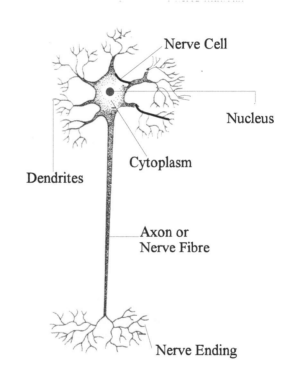

Neurons are classified into three functional types according to the direction in which they conduct impulses. These include:

1)   Sensory (or Afferent) neurons
These are responsible for conducting impulses from receptors in the body to the CNS.
They pick up sensations such as touch, pressure, pain, joint position, muscle tension, etc.

2)   Motor (or Efferent) neurons
These direct command impulses from the CNS to the muscles via the motor end plate (a band of fibres that flow into the sheath of the muscle) and releases a neurotransmitter to induce muscle action.

3)   Inter-neurons
These are found within the central nervous system. They carry information throughout the CNS and help transmit impulses from sensory neurons to motor neurons.

Nerves have a specific type of nerve fibre. There are two types of peripheral nerve fibres.

1.   White nerve fibres which are myelinated (enclosed in a sheath) . The function of the myelin sheath is to increase the speed of the nerve impulse and to insulate and maintain the nerve fibre (axon).
2.   Grey nerve fibres which are un-myelinated (without a sheath).

A nerve impulse is required to conduct information from one neuron to another until it reaches the required destination. Neurons do not have contact with one another. There is a space between them. This gap must be crossed. It is done through a *"bridging of the synapsis gap"*. This involves the nerve endings to liberate chemical substances which stimulate the adjacent cell to start a fresh impulse along its own fibre. This process continues throughout the nerve network. (See diagram below)

Example:
A hand is placed on a hot stove. The sensory neurons and the pain receptors of the peripheral nervous system register the excessive heat and conducts a message through the neurons to the central nervous system and the brain. The brain processes the information and sends a message back down the spine, out of the CNS, through the motor neurons of the PNS, which in turn will transmit the information to the muscles of the hand in order to contract the muscles to pull away from the heat.

Diagram of synapsis

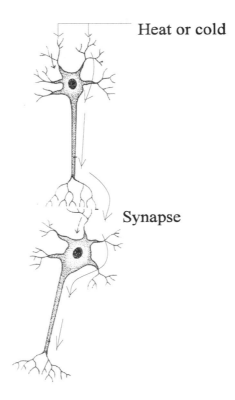

Heat or cold

Synapse

The chemical mediators used to create synapsis include acetylcholine and adrenaline (*epinephrine and norepinephrine*).

Acetylcholine is a skeletal muscle chemical mediator. This neurotransmitter is widely distributed in the body tissues. After it has been utilized, it is then destroyed by an enzyme called acetylcholinesterase. Its function is to inactivate the acetylcholine released during nerve impulses and further prevent accumulation by breaking down the acetylcholine into acetate and choline. Both acetylcholine and adrenaline are autonomic neurotransmitters.

When we consider the autonomic system, we shall see that chemical agencies play a very large part in regulating internal organs and blood vessels and that certain endocrine glands, like the adrenal glands, can secrete the same substances into the blood as hormones to secure a rapid response in emergencies.

AUTONOMIC NERVOUS SYSTEM
(a part of the peripheral nervous system)

The autonomic nervous system functions without conscious control. Its role is to maintain homeostasis within the body by manipulating the activity of the visceral organs over which we have no voluntary control. The autonomic nervous system will either increase or decrease activity according to changing internal conditions. Some of the functions it is responsible for include regulation of the heart rate, body temperature, blood pressure, etc.

It is divided into two separate parts: The sympathetic system and the parasympathetic nervous system.

TABLE OF AUTONOMIC FUNCTIONS		
EFFECTOR	SYMPATHETIC CONTROL	PARA SYMPATHETIC CONTROL
Heart muscle	Accelerates heartbeat	Slows heart beat
Smooth muscle of most blood vessels	Constricts blood vessels	None
Smooth muscle of blood vessels in skeletal muscles	Dilates blood vessels	None
Smooth muscle of the digestive tract	Decreases peristalsis & inhibits defecation	Increases peristalsis
Smooth muscle of the anal sphincter	Stimulates - closes sphincter	Inhibits - opens sphincter for defecation
Smooth muscle of the urinary bladder	Inhibits - relaxes bladder	Stimulates - contracts bladder
Smooth muscle of the urinary sphincter	Stimulates - closes sphincter	Inhibits - opens sphincter for urination
Smooth muscle of the iris	Stimulates radial fibres - dilation of pupil	Stimulates circular fibres - constriction of pupil
Smooth muscle of the ciliary	Inhibits - accommodation for far vision (flattening of lens)	Stimulates - accommodation for near vision (bulging lens)
Smooth muscle of hairs (pilomotor muscles)	Stimulates - goose bumps	No parasympathetic fibres
Adrenal medulla gland	Increases epinephrine secretion	None
Sweat glands	Increases sweat secretion	None
Digestive glands	Decreases secretion of digestive juices	Increases secretion of digestive juices

All the internal organs have a double nerve supply from the sympathetic and parasympathetic systems and their effect is opposite. A sympathetic nerve has the effect of increasing body activity and speeding it up, whereas the parasympathetic, on the contrary, slows down body activity.

The sympathetic system is comprised of a ganglionic cord which runs anteriorly on either side of the vertebral column. The principal plexus of this system is the cardiac plexus. This supplies all the thoracic viscera and the thoracic vessels. The coeliac or solar plexus supplies all the abdominal viscera and the hypogastric plexus supplies the pelvic organs. The effects of sympathetic stimulation is increased body activity in relation to fear, flight or fight, aided by adrenaline secreted by the adrenal gland.

Sympathetic stimulation
1.   Constricts the blood vessels of the skin, which raises the blood pressure
2.   Shunts blood to the heart and brain
3.   Speeds and strengthens the heartbeat
4.   Dries up glandular secretions
5.   Dilates the pupils
6.   Stands the hair on end
7.   Initiates sweating
8.   Mobilizes glucose and relaxes the walls of the hollow viscera

The sympathetic system provides for today's work and its action increases when involved with physical activity.

The parasympathetic nervous system consists mainly of the vagus nerve. This branches off to the organs of the thorax and abdomen, but also includes branches from other cranial nerves. These include mainly the third, seventh, and ninth as well as nerves in the sacral region of the spinal column.

The parasympathetic system produces relaxed states, it dilates the peripheral vessels, slows the heart and lowers the blood pressure and excites secretion and peristalsis. The parasympathetic system looks after tomorrow, being mainly concerned with the changes that takes place during rest.

In some people, the sympathetic nerves are stronger and hold the balance in the body. The sympathetic nerves are stimulated by strong emotions such as fear, anger and excitement. The adrenals are one of the glands which the sympathetic system stimulates and the liberation of adrenalin is one of the body's responses to strong emotions.

In other people, the parasympathetic nerves are stronger and hold the balance in the body. These people have a placid disposition, good digestion and are not very easily disturbed. These are known as vagotonic types. In other people, the sympathetic nerves are the stronger and these people are more emotional, less stable and their digestion is more readily disturbed. These are known as sympatheticotonic types.

Within the autonomic nervous system, there are peripheral ganglia. These ganglion connect a paired unit of autonomic motor systems. One neuron from the central nervous system and one from the peripheral nervous system. These are divided into pre-ganglionic fibres (they enter the ganglion) and post ganglionic (they exit the ganglion).

Pre-ganglionic fibres of the sympathetic and parasympathetic systems secrete acetylcholine (epinephrine), but sympathetic postganglionic chemical neurotransmitters secrete norepinephrine (adrenaline) while the parasympathetic secrete acetylcholine.

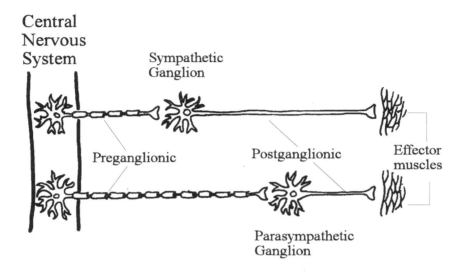

DERMATOMES

Dermatomes are areas of the skin that are supplied with sensory receptors that are connected and enervated by a specific spinal nerve. These dermatomes only communicate cutaneous pain and any pain that is referred to the skin.

If the nerve supply is interrupted, there may be a loss of sensation in that area. However, many dermatomes overlap in certain areas (especially in the trunk), therefore there may be no loss of sensation.

Many professional practitioners know which spinal nerves are associated with each dermatome. With this knowledge, it is possible to determine which spinal nerve is not functioning appropriately by stimulating a dermatome area. If the client/patient feels no sensation, it may be that the nerves supplying that dermatome are involved.

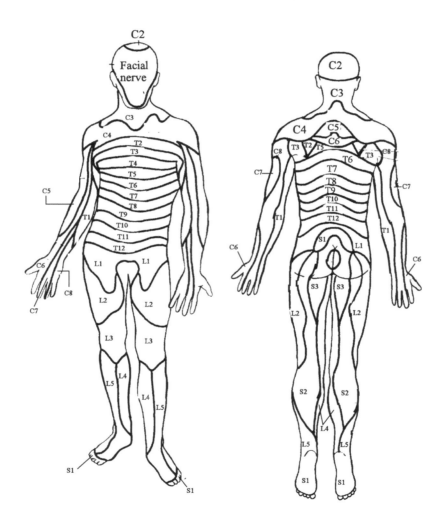

THE BRAIN

At the centre of the nervous system is the brain. The brain is well protected from the outside by the hard bone structure of the skull. Inside the brain is protected externally by three enveloping membranes known as the meninges.

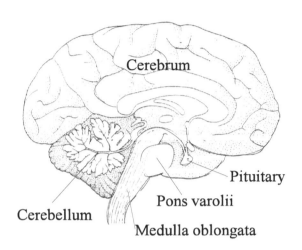

The outer layer is known as the dura-mater or strong or hard mother. A tough loosely applied protective envelope, in the cranium, it also forms the lining periosteum of the skull.

The middle layer is known as the arachnoid. This fits closely inside the dura, but there is a sub-arachnoid space separating it from the pia, filled with cerebrospinal fluid and traversed by spidery connective tissue.

The inner layer is called the pia mater or soft mother, a fine membrane closely applied to the brain and cord, following every cleft and crevice and carrying with it the fine blood vessels.

The outer meninges (the dura mater) is constructed of strong fibrous tissue anchored to the skull. The middle tissue, or arachnoid, is much more delicate and is not anchored to the skull, thus allowing the brain to expand. Under it lies the big reservoir of cerebral spinal fluid by which the whole of the brain is surrounded and on which it rests. Then comes the pia mater which is in contact with the grey matter of the brain itself and dips deep down between the brain convolutions.

When we speak of the brain, we are really considering three quite different structures.

The CEREBRUM, the CEREBELLUM and the MEDULLA OBLONGATA.

The adult human brain weighs rather more than three pounds and is so full of water that it tends to slump rather like a jelly if placed without the support of a firm surface. It is estimated that it has twelve billion neurons or nerve cells.

THE CEREBRUM

The cerebrum consists of two symmetrical hemispheres. The outer layer of the cerebrum is known as the cortex and this is arranged in convolutions. These are deep irregular shaped fissures or indentations. This is the grey matter of the brain. Underneath the cortex lies nerve fibre or white matter.

The function of the cerebrum is to control voluntary movement, to receive and interpret conscious sensations. It is the seat of the higher functions such as the senses, memory, reasoning, intelligence, and moral sense.

THE CEREBELLUM

The cerebellum is much smaller in size and lies below and behind the cerebrum. It too has grey matter under which is white matter. Its function is to control muscular co-ordination and balance.

THE MEDULLA OBLONGATA

The medulla oblongata is about 32 mm long, tapering from its greatest width of 19 mm and connects the rest of the brain with the spinal cord with which it is continuous. It is made up of interspersed white and grey matter. The medulla oblongata not only acts as the link between the brain and the central nervous system of the body, but it is also the centre of those parts of the autonomic nervous system which controls the heart, lungs, processes of the digestion, etc.

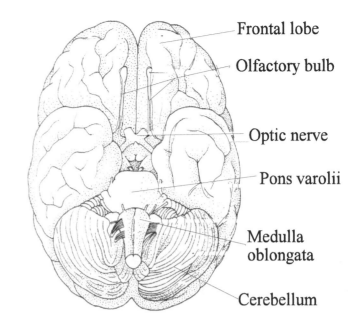

Frontal lobe
Olfactory bulb
Optic nerve
Pons varolii
Medulla oblongata
Cerebellum

THE SPINAL CORD

The spinal cord, which is continuous with the medulla oblongata, extends downwards through the vertebrae of the spinal column. The cord itself is cylindrical in shape with an outer covering of supporting cells and blood vessels and an egg-shaped core of nerve fibres. It has two swellings, the cervical and lumbar enlargements, which are the origins of the roots of the brachial and lumbar plexuses for the upper and lower limbs. It extends through four-fifths of the spinal column and averages between sixteen and seventeen inches in length.

SPINAL CHART

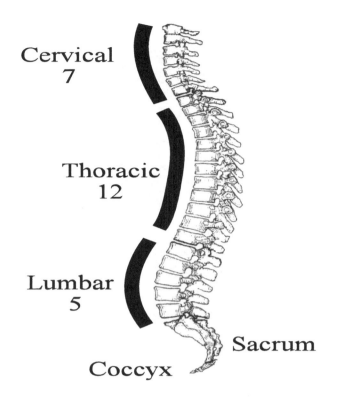

Cervical
7

Thoracic
12

Lumbar
5

Sacrum

Coccyx

STRUCTURE GOVERNS FUNCTION;
           C=CERVICAL   T=THORACIC   L=LUMBAR

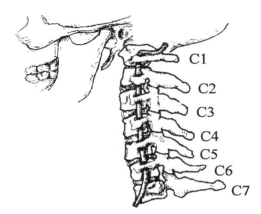

VERTEBRAE	AREA AFFECTED	SYMPTOMS
C1	Blood supply to the head pituitary gland & brain, sympathetic nervous system, ear both middle and inner.	Headaches, nervousness. insomnia, mental conditions. amnesia, epilepsy, tiredness. Dizziness, St. Vitus Dance
C2	Optic & auditory nerve sinuses, mouth, forehead	Allergies, deafness eye trouble, earache, fainting spells
C3	Cheeks, outer ear, face bones, teeth, trifacial nerve	Neuralgia, acne, neuritis eczema
C4	Nose, lips, mouth hearing, adenoids eustachian tube	Hay fever, catarrh, ear ache, sore throat
C5	Vocal cords, neck glands	Laryngitis, throat conditions
C6	Neck muscles, shoulders tonsils	Stiff neck, upper arm pain, tonsillitis, cough & croup
C7	Thyroid	Bursitis of the shoulder or elbow, colds, thyroid conditions, goitre.

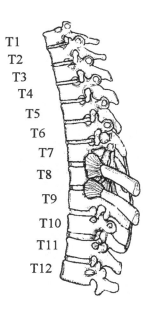

T1
T2
T3
T4
T5
T6
T7
T8
T9
T10
T11
T12

VERTEBRAE	AREA AFFECTED	SYMPTOMS
T1	Lower arms, oesophagus trachea	Asthma, cough, difficult breathing, pain in lower arm and hands.
T2	Heart & valves coronary arteries	Functional heart conditions, chest pains
T3	Lungs, bronchial tube pleura, chest, breast	Bronchitis, congestion, flu, pleurisy, grippe, pneumonia
T4	Gall bladder, common duct	Gall bladder conditions jaundice, shingles.
T5	Liver, solar plexus blood pressure	Liver conditions, fever, arthritis, anaemia, poor circulation,
T6	Stomach	Heartburn, dyspepsia, indigestion, stomach troubles
T7	Pancreas, duodenum	Diabetes, ulcers, gastritis
T8	Spleen, diaphragm	Leukaemia, hiccoughs.
T9	Adrenals	Allergies, hives
T10	Kidneys	Kidney troubles, hardening of the arteries, chronic tiredness, nephritis, pyelitis
T11	Kidneys, ureters	Skin conditions like acne & eczema
T12	Small intestines, fallopian tubes,	Rheumatism, flatulence

lymph circulation

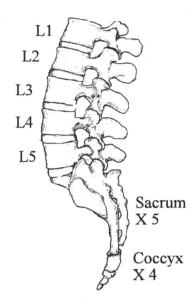

L1
L2
L3
L4
L5

Sacrum
X 5

Coccyx
X 4

VERTEBRAE	AREA AFFECTED	SYMPTOMS
L1	Large intestines	Constipation, colitis, hernia, diarrhea, etc.
L2	Appendix, abdomen, Upper leg, caecum	Appendicitis, varicose veins, cramps, difficult breathing
L3	Sex organs, uterus, bladder, knee	Bladder troubles, menstrual troubles, miscarriages, bed wetting, impotency, change of life symptoms, knee pains.
L4	Prostrate gland muscles of the lower back, sciatic nerve	Sciatica, lumbago, backache
L5	Lower legs, ankles, feet, toes, arches, sacrum, buttocks, hip bones, spinal curvatures, coccyx, rectum anus.	Poor circulation in the legs, swollen & weak ankles, cold feet, weak legs, sacro-Iliac conditions, haemorrhoids, pruritus or itching, pain at the end of the spine

DIAGRAM OF NERVES OF THE BODY

Anterior view

Posterior view

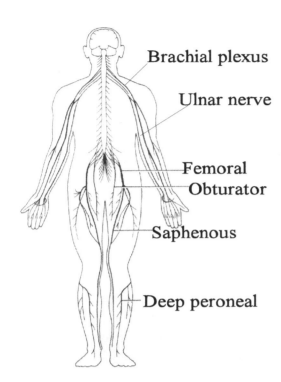

Brachial plexus

Ulnar nerve

Femoral
Obturator

Saphenous

Deep peroneal

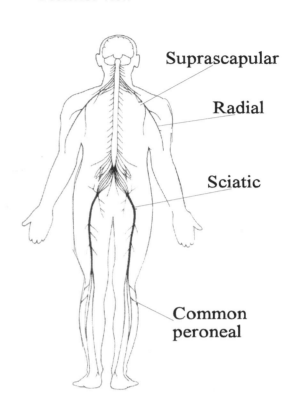

Suprascapular

Radial

Sciatic

Common
peroneal

Common Diseases or Disorders

Disease or Disorder	NEUROPATHY
Description	Neuropathy is inflammation or degeneration of a single peripheral nerve (mononeuropathy), two or more nerves in a separate area (multiple mononeuropathy), or many nerves (polyneurpathy). Symptoms include loss of sensory perception, and muscle activity and even the possibility of a loss of function of internal organs. Tingling, numbness, pain and/or swelling may be present with neuropathy. Common causes include physical injury to a single nerve. An example of this mononeuropathy problem would include carpal tunnel syndrome. Polyneuropathy on the other hand has many causes including infections, cancer, nutritional deficiencies and metabolic disorders, diabetes, and kidney failure. In the case of polyneuropathy, temperature changes and/or pain may not be registered due to the degeneration of the nerve. Burns, open sores and other injuries may occur in people with this disorder.
Possible Allopathic Treatment	Mononeuropathies, such as carpal tunnel, that stem from entrapment of the nerves may be given corticosteroid injections or if required, surgery may be performed in order to release the compression. Polyneuropathy that stem from a systemic disorder, should be treated accordingly to help halt the progression and potentially improve the condition.
Possible Holistic Aromatherapy Treatment	Auto-immune enhancers like; *Cinnamon leaf, Clove bud, Frankincense.* Sedative oils like; *Clary sage, Chamomile, Jasmine, Lavender, Marjoram, Benzoin, Cedarwood, Frankincense, Myrrh, Rose, Sandalwood and Ylang ylang.* Anti-inflammatory essential oils like; *Caraway, Teatree, Camphor, Chamomile, Fennel, Geranium, Jasmine, Peppermint, Benzoin, Frankincense, Myrrh and Patchouli.* Pain-killing analgesic oils like; *Bergamot, Cajeput, Coriander, Eucalyptus, Lemon-grass, Niaouli, Black-pepper, Chamomile, Jasmine, Lavender, Marjoram, Peppermint, Rosemary and Ginger.* Anti-depressant essential oil like; *Basil, Bergamot, Lemongrass, Clary Sage, Geranium, Jasmine, Lavender, Melissa, Orange Blossom, Patchouli, Rose, Sandalwood and Ylang Ylang.*

Disease or Disorder	BELL'S PALSY (FACIAL PARALYSIS)
Description	Bell's palsy is an inflammation of the facial nerve, causing neuritis type symptoms. It is named after the Scottish surgeon Charles Bell. Often caused by a viral infection, trauma, lack of blood supply or compression of the nerve as it passes through a tiny opening in the skull inferior and anterior to the ear. Symptoms include an inability to close an eye or control salivation on one side of the face. The condition is unilateral and can be transient or permanent. The extent of the nerve damage will determine the recovery outcome. Complete recovery within 2 months is not uncommon with mild or partial paralysis. The recovery of total paralysis varies from case to case, provided the nerve retains its excitability to maximise electrical stimulation then 90% of those afflicted will eventually recover.
Possible Allopathic Treatment	Methylcellulose drops and eye patches. Corticosteroids such as prednisone have been used to help relieve acute pain and reduce residual paralysis on occasion. Faradic stimulation of the nerve and physical therapy are useful in provoking muscle motion and preventing muscle contraction.
Possible Holistic Aromatherapy Treatment	Anti-inflammatory essential oils like; *Caraway, Teatree, Camphor, Chamomile, Fennel, Geranium, Jasmine, Peppermint, Benzoin, Frankincense, Myrrh and Patchouli.* Pain-killing analgesic oils like; *Bergamot, Cajeput, Coriander, Eucalyptus, Lemon-grass, Niaouli, Black-pepper, Chamomile, Jasmine, Lavender, Marjoram, Peppermint, Rosemary and Ginger.* Anti-depressant essential oil like; *Basil, Bergamot, Lemongrass, Clary Sage, Geranium, Jasmine, Lavender, Melissa, Orange Blossom, Patchouli, Rose, Sandalwood and Ylang Ylang.* Neurological stimulators: *Basil, Bergamot, Camphor wood, Chamomile (m), Cinnamon, Clary sage, Coriander, Cypress, Frankincense, Marjoram Sweet, Neroli, Nutmeg, Peppermint, Petitgrain, Pine, Rose Otto, Rosemary.* Auto-immune enhancers like; *Cinnamon leaf, Clove bud, Frankincense. Sedative oils like; Clary sage, Chamomile, Jasmine, Lavender, Marjoram, Benzoin, Cedarwood, Frankincense, Myrrh, Rose, Sandalwood and Ylang ylang.*

Disease or Disorder	PARKINSONS
Description	This is an extremely common neurological disorder beginning in middle life, caused by degenerating nerve cells in the basal ganglia. Parkinsons is a slow progressing disorder of the nervous system. The chief symptoms of this illness are resting tremors, muscular rigidity or stiffness, postural instability and slowness of movement. Eventually the face may lose much of its expression. Although most individuals with Parkinsons maintain their intellect, many may develop dementia. There is a condition known as Secondary Parkinsonism. This results from a loss or interference of dopamine within the basal ganglia. The most common cause of this disorder is the ingestion of anti-psychotic drugs that block dopamine receptors.
Possible Allopathic Treatment	Drug therapy is normally prescribed to treat Parkinsons. Levodopa is a commonly prescribed drug that converts to dopamine in the brain. Unlike dopamine, Levodopa is able to cross the blood-brain barrier into the basal ganglia, where it will replace the missing neural transmitter. Tricyclic antidepressants are often used to deal with the secondary effects of depression. None of the drugs used will cure or stop the disease, but they appear to prolong the quality of life.
Possible Holistic Aromatherapy Treatment	Pain-killing analgesic oils like; *Bergamot, Cajeput, Coriander, Eucalyptus, Lemon-grass, Niaouli, Black-pepper, Chamomile, Jasmine, Lavender, Marjoram, Peppermint, Rosemary and Ginger.* Anti-depressant essential oil like; *Basil, Bergamot, Lemongrass, Clary Sage, Geranium, Jasmine, Lavender, Melissa, Orange Blossom, Patchouli, Rose, Sandalwood and Ylang Ylang.* Warming (Rubefacient) essential oils like; *Bergamot, Eucalyptus, Thyme, Black Pepper, Camphor, Juniper, Lavender, Peppermint, Pine and Ginger.* Neurological stimulators: *Basil, Bergamot, Camphor wood, Chamomile (m), Cinnamon, Clary sage, Coriander, Cypress, Frankincense, Marjoram Sweet, Neroli, Nutmeg, Peppermint, Petit grain, Pine, Rose Otto, Rosemary.* Auto-immune enhancers like; *Cinnamon leaf, Clove bud, Frankincense.* Sedative oils like; *Clary sage, Chamomile, Jasmine, Lavender, Marjoram, Benzoin, Cedarwood, Frankincense, Myrrh, Rose, Sandalwood and Ylang ylang.*

Disease or Disorder	SCIATICA
Description	Sciatica is an inflammation of the great sciatic nerve. This is the longest single nerve in the body. Sciatica is often a form of rheumatic neuritis but can also be caused by compression by an arthritic spur or a slipped disc, marked by pain & tenderness along the length of the nerve. Recovery from a single acute attack is common, but attacks that recur often become chronic. Acute low back pain following strain or over use of muscles are characterized by muscle tightening, tenderness or spasm.
Possible Allopathic Treatment	In the first instance bed rest to relieve muscle spasm, localised heat pads, massage, oral analgesics, NSAIDs, muscle relaxants. Chronic pain treatment may involve wearing lumbosacral corsets, muscle strengthening exercises and weight loss diets.
Possible Holistic Aromatherapy Treatment	Anti-inflammatory essential oils like; *Caraway, Teatree, Camphor, Chamomile, Fennel, Geranium, Jasmine, Peppermint, Benzoin, Frankincense, Myrrh and Patchouli.* Pain-killing analgesic oils like; *Bergamot, Cajeput, Coriander, Eucalyptus, Lemon-grass, Niaouli, Black-pepper, Chamomile, Jasmine, Lavender, Marjoram, Peppermint, Rosemary and Ginger.* Anti-depressant essential oil like; *Basil, Bergamot, Lemongrass, Clary Sage, Geranium, Jasmine, Lavender, Melissa, Orange Blossom, Patchouli, Rose, Sandalwood and Ylang Ylang.* Warming (Rubefacient) essential oils like; *Bergamot, Eucalyptus, Thyme, Black Pepper, Camphor, Juniper, Lavender, Peppermint, Pine and Ginger.* Antispasmodics; *to prevent or relieve muscle spasms like Chamomile (M)* *Cardamon, Clary sage, Ginger, Marjoram Sweet, Orange.* Auto-immune enhancers like; *Cinnamon leaf, Clove bud, Frankincense.* Sedative oils like; *Clary sage, Chamomile, Jasmine, Lavender, Marjoram, Benzoin, Cedarwood, Frankincense, Myrrh, Rose, Sandalwood and Ylang ylang.*

Disease or Disorder	EPILEPSY
Description	Epilepsy is a neurological disorder that produces excessive activity in some area of the brain characterized by convulsive fits or seizures, sensory disturbances, loss of consciousness and/or abnormal behaviour. Seizures are categorized by their characteristics. The frequency of occurrence could range from a few a day to one every few years. Epileptic seizures can be triggered by flashing lights, repetitive sounds, drugs, hypoglycaemia or low levels of blood oxygen.
Possible Allopathic Treatment	Drug therapy in the form of anticonvulsants is commonly prescribed. In 1/3 of the patients, seizures will be completely eliminated, while another 1/3 will experience a reduction in the frequency of the fits. However, there is no one single drug that is able to control all the various types of seizures and different drugs are required for each individual patient. Some of the anti-seizure drugs include carbamazepine, ethosuximide, gabapentin, phenobarbital, primdone and phenytoin.
Possible Holistic Aromatherapy Treatment	Anti-inflammatory essential oils like; *Caraway, Teatree, Camphor, Chamomile, Fennel, Geranium, Jasmine, Peppermint, Benzoin, Frankincense, Myrrh and Patchouli.* Anti-depressant essential oil like; *Basil, Bergamot, Lemongrass, Clary Sage, Geranium, Jasmine, Lavender, Melissa, Orange Blossom, Patchouli, Rose, Sandalwood and Ylang Ylang.* Antispasmodic essential oils; *Aniseed, Basil, Bergamot, Black Pepper, Cajeput, Chamomile, Clary-Sage, Coriander, Cypress, Fennel, Ginger, Hyssop, Jasmine, Juniper, Lavender, Marjoram, Melissa, Orange, Peppermint, Patchouli, Petit grain, Rosemary, Thyme.* Auto-immune enhancers like; *Cinnamon leaf, Clove bud, Frankincense. Sedative oils like; Clary sage, Chamomile, Jasmine, Lavender, Marjoram, Benzoin, Cedarwood, Frankincense, Myrrh, Rose, Sandalwood and Ylang ylang.* Sedative: *Benzoin, Cedarwood, Clary sage, Chamomile, Frankincense, Jasmine, Lavender, Marjoram, Melissa, Myrrh, Neroli, Rose, Sandalwood and Ylang Ylang.*

Essential Oils

BASIL

Latin name: *ocimum basilicum*   Botanical family: *Labiatae*

Three main areas where this oil can help:

1.   Respiratory disorders
2.   Nervous disorders
3.   Digestive problems

Properties   Uses

Expectorant	Colds, coughs, catarrh, emphysema, whooping cough, influenza, sinus congestion, bronchitis
Digestive	Dyspepsia, nausea, vomiting, colitis, flatulence, gastric spasm, cramps
Cephalic	Mental stimulant, lethargy, fatigue, headaches, adrenal cortex stimulant
Nervine	Paralysis, MS, fainting, anxiety, depression, hysteria
Antiseptic	Infections, influenza, fevers,

Place of Origin
Basil was historically recorded in India, Asia, Africa, where it has a long history of use as a traditional Indian medicine. Basil grows wild all over the Mediterranean area. Today it is found in most countries, although the main essential oil producer is France. There are a number of varieties varying in height, colour of the leaves, etc. The variety most commonly used in aromatherapy has a pale pink flower with hairy oval leaves.

Method of Extraction
The essential oil is extracted by means of steam distillation of the flowering tops and leaves. Some of the chemical constituents include borneone, methyl chavicol, linalool, cineol, eugenol, limonene, citronellol, pinene and camphor. The essence is a light greenish-yellow and has a clear refreshing odour.

Traditional Uses
The basil plant takes its name from the Greek word for royalty "Basilicos". Basil is highly regarded in India, where it is worshipped more than a king. A sacred herb that was once used to protect the dead from the evil spirits who may block their entrance to paradise

Herbal Medicine

A popular culinary herb, basil has antispasmodic properties that will assist in digestive disorders such as cramps and flatulence. Traditionally used in the treatment of bee and wasp stings, or venomous bites, it has a drawing action on the poisons.

Aromatherapy

Cephalic in nature, basil like rosemary, is an extremely effective adrenal cortex stimulant. It is beneficial in cases of loss of memory, mental fatigue and anxiety. Basil has been regarded as one of the best nerve tonics in aromatherapy. Strengthening and reviving, it is considered an up-lifter. It will stimulate the sympathetic nervous system and strengthen the adrenal cortex. These effects on the cerebrospinal system make it useful for paralysis, and MS.

Headaches, especially those brought on by stress, insomnia and nervousness respond well with the treatment of this essence. Basil can be utilized in all types of nervous disorders and is particularly valuable in treating people suffering from anxiety, depression or hysteria.

Combined with the antispasmodic properties, stress or nervous related disorders of the digestive system will find relief. Indigestion, nausea, vomiting, dyspepsia, or other stomach ailments are indicated uses for basil. Use a topical application in a cream or oil base and apply on the abdomen in a clockwise direction. Menstrual pain may also show improvement with this application method. It appears that basil has a cleansing ability on both the kidneys and intestines.

Basil has a strong affinity for the respiratory tract and has been used since antiquity for chest infections. It is a good antiseptic, expectorant and neurotrophic antispasmodic which makes it useful in treating asthma, bronchitis, emphysema and whooping cough. One of the most effective mediums in which to use basil is in a steam inhalation. Two drops in a bowl of hot water will suffice. Place a towel over the head to cover it and inhale the vapour for 5- 10 minutes.

This essence is said to help restore the sense of smell caused by problems like sinusitis, rhinitis and other disorders. Psychologically, essential oil of basil is restorative. It is soporific -especially for insomnia and as an antidepressant. By strengthening the nerves, basil elicits a calming effect for high stress individuals who are bordering on "burn-out".

Warning: *Possible toxic with prolonged use (Use 2-3 weeks at a time)*
             Emmenagogic - avoid use during pregnancy.

BERGAMOT

Latin name: *citrus bergamia*   Botanical family: *Rutaceae*

Three main areas where this oil can help:

1.   Urinary tract infections
2.   Depression
3.   Skin care

Properties   Uses

Antidepressant	Anxiety, depression, sadness
Antispasmodic	Dyspepsia, colic, indigestion
Antiseptic	Sore throats, eczema, psoriasis, acne, boils, abscesses, wounds, shingles, scabies, urinary tract infections, cystitis, urethritis
Expectorant	Colds, coughs, bronchitis, respiratory infections, tuberculosis
Sedative	Nervous tension, anger, irritability

Place of Origin
Christopher Columbus was said to have brought this tree from the Canary Islands to Spain and Italy. Bergamot takes it name from the small town in the City of Bergamo in northern Italy. The fruit has the appearance of a small pear-shaped orange. The oil has a greenish-yellow colour. The smell is citrus and sweet with a slight hint of floral. However, the taste is bitter.

Method of Extraction
Bergamot oil is obtained by expression of the fruit rind. Cold pressed bergamot oil is precious, so some manufacturers will steam distill the peel after the expression, as this releases even more essential oil, although it is of a poorer quality. The active constituents include linalool, nerol, terpineol, linalyl acetate, bergaptene, limonene and dipentene.

Traditional Uses
An Italian folk remedy for the treatment of fever and/or infection. This product has commonly been used in the perfume industry as a main ingredient in perfumes and eau de cologne.

Herbal Medicine
Other than herbal tea, there is no other use for bergamot in herbal medicine.

Aromatherapy

Bergamot is an essential oil that has antiseptic properties that are invaluable in the treatment of urethritis, cystitis, urinary tract infections, or genito-urinary infections with heat and inflammation present. A bath or topical application *(do not use neat on the skin and make sure to dissolve in a carrier for the tub)* proves extremely useful for those individuals suffering from these problems.

The same antiseptic properties make it an ideal oil to use in skin care ailments like eczema, psoriasis, boils, acne, wounds and more. When combined with eucalyptus, shingles and herpes respond favourably to the treatment.

Due to its ability to decrease the action of the sympathetic nervous system while increasing the response of the para-sympathetic nervous system, stress related conditions show improvement.

Its uplifting yet sedative qualities blend well to help both mental and psychological problems. Anxiety, tension, depression, sadness and irritability show a positive response. It is refreshing (as are most citrus oils) and seems to lift the spirits.

Reports suggest that bergamot oil has been successfully used as an appetite regulator, possibly because it directly influences the appetite-control centre in the brain. By interacting with the underlying tensions that have provoked the under *(anorexia)* or over-eating, it enables the sufferer to return to a normal weight and eating pattern. Some aromatherapy magazines report that not only is it useful for casting out intestinal parasites, but it will also diminish gall stones.

The expectorant properties of essential oil of bergamot prove useful for respiratory problems. Traditional complaints of problems associated with breathing such as bronchitic, tuberculosis, coughs and respiratory infections benefit from the action on this system. An excellent insect repellant as well as deodorant.

Warning: *Photo toxic due to the chemical constituent of bergaptene. Avoid sun exposure after use of this essential oil.*
May irritate sensitive skin

JUNIPER

Latin name: *juniperus communis*   Botanical family: *Cupressaceae*

Five main areas where this oil can help:

1.   Diuretic for urinary tract infections
2.   Chronic skin disorders
3.   Digestive problems
4.   Strengthening effect on the nerves
5.   Detoxifier

Properties   Uses

Detoxifier	Hangovers, arthritis, rheumatism, gout, cirrhosis
Diuretic	Water retention, cystitis, kidney stones, cellulite, urine retention
Astringent	Haemorrhoids, acne, oily skin
Tonic	Pancreas, adrenals
Emmenagogic	Amenorrhea, dysmenorrhea

Place of Origin
Juniper is a small evergreen tree or shrub with short, spiny needle-like leaves, closely arranged in whorls of three. It grows four to six feet in height and is commonly found in chalky soils. This small hardwood bush is found in Central and Southern Europe, Sweden and Canada.

Method of Extraction
Essential oil of juniper is steam distilled from the berries which are small like blackcurrants. They turn from green to a deep purple-blue or almost black when they are ripe. There is an oil that is obtained from the wood of the plant, but it has little if any therapeutic value. It is slightly greenish-yellow. Juniper is bitter to taste. This makes sense when you know that it is an ingredient found in gin. The chemical constituents are: alpha pinene, borneol and isoborneol, cadinene, camphene, pinene, and terpineol.

Traditional Uses
Historically, juniper has been known for its antiseptic and diuretic properties. The French were known to burn juniper twigs and rosemary leaves in hospital wards and sick rooms to purify the air. It has consistently, through out the ages, guarded against infections and contagious disease.

Herbal Medicine
Juniper has been used to help alleviate problems that have uric acid retention. It is thought that it is high in natural insulin and possesses the ability to restore the pancreas. However, this is only in cases where there has been no permanent damage to the pancreas.

Aromatherapy

Juniper is one of the top essential oils to utilize should there be a need to throw off any toxic waste found within the body. It is able to reduce uric acid build up that is commonly found in the joints in cases of arthritis, rheumatism and gout. Poor elimination is one of the root causes of these disorders and juniper should be considered as an effective way of improving this elimination process.

The diuretic properties of this essence will make it invaluable in the treatment of cellulite. Remember that accumulated toxins are associated with fluid retention. The detoxifying and diuretic actions together are an added benefit in the fight against this common disorder.

In cases of water retention and problems associated with the kidneys such as stones and cystitis, this is one of the best oils to choose. It will also relieve urine retention which often occurs in men when the prostrate is enlarged. Juniper has a special affinity with the genito-urinary tract, being tonic, purifying, antiseptic and stimulant.

One of the main actions of juniper is on the kidney and liver. It will help detoxify the liver in cases of hangovers and further helps with more severe problems such as cirrhosis. However, as a word of caution, *prolonged use may overstimulate the kidneys and should be avoided when dealing with severe kidney disease.*

Light menstrual flow or missed periods can be treated with juniper due to its emmenagogic properties. Painful periods are another area to utilize this oil. Apply either topically or better yet, use in a bath blend to help ease pain and tension.

Skin conditions like eczema, dermatitis, acne and oily skin will be helped through not only the detoxifying action, but also of the astringent action of Juniper. An external application for the treatment of haemorrhoids - either as a spritzer/wash or bath blend with frankincense- is ideal in this situation

Warning: *Emmenagogic - do not use with pregnancy*

ROSEMARY

Latin name: *rosmarinus officinalis*   Botanical name: *Labiatae*

Three main areas where this oil can help:

1.   Stimulates the nervous system
2.   Skin and scalp care
3.   Respiratory disorders

Properties   Uses

Nervine/Cephalic	Debility, epilepsy, fainting, hysteria, mental fatigue, nervous disorders, memory loss, lethargy, paralysis
Analgesic	Headaches, migraines, aches and pains, arthritis, rheumatism, gout
Hepatic	Cirrhosis, jaundice, hepatitis, gallstones
Stimulant	Circulatory system, low blood pressure, arteriosclerosis, poor circulation, baldness
Tonic	Digestive system, respiratory system

Place of Origin
The name rosemary comes from the Latin "ros marinus", meaning "dew of the sea". This comes from the plants original location near the Mediterranean coast. It is a well known perennial herb with long, straight stems studded with one-inch long narrow pointed leaves. It grows up to six feet in height. Commonly found throughout Europe, it favours locations near the sea.

Method of Extraction
Rosemary, unlike some essential oils, is steam distilled from the whole plant. Its chemical constituents include: borneol, camphene, camphor, cineol, lineol, pinene, resins and saponin.

Traditional Medicine
In ancient Greece, students believed that rosemary would help their memory. While they would study for exams, they would wear rosemary garlands on their head.
The same plant, was one of the earliest and renowned of English herbs, although it was not native to the country. Sprigs of rosemary would be used as incense, as well as to drive away any evil spirits.
France used it to fumigate hospitals and sick wards. The practice of burning rosemary in the hospital wards persisted into this present century. Ironically is was abandoned at about the same time that modern research proved its antiseptic properties.

Herbal Medicine

Rosemary has long been included in many herbal remedies. Treatments in the form of infusions or linaments for conditions such as muscle spasms, rheumatism, sores, headaches and depression. It is a tonic to the scalp and an infusion can be used for washing the hair

Aromatherapy

Essential oil of rosemary is an adrenal cortex stimulant. It is known for its ability to increase the blood circulation to the brain and the nervous system. Because of this known effect on the central nervous system, many wasting diseases like atrophy, temporary paralysis, debility, MS and possible even chronic fatigue syndrome will show a marked improvement. The use of rosemary responds to common complaints such as mental fatigue, fainting, loss of memory, anxiety, poor concentration, headaches and migraines.

The circulatory stimulant properties make it a tonic to the heart, a wise treatment for low blood pressure and arteriosclerosis. When adding the analgesic properties of this oil, arthritis, rheumatism, gout and general aches and pains will be eased. It also helps to lower blood cholesterol levels. A liver tonic, rosemary helps to regulate bile production. Use of this essence is favourable in cases of cirrhosis, gallstones, jaundice, alcoholism, hepatitis and other liver disorders.

The sharp quality of rosemary, along with the antiseptic properties, makes it a valuable oil in respiratory complaints like sinusitis, colds, bronchitis and influenza. Individuals with chronic lung disorders will benefit from these tonic properties. The antispasmodic properties can be used to treat digestive complaints like diarrhea, colitis and other gastrointestinal complaints, especially for those who have a weak disposition that seems to arise in tense, nervous people. Baldness, dandruff and thinning hair benefit from the stimulating action of rosemary while skin disorders (eczema, dermatitis, wrinkles, etc.) benefit from its astringent qualities.

Warning   *Emmenagogic do not use with pregnancy. Heavy or prolonged use could result in nervousness or other nerve problems due to its effects of the nervous system and adrenal glands. May cause epileptic type fits if used too often or in large quantities and may antidote homeopathic remedies. Avoid with high blood pressure.*

Linden Blossom

Latin name: *telia euripi*   Botanical name: *Telic*

Three main areas where this oil can help:

1.   Nervous disorders/uplifter
2.   Respiratory problems
3.   Digestive disorders

Properties   Uses

Properties	Uses
Nervine	Neuralgia, irritability, anxiety
Diuretic	Water retention, urine retention, kidney disorders
Sedative	Insomnia, anger, nervous tension
Decongestant	Respiratory infections, allergies, coughs, catarrh, pleurisy, bronchitis
Antidepressant	Depression, sadness, grief

Place of Origin
Linden Blossom is native to the European countries. It is commonly found in England, France , Holland and Germany. A tall graceful tree that can grow upwards to over 100 feet in height. The flowers, yellowy-white in colour are almost completely hidden by the leaves which are similar in colour.

Method of Extraction
Obtained by solvent extraction or enfleurage of the flowers, linden blossom results in an absolute form. Today, this oil is frequently adulterated. Make sure to purchase it from a reputable supplier. Its main principal chemical constituent is farnesol.

Traditional Uses
Culpepper regarded linden blossom as 'a good cephalic and nervine, excellent for apoplexy, epilepsy, vertigo and palpitations of the heart.' Large amounts of these flowers were collected for use during World War II.

Herbal Medicine
Infusion of these blossoms are used as a nerve tonic for the treatment of tension headaches, hysteria or any other problems that are caused by nervous tension. This plant is used as an effective sleep aid as well as being used to quiet coughs.

Aromatherapy

As with herbal medicine, linden blossom is considered a terrific nerve tonic that alleviates a wide variety of nervous disorders especially those that arise from stress. Irritability, nervous tension, apprehension, neuralgia, headaches and anxiety respond well to the use of this flowery essential oil.

A sedative essential oil, it may show positive results for the hyperactivity in children that is such a concern for parents and teachers today. Diffusion of linden blossom oil, or topical application would be applicable. This essential oil seems to have a thinning action on the blood and may help in case of arteriosclerosis, anaemia and high cholesterol levels.

Due to its sudorific properties, this oil is effective against chronic catarrhal conditions. It will help reduce temperature by increasing perspiration. Most respiratory illnesses including coughs, bronchitis, congestion and pleurisy respond well, especially through inhalation.

Digestive disorders like indigestion, cramps and diarrhea will benefit. Linden blossom's diuretic action is beneficial for kidney disorders, while its detoxifying effect on the liver and its ability to clear an excess build up of urea will lead to a general tonic effect on the body as a whole.

As with many base notes and "flower" essential oils, Linden blossom serves as a powerful uplifter. It is a very "heady' oil and appears to bring down the barriers created within, while calming the mind and uplifting the spirits.

Question and Answer Sheets

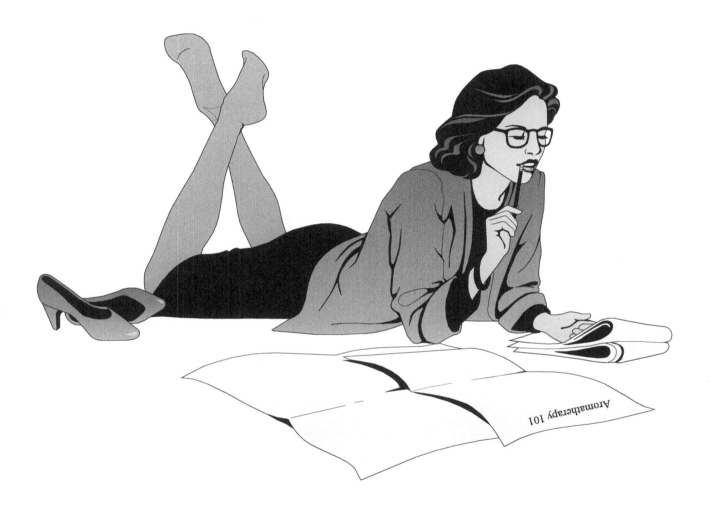

Please keep the questions for review.
Circle the correct answer/s on the Answer Sheets at the back of the book and
<u>return these sheets only</u> to your instructor.

Questions - Lesson #6

1. Which of the following constituents are found in essential oils?
a. lactides
b. monoterpenes
c. ethers
d. triterpenes
e. lactones
f. aldetones
g. aldehydes
h. ketones
i. ketides
j. esters

2. In general, most alcohols are;
a. digestive stimulants
b. nerve tonics
c. immune enhancers
d. anti-inflammatory

3. Eucalyptol, also know as cineole,is;
a. mucolytic
b. sedative
c. stimulant
d. hypotensive

4. Many essential oils are commonly adulterated. List your own reasons why it is important to purchase a professional quality product.

5. In your opinion, should you choose essential oils based on "chemotyping?" Explain why or why not.

6. The neurological system has three main functions, they are?
a. sensory perception
b. nervous perception
c. motor control/functions
d. integrative functions

7. The neurological system has two main divisions. These are;
a. central nervous system
b. cerebral nervous system
c. cranial nervous system
d. peripheral nervous system

8. Describe the nerve cell or neuron.

9. The two kinds of peripheral nerve fibre are?
a. white or myelinated
b. white or unmyelinated
c. grey or myelinated
d. grey or unmyelinated

10. The difference between white and grey nerve fibres is:
a. white nerve fibres are to organs and grey nerve fibres are to muscles
b. white nerve fibres are enclosed in a sheath or myelin and grey nerve fibres are finer and not enclosed in a sheath
c. white nerve fibres run from the brain and grey nerve fibres return to the brain
d. grey nerve fibres are enclosed in a sheath or myelin and white nerve fibres are finer and not enclosed in a sheath

11. Which chemical(s) are produced to assist with synapses between nerve endings?
a. noradrenaline
b. acetylcholine
c. endocrine
d. adrenaline

12. What does the word "preganglionic" mean?
a. a nerve fibre that enters a sympathetic or parasympathetic ganglion
b. a nerve fibre that senses temperature
c. a nerve fibre that exits a sympathetic or parasympathetic ganglion
d. a nerve fibre controlling contraction of an organ

13. What does the word "postganglionic" mean?
a. a nerve fibre that enters a sympathetic or parasympathetic ganglion
b. a nerve that senses temperature
c. a nerve fibre that exits a sympathetic or parasympathetic ganglion
d. a nerve fibre controlling contraction of an organ

14. In relation to the fear, fight or flight syndrome, adrenaline does what to the body?

a. produces relaxed and constructive activities in tranquillity

b. raises blood pressure, increasing speed of both brain and heart beat and dilates the pupils

c. lowers blood pressure, slows the heart and brain activity and increases digestive processes

d. raises blood pressure, increasing speed of nerve reaction and increases sweat processes

15. How does parasympathetic stimulation affect the body?

a. produces relaxed and constructive activities in tranquillity

a. raises blood pressure, increasing speed of both brain and heart beat and dilates the pupils

c. lowers blood pressure, slows the heart and brain activity and increases digestive processes

d. raises blood pressure, increasing speed of muscle reaction and increases sweat processes

16. Draw and label a diagram of a neuron.

17. The central nervous system;

a. controls only voluntary muscle movement

b. is composed of a network of cranial and spinal nerves

c. controls the entire body

d. controls the autonomic nervous system

18. The peripheral nervous system;

a. controls only voluntary muscle movement

b. is composed of a network of cranial and spinal nerves

c. controls the entire body

d. controls the autonomic nervous system

19. The basic structure of the nervous system is;

a. the dendrite

b. the axon

c. the nucleus

d. the neuron

20. The three different types of nerve cells include;

a. inter-neurons

b. tactile neurons

c. motor neurons

d. sensory neurons

e. temperature neurons

f. periphery neurons

21. The brain is protected by three enveloping membranes collectively known as?

a. meninges

b. dura-mater

c. arachnoid

d. pia mater

e. cerebral cortex

22. Describe each of the three answers to question 21 and give a brief description of each one.

23. The brain is divided into three structures, the cerebrum is one, the other two are?

a. meninges

b. cerebellum

c. central nervous system

d. medulla oblongata

24. Describe the adult human brain.

25. Draw and label a diagram of the brain.

26. Describe the cerebrum.

27. Describe the cerebellum.

28. Describe the medulla oblongata.

29. Describe the spinal cord.

30. What does the "autonomic nervous system" control?

a. all body structures over which we have no voluntary control

b. all body structures over which we have voluntary control

c. all body structures involved with the immune system

d. all body structures involved with the hormonal system

31. The autonomic nervous system is divided into separate parts, they are?

a. the sympathetic

b. the preganglionic

c. the ganglionic

d. the parasympathetic

32. What is the difference between the two answers to question #31?

33. Which of the following effects occur with sympathetic stimulation?
a. pupils constrict
b. digestion increases
c. sweating occurs
d. blood vessels constrict
e. glandular secretions dry up
f. blood pressure lowers

34. A vagotonic person is one who?
a. the sympathetic nerves are stronger and hence this person has a more placid disposition and a good digestion
b. the parasympathetic nerves are stronger and hence this person has a more placid disposition and a good digestion
c. the sympathetic nerves are stronger and hence this person is more emotional and the digestion is more readily disturbed
d. the parasympathetic nerves are stronger and hence this person is more emotional and the digestion is more readily disturbed

35. A sympatheticotonic person is one who?
a. the sympathetic nerves are stronger and hence this person has a more placid disposition and a good digestion
b. the parasympathetic nerves are stronger and hence this person has a more placid disposition and a good digestion
c. the sympathetic nerves are stronger and hence this person is more emotional and the digestion is more readily disturbed
d. the parasympathetic nerves are stronger and hence this person is more emotional and the digestion is more readily disturbed

36. The sympathetic post-ganglionic chemical neurotransmitters secrete which substance(s)?
a. acetylcholine
b. norepinephrine
c. both of the above

37. The para-sympathetic post-ganglionic chemical neurotransmitters secrete which substance(s)?
a. acetylcholine
b. norepinephrine
c. both of the above

38. What is "neuritis"?
a. a disturbance of a peripheral nerve
b. an inflammation of a nerve
c. a degeneration of a nerve root
d. a disturbance of the facial nerve

39. What is "Bell's Palsy"?
a. a disturbance of a peripheral nerve
b. an inflammation of a facial nerve
c. a degeneration of a nerve root
d. a disturbance of the facial nerve

40. What are the symptoms or effects of neuralgia?
a. an inflammation of a nerve due to degeneration of a nerve root
b. a lot of pain in a nerve due to irritation or inflammation
c. a lot of pain in a nerve due to an arthritic spur or slipped disc
d. tremors, rigidity and slowness of movement

41. What are the main symptoms of "Parkinsons' Disease"?
a. an inflammation of a nerve due to degeneration of a nerve root
b. a lot of pain in a nerve due to irritation or inflammation
c. a lot of pain in a nerve due to an arthritic spur or slipped disc
d. tremors, rigidity and slowness of movement

42. Name some of the causes of "sciatica".
a. poor muscle condition
b. compression of the nerve by an arthritic spur
c. compression of the nerve by a slipped disc
d. inflammation of the nerve due to degeneration of the nerve root

43. Label the diagram of nerves.
(SEE ANSWER SHEET FOR DIAGRAM)

44. What are dermatones?
a. post-ganglionic fibres
b. spinal nerves
c. skin areas that are innervated by a specific spinal nerve
d. dermal areas of the skin

45. What is epilepsy"?
a. a neurological condition characterized by numbness
b. a neurological condition characterized by seizures
c. a skeletal condition characterized by numbness
d. a muscular condition characterized by seizures

46. What part of the plant is used to obtain essential oil of basil?

a. the flowering tops
b. the rind of the fruit
c. the leaves
d. the wood

47. What three main areas will basil help most?

a. urinary tract infection and mucous membranes
b. digestive tract
c. nervous system tonic
d. skin care
e. respiratory infections or problems

48. What do you have to be careful of when using basil?

a. during pregnancy
b. possible toxicity with extended use
c. photo sensitivity
d. mucous membrane irritant

49. What part of the plant is used to obtain essential oil of bergamot?

a. the flowering tops
b. the rind of the fruit
c. the leaves
d. the wood

50. What three main areas will bergamot help the most?

a. urinary tract infection and mucous membranes
b. arthritis
c. depression and anxiety
d. skin care
e. respiratory infections or problems

51. What do you have to be careful of when using bergamot?

a. during pregnancy
b. people want to drink it
c. photo sensitivity
d. mucous membrane irritant

52. What part of the plant is used to obtain essential oil of juniper?

a. the seeds of the plant
b. the leaves
c. the flowering tops
d. the roots
e. the fruit or berries of the plant
f. the wood

53. How is juniper obtained?

a. distilled
b. extracted
c. maceration
d. enfleurage

54. What five main areas will juniper help most?

a. detoxifying the body
b. for chronic skin infection
c. headaches and migraines
d. treatment of sore throats
e. diuretic for genito-urinary infections
f. strengthening on nervous system
g. digestive problems
h. high blood pressure

55. When should you not use juniper?

a. low blood pressure
b. high blood pressure
c. epilepsy
d. diabetes
e. pregnancy

56. What part of the plant is used to obtain essential oil of rosemary?

a. the seeds of the plant
b. the leaves and flowering tops
c. the fruit or berries of the plant
d. the wood
e. the whole plant

57. What three main areas will rosemary help most?

a. stimulating to the nervous system
b. tonic to the respiratory system
c. healing in skin and scalp care
d. analgesic on skin and muscles
e. calming to the genito-urinary system

58. What do you have to be careful of when using rosemary?

a. pregnancy
b high blood pressure
c. epilepsy
d. anti-dote to homeopathic remedies
e. all of the above

59. How is linden blossom obtained?

a. distilled
b. extracted
c. maceration
d. enfleurage

60. What three main areas will linden blossom help most?
a. digestive problems
b. skin disorders
c. respiratory problems
d. nervous disorders/uplifter
e. low blood pressure

61.   What do you have to be careful of when using linden blossom?
a. pregnancy
b. high blood pressure
c. epilepsy
d. all of the above
e. none of above

Answer Sheet - Lesson #6

(Keep the questions for review. Circle the correct answer/s and return these sheets only to your instructor.)

1. A   B   C   D   E   F   G   H   I   J

2. A   B   C   D

3. A   B   C   D

4. It is important to use professional quality product in aromatherapy because _____

_____

_____

_____

_____

5. Chemotyping should/should not be used because _____

_____

_____

_____

_____

6. A   B   C   D

7. A   B   C   D

8. Describe a neuron.

_____

_____

_____

_____

9. A   B   C   D

10. A   B   C   D

11. A   B   C   D

12. A   B   C   D

13. A   B   C   D

14. A   B   C   D

15. A   B   C   D

16. Label the diagram of a neuron.

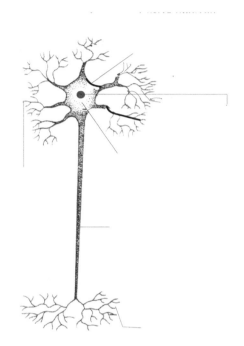

17. A   B   C   D

18. A   B   C   D

19. A   B   C   D

20. A   B   C   D   E   F

21. A   B   C   D   E

22. The following is a description of each of the three enveloping membranes are:

1._____

_____

2._____

_____

3_____

_____

23.   A   B   C   D

24.   The adult brain_____

_____

_____

25.   Label the diagram of the brain

26.   The cerebrum consists of _____ symmetrical hemispheres, the outer layer is known as the

_____under this lies the _____. The function of the cerebrum is to control

_____ and is the seat of the _____ dealing with

_____ _____ and_____

27.   The cerebellum is _____ in size, it lies _____ the cerebrum.

       Its function is to _____

28.   The medulla oblongata connect the _____ to the _____ .

29.   The spinal cord extends down the _____. It has two swellings the _____

and _____.

_____

30.   A   B   C   D

31.   A   B   C   D

32.   The difference is _____

_____

_____

_____

33.   A   B   C   D   E   F

34.   A   B   C   D

35.   A   B   C   D

36.   A   B   C

37   A   B   C

38.   A   B   C   D

39.   A   B   C   D

40.   A   B   C   D

41.   A   B   C   D

42.   A   B   C   D

43.   Label the diagrams of the nerves
       Posterior view

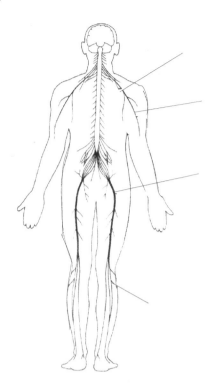

Anterior view

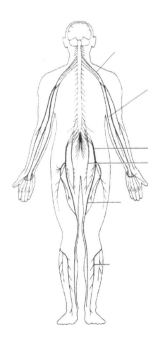

44.   A   B   C   D

45.   A   B   C   D

46.   A   B   C   D

47.   A   B   C   D   E

48.   A   B   C   D

49.   A   B   C   D

50.   A   B   C   D   E

51.   A   B   C   D

52.   A   B   C   D   E   F

53.   A   B   C   D

54.   A   B   C   D   E   F   G   H

55.   A   B   C   D   E

56.   A   B   C   D   E

57.   A   B   C   D   E

58.   A   B   C   D   E

59.   A   B   C   D

60.   A   B   C   D   E

61.   A   B   C   D   E

LESSON SEVEN

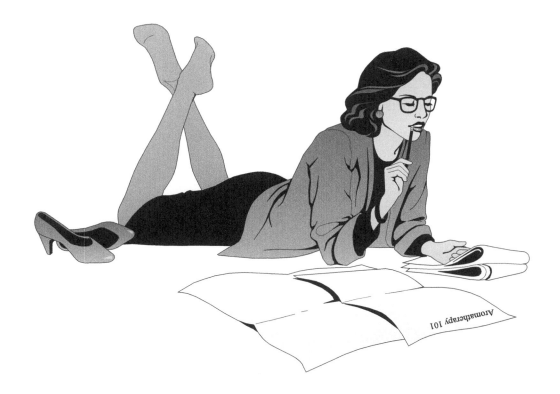

Lesson #7

Table of Contents

Carrier Oils

WHAT IS A CARRIER OIL?

A carrier oil is a massage oil that can be used to dilute essential oils. Most essential oils should not be used straight from the bottle and placed directly onto the body. They are far too powerful and may cause irritation. Carrier oils provide a natural medium to dilute the essential oils to allow them to penetrate safely, while acting as a lubricant to assist the hands to glide effortlessly over the body without resistance. These massage oils should be light and non-sticky so the essential oils may penetrate into the skin. They should be low in odour so the aroma of the blend will have its full effect instead of the carrier oil taking precedence.

Carrier oils are sometimes referred to as *"fixed oils"*. They should be 100% pure, unrefined, unbleached and cold pressed. Mineral oil (baby oil) should be avoided as it does not absorb into the skin and leaves a greasy residue. Mineral oil, a petroleum by-product, acts as a barrier to the skin and therefore restricts the absorption of the essential oils.

A fixed oil is a compound of glycerol and fatty acids.

▸   Glycerols are: An alcohol that is a component of fats. Most carrier oils are yellowish in colour and they have a tendency to go rancid or oxidize. Oxidation is a process that occurs when the glycerol in the oil turns to fatty acid when it is exposed to air.

▸   Fatty acids are: An organic acid produced by the hydrolysis *(decomposition or alteration of neutral fats)*. Essential fatty acids are not produced by the body and must be supplemented by healthy eating in a balanced diet. An example of an essential fatty acid is linoleic acid.

Carrier oils are called a fixed oil because they do not evaporate. Essential oils on the other hand, evaporate on contact with air or when warmed. Massage carrier oils used in aromatherapy are made from vegetable sources and educated professional aromatherapists do not use those that are made from animal sources or petro-chemical products. Individuals who are unaware of the quality of these oils will often purchase inferior oils due to the price. They are unaware that *you use much more of the cheaper massage oils and it tends to cost more in the long run.*

How are they made ?
Carrier oils used in aromatherapy are of vegetable origin and many of them contain therapeutic properties of their own. They should be cold pressed to ensure that the vitamins and therapeutic fatty acids are not destroyed during the manufacturing process. One commonly occurring problem with cold pressing is the creation of internal heat. This occurs when the seeds or nuts are placed on a press. A large screw is turned causing the pressure to build up on the seeds or nuts, thus releasing the oils. Heat is naturally produced using this technique because of the friction between the seeds during compression. A careful watch must be kept to ensure that the temperature doesn't exceed 30 degrees Celsius.

It appears that at present only a handful of suppliers follow this method because of the time and cost involved with monitoring the presses. In France they are more willing to limit the process and maintain this temperature. After pressing, the oil is then filtered.

Many companies sell "pure" cold pressed carrier oils. Labelling laws are not stringent in most countries and there is no clarification as what constitutes a "pure" oil. Many producers heat-up the carrier oil to clarify the final look of the oil. Heating a carrier oil will make the oil appear clear/clean but unfortunately it will also kill all of the vitamins that naturally occur in the carrier oil and render it useless as a natural therapeutic agent.

Most inexpensive vegetable carrier oils are intended for commercial use or for cooking. They are obtained by a cheaper method called solvent extraction and later refined or clarified. This method kills the beneficial therapeutic properties and renders it unsuitable for aromatherapy.

Be warned, *only the best and most reliable oils should be used by professionals* and these are normally only available to aromatherapists and other educated professionals. Oils that are available for public purchase should be checked out thoroughly. Inferior products, whether essential oils or carrier oils, commonly cause allergic reactions due to the additives and preservatives.

Infused Oils

Infusion is a method of making therapeutic carrier oils, by immersing the plant material (or flowers) in a warm vegetable oil, *(ie. carrier oils such as St Johns Wort, also known as hypericum)*. The chosen plant is chopped up into small pieces and added to the warm oil and left to soak. The therapeutic nutrients are absorbed into the carrier oil for about 1-2 weeks. When this process is complete, the infused oil is filtered to remove the remaining plant matter and bottled.

Thousands of years ago infused oils were used by ancient civilizations like Egyptians and the Greeks for their well known therapeutic properties. Today, we are able to use this method to enhance an aromatherapy treatment. Simply add a 5% solution of infused oil to the regular carrier and essential oil preparation for the clients added benefit..

How to Store Them

Carrier oils should be stored in a cool environment *(not a fridge)*. If they are kept properly, they will keep for approximately 12-18 months. The shelf life will depend on how fresh the oil is *(the time between cold pressing and you purchasing it)* and the content of saturated fatty acids compared to unsaturated fatty acids. If they are high in saturated fatty acids *they will be more stable* compared to those that are higher in unsaturated fatty acids *(which are less stable)*.

FIXED OILS OF VEGETABLE ORIGIN (CARRIER OILS)

Sweet Almond Oil (*prunus amygdalus*)

Obtained from: The kernel of the sweet almond tree.

Best used for: 1.   Relieving itching caused by eczema
2.   Dry skin
3.   Inflammation

The oil is pale yellow in colour, and slightly viscous. It is drawn from the kernel of the sweet almond tree. Almonds are cultivated in Asia Minor, Greece, Italy, France, Portugal and Spain.

Sweet almond oil is rich in proteins, glucosides, minerals, and contains vitamin A, B1, B2, B6, a small amount of vitamin E and is high in polyunsaturated fatty acids. Because it has a small amount of vitamin E (a natural preservative), it will keep for longer periods of time and will not easily go rancid.

The fixed oil, or carrier oil of almond is expressed from both the bitter and sweet almonds. The best results are obtained from cold pressed sweet almond oil.

As much as *40-46%* of the total weight of the kernels will result in carrier oil, if obtained by using solvents. This is, of course the cheaper oil.   Whereas the method of crushing will not produce anywhere near that amount, it will be a superior oil.

Due to its rich content of proteins, it is a good oil to choose for dry skin types (*although it is very oily*). The smell is almost nonexistent which makes it a good fixed oil to use becaue it will not affect the smell of the aromatherapy blend. Almond oil will give protection and nourishment to the skin. It is also beneficial for relieving itching caused by eczema.

One great advantage that these oils have over other oils is that it won't go rancid so easily.

For therapeutic purposes, it is best to avoid any carrier oil derived from "nuts" on people with nut allergies.

Note: *There is also an* <u>*essential oil*</u> *of almond, but this is made from bitter almonds and is never used in aromatherapy. When bitter almond essential oil is extracted by steam distiallation, prussic acid is formed. Prussic acid is also known as hydrocyanic acid or cyanide. This acid is not formed during the crushing process to extract the carrier oil.)*

Apricot Kernel Oil (*Prunus armeniaca*)

Obtained from: Expressed from the avocado pear kernel.

Best used for: 1.   Mature skin/ premature aged skin
               2.   Dry skin or sensitive skin
               3.   Inflammation

Apricot oil is obtained from the kernel of apricots. It is pale yellow in colour and contains desirable levels of essential fatty acids. One of the drawbacks of using this oil is due to its light texture. Apricot oil is absorbed very quickly by the skin and is beneficial for all skin types, especially prematurely aged, sensitive and inflamed skin.   As an added benefit, it can be added to almond or grapeseed oil as an addition to suit your own particular requirements, or it may be used as the main carrier oil.

Apricot is very similar in effect to peach or sweet almond oil. Apricot and peach tend to be more expensive. Some unethical suppliers may offer almond oil and call it apricot or peach as it is very hard to tell the difference because the effects are so similar.

Avocado Oil (*Persea americana*)

Obtained from: The dried and sliced flesh of the fruit.

Best used for: 1.   Eczema
               2.   Dehydrated or dry skin
               3.   Deep penetrating oil

Expressed from the dried fruits of the avocado pear that have been damaged and are unfit for marketing as fresh fruit. They are often dehydrated and sliced before pressing.

Avocado oil is deep green in colour. *Any clear or pale green avocado oil has been bleached and should not be used therapeutically.* The extraction of avocado oil can be difficult and pure avocado oil is comparatively expensive. Cold pressed-unrefined avocado oil has a slight odour and a deep green to slight brownish colour, due to its chlorophyll content.. Occassionally avocado oil has a slightly cloudy appearance and you may find a residue at the bottom. This is usually a good sign, indicating that the oil has not been refined, which means that it will be rich in vitamins and therefore nourishing to the skin.   It does not go rancid very easily as it has a in-built antioxidant characteristics

A refined oil is often pale yellow and should be avoided. Unfortunately, when avocado oil is refined this removes most of the therapeutic properties as well as killing the naturally occurring
vitamins found in the oil.

Refined avocado oil is easily recognised by its pale golden colour, lack of odour and cheap sale price. If this oil is kept chilled, some of the therapeutic components will separate. If this does happen and the oil goes cloudy, place the bottle in a warm place and the avocado oil will return to its original state without any harmful effects.

Because it is a good penetrating oil it is valuable in massage for muscle preparations when dealing with aches and pains, rheumatism and arthritis. The skin healing properties of avocado oil are well publicised, being rich in lecithin and vitamins, A, B and D.

Borage Seed Oil (*Borago officinalis*)

Obtained from: The seeds

Best used for: 1.   Eczema/psoriasis
             2.   Regenerating and stimulating all skin types
             3.   Inflammation and bruising

The oil is extracted from the seeds and can be used as an alternative to evening primrose oil. Borage oil is very rich in gamma-linolenic acid (GLA), vitamins and minerals. Research shows that borage oil can contain up to *25% GLA.*

The great herbalist *John Gerard* quotes *"the old tag ego borago gaudia semper ago"* (*I borage, always bring courage*). Modern research shows that the plant is now known to stimulate the adrenal glands, because it will encourage the production of adrenaline, which is the fight or flight hormone.   This gears the body for action in stressful situations, as well as proving beneficial for chronic conditions like *"arthritis"*.

Borage was used in the middle ages in England as an anti-inflammatory oil to treat both rheumatism and heart disease. Modern aromatherapists can add a *5% solution* of borage oil to massage oil blends for arthritis, rheumatoid arthritis and all types of muscular aches and pains.

Calendula Oil (*Calendula officinalis*)

Obtained from: An infusion of the Marigold flowers.

Best used for: 1.   Chapped and cracked skin
                2.   Varicose veins or skin ulcers
                3.   Reduces skin inflammation

This oil is also known as *"Marigold oil"*. Calendula oil is obtained from an infusion of marigold petals soaked in vegetable oil.

Calendula oil has a favourable effect on the skin in all cosmetic preparations and has been proved highly successful in protection against chapped and cracked skin.
It is an anti-inflammatory, anti-spasmodic, choleretic (*assists bile production*) and helps heal wounds "vulnerary". Bed sores and diaper rash respond well, as do broken veins or varicose veins, bruises, and mouth infections. The British Herbal Pharmacopoeia infers that it would be useful for inflamed lymph nodes, sebaceous cysts or inflamed skin lesions.

Carrot Oil (*Daucus carota*)

Obtained from: By maceration of the finely chopped traditional carrot root.

Best used for: 1.   Rejuvenating for premature-aged or mature skin
                2.   Psoriasis and eczema or acne
                3.   Reduces scarring

Carrot oil consists mainly of water. The oil is present only in tiny quantities. Extraction of this carrier oil requires expert attention. It is not readily available. The oil is rich in vitamins, A, B, C, D, E, and F. As it will rejuvenate and act as a tonic for the skin it, is sought after as a particularly good oil with which to massage the neck. This oil will have a tonic action on the liver and gall bladder, which will make it useful for the treatment of jaundice, urine retention, colic, kidney disorders. In Chinese traditional medicine the plant matter is used to treat dysentery and to expel worms.

Coconut Oil (*Cocos nucifera*)

Obtained from: The white flesh of the coconut.

Best used for: 1.   Suntan lotion base
             2.   Helps water absorption of dry skin
             3.   Helps maintain hair colour

Coconut oil is obtained by hot extraction from the white flesh found inside the shell of the husk. This is a white, solid, crystalline fatty oil, having a well recognized odour, and is used often as an emollient for the skin and as a pomade for the hair. The deodorized fat has been used as a substitute for butter, and in the manufacture of margarine. It is worth mentioning that tropical races who anoint the hair with coconut oil from childhood seldom go grey or bald. It makes the skin smooth to the touch. The oil also aids tanning and does not filter the sun's rays.
Please note: On some people it will cause a rash.

Evening Primrose Oil (*Oenothera biennis*)

Obtained from: The seed.

Best used for: 1.   All skin conditions
             2.   Hormonal imbalances
             3.   Multiple sclerosis

Evening primrose oil is cold pressed from the seed. It contains linoleic acid (vitamin F), a polyunsaturated fatty acid and approximately 8-10% gamma linolenic acid (compared to that of borage oil which contains 25%GLA), an essential fatty acid which the body uses to manufacture hormone-like substances called *"prostaglandins"*.

Prostaglandins are involved in the healthy functioning of many types of body tissue, in areas as different as combatting pain and inflammation, to regulating the menstrual cycle and controlling blood cholesterol levels. They appear to have a beneficial effect on the immune system and on the brain, particularly for people who are unable to make sufficient prostaglandins for their body's needs, for a variety of reasons, which may include poor nutrition, viral infection, alcohol and hereditary factors.

The gamma linolenic acid in evening primrose oil makes good the deficiency, and in this way relieves the symptoms, caused by a lack of prostaglandins in the body. The oil of evening primrose is not an essential oil, but is a valuable oil in many ways and has proved useful for helping conditions like menstrual and pre-menstrual problems, eczema and psoriasis.

There is a great deal of on-going research projects into the effects of evening primrose oil, and these suggest that it may also be beneficial in multiple sclerosis, rheumatoid arthritis, heart disease and psychological disturbances, ranging from schizophrenia to hyperactivity in children.

Grapeseed Oil (*Vitis vinifera*)

Obtained from: The seed.

Best used because: 1.   Its tasteless, colourless and odourless
                         2.   Hypo-allergenic
                         3.   Inexpensive

This oil was first produced in France as a substitute for the more expensive olive oil. The grape seeds are washed, dried, ground and warm-pressed (this means that as the seeds are compressed heat is naturally generated, this also helps to express or release the oil from the seed). The temperature is closely monitored and should not exceed 60 degrees Celsius to preserve the vitamin content . This oil is tasteless and odourless, with a pale green colour, and has no allergic effect on the skin (hypo-allergenic). It contains linoleic acid, vitamin F, E, and minerals.

It keeps fairly well, but the addition of an anti-oxidant *(wheatgerm)*, is recommended if mixed with essential oils and kept for a long time. Grapeseed oil is the most popular fixed oil that does not contain cholesterol and is therefore ideal for culinary use in cases of hypertension and arteriosclerosis. Grapeseed oil leaves the skin with a smooth satin finish without being greasy, and is the favourite oil of all aromatherapists.

Hazelnut Oil (*Corylus avellana*)

Obtained from: The kernel.

Best used for: 1.   Acne/ oily skin
                   2.   Dry skin
                   3.   Stimulates skin circulation

Hazelnut oil is a cold pressed oil derived from the kernel. The colour of this oil is an amber-yellow and it has a pleasant nutty aroma. Very nourishing to the skin, it has the advantage of possessing deep penetration properties. Because of the astringent action of this oil, it will stimulate the circulation and is a good choice to use in cases of acne.

St. Johns Wort (*Hypericum perforatum*)

Obtained from: Maceration (infusion) of the blossoms.

Best used for: 1.   Multiple sclerosis
              2.   Wounds and bruises
              3.   Inflammation and burns

St. Johns Wort carrier oil is derived from the infusion of the blossoms. The colour is a rich reddish ruby hue. The natural anti-inflammatory properties of this oil makes it useful for wounds, while soothing inflamed nerves or skin conditions. Any cases where there is damage to nerve tissue would make it a valuable oil to choose. Neuralgia, sciatica or fibrositis respond well as do sprains, burns or bruises.

Traditionally, St. Johns Wort has been used as an antispasmodic for muscles.. When diluted (5%) with your regular carrier oil it is very healing for sprains and strains related to sports injuries. I have found rapid healing takes place with broken bones when gently massaged on and around the area of injury, also at a higher (50%) dilution inflamed neurological conditions show a marked improvement as well.

Jojoba Oil (pronounced hohoba) (*Simmondsia chinesis*)

Obtained from: The bean

Best used for: 1.   Acne/oily skin
              2.   Psoriasis or eczema
              3.   Inflamed skin

Jojoba oil is derived from a desert plant, native to semi-arid regions in South California, Arizona, Israel and Australia. Although it is used as a carrier oil, jojoba oil is a liquid wax. It is very stable. Chemically it resembles the skins natural lubricant "*sebum*" and when massaged into the skin it helps unblock pores, and, like hazelnut is very good for acne as it dissolves sebum. Jojoba dissolves rapidly into the skin and actually mimics collagen in its action and has excellent moisturising properties. Jojoba contains an acid (*myristic acid*) which has anti-inflammatory properties, helpful with psoriasis, eczema , acne, most skin disorders, rheumatism and arthritis. Jojoba oil is used as a base for aromatherapy perfumery blends.

Macadamia Oil (*Macadamia intergrifolia*)

Obtained from: The nut

Best used for: 1.   Beauty care treatments
              2.   Nourishing for dry or mature skin
              3.   Sunburn

Macadamia oil is derived from the macadamia nuts that are grown in Australia. Until recently this carrier oil was relatively unheard of, originally grown in New South Wales and Queensland. It is high in palmitoleic acid (*a mono-unsaturated fatty acid*) that does not occur in any other plant oil, but is found in human sebum. As we age, the skin tends to lose the palmitoleic acid so regular use of macadamia carrier oil will help reduce the signs of aging.

This oil is fairly stable and if unrefined appears as a soft golden colour with only a small hint of an aroma. Refined oil is pale yellow and has no smell at all.

Olive Oil (*Olea europaea*)

Obtained from: Cold pressed fruit.

Best used for: 1.   Sprains and bruises
              2.   Soothing to inflamed skin
              3.   Calming and emollient

Sometimes referred to as *"Florence Oil"*, it is a non-drying oil cold pressed from the fruit with a pale yellow-greenish colour, with a little odour and a pleasant taste. Olive oil is slightly green due to the retention of minute amounts of chlorophyll.

When taken internally this oil acts as a mild laxative. Topically as an emollient, it will relieve pruritus in skin diseases, soothing to inflamed skin and good for sprains and bruises. This oil has been in use since ancient times. Cultivation of the olive trees are recorded from the earliest times, and the chief centres of olive oil cultivation are Italy, Southern France, Spain, Portugal, Greece, Asia Minor, Palestine, Morocco and Tunis.

The picked fruits are exposed under the sun until they begin to ferment. At this time they are crushed and pressed. The first portion is known as "virgin oil". Water is then mixed with the pulp and again pressed to obtain an oil of second quality.

The refuse is allowed to accumulate in pits and the oil extracted by boiling or by solution in carbon disulphide and recovery of the solvent. Such oil is only fit for the very roughest purposes, such as a low quality soap. Care is taken to separate the oil from the water, in order to avoid the development of acidity. The fruits yield about *18-20%* of oil. At one time this oil was frequently adulterated with cotton-seed oil.

Olive oil is prone to congeal when cooled. Occasionally, a genuine olive oil is found that is not recognized by taste or colour. This is the result of chemical refining process, which gives a once genuine olive oil a bad quality. Olive oil used in aromatherapy should always be specified as cold pressed, first pressing. It has calming and emollient propertis, and although it is considered a good oil for massage, the characteristic odour is not always acceptable to the client or the therapist, and can overpower the scent of the essential oils.

Peach Kernel Oil (*Prunus Persica*)

Obtained from: The kernel

Best used for: 1.   Mature skin/premature aged skin
              2.   Dry skin or sensitive skin
              3.   Inflammation

Due to the similarity in chemical composition to apricot oil, peach kernel exhibits the same beneficial properties, but with greater expensive. Like apricot, this oil is also very light and quickly absorbed making it excellent for facial care. It contains essential fatty acids and vitamins A & E. This carrier oil enhances skin suppleness and elasticity, and makes an excellent face massage oil. Both peach and apricot oil are often used in the manufacture of good quality moisture creams and lotions.

Peanut Oil (*Arachis hypogeae*)

Obtained from: The seed.

Best used for: 1.   Slows down the absorption of massage oils
              2.   Dry skin
              3.   Sunburnt skin

(*Groundnut oil, Katchung oil, Arachis oil*). Expressed oil of the seeds are used as a cheap substitute for almond oil. Peanut oil has a distinctive odour and for massage is perhaps too "oily". It tends to go rancid very quickly and is not as stable as most carrier oils. It is a good oil to add to grapeseed oil if prolonged massage is indicated as it will slow down the absorption rate of the other carrier oil and allow more time in deep muscle massage work. Rich in vitamin E and unsaturated fatty acids.

Rosehip Oil (*Rosa Casina*)

Obtained from: Rosehip seed

Best used for: 1.   Nourishing to the skin
          2.   Burns
          3.   Scars

Obtained mostly from wild or organic plants, this oil takes on a regal red appearance. This oil has recently been used in clinical trials in Chile, where it has been shown to be highly effective in the reduction of scar tissue and wrinkles. Other trials are being held in hospitals that specialize in the treatment of burns with some very encouraging results. The strong rejuvenating properties are more than likely due to the high level of unsaturated fatty acids that rosehip oil contains.

This oil certainly makes an excellent night treatment because it is very easily absorbed, making the skin feel smooth and silky at the same time helping to minimise wrinkles. Rosehip oil can also be added to day and night creams to make them more nourishing to the skin.

Sesame Oil (*Sesamum indicum*)

Obtained from: The seed.

Best used for: 1.   Psoriasis and eczema
          2.   Rheumatism or arthritis
          3.   Inflammation skin conditions

Sesame oil has more colour and odour than nut oil, but it is very useful where colour and odour are no objection. Many of these oils are obtained in the "bleached" condition, but such oils are prone to be somewhat acid and fairly pale. Sesame oil can also be extracted by solvents, and this is used for soap manufacture.

It is advisable to choose the pressed oil for aromatherapy as it is rich in vitamins A and E. Vitamin E stimulates muscular activity, and vitamin A acts to protect the skin. Sesame oil is noteworthy for its stability, as some of its components act to give an antioxidant effect.

Aromatherapists in Scandinavia use it in cases of psoriasis and dry eczema. It will also protect the skin to a certain extent from the harmful rays of the sun. This is an excellent oil for massage, but the odour can be a little strong.

Sunflower Oil (*Helianthus anuus*)

Obtained from: The seed.

Best used for: 1.   Mature skin/premature aged skin
              2.   Dry skin or sensitive skin
              3.   Eczema

Sunflower oil is cold pressed from the seeds and contains vitamin F, and pseudo vitamins which are made of fatty acids along with vitamins A, B, D and E. Most sunflower oil is produced by solvent extraction, so make sure that yours is obtained by cold pressing.

Particularly useful in cases of skin disease, the prophylactic effects on the skin helps heal bruises and skin ulcers that are common to most skin diseases. The consistency of the oil is similar to grapeseed in feel and use. The small, but never-the-less apparent, diuretic properties along with its expectorant constituents *(inulin)* make sunflower oil useful to assist in the treatment of asthma or bronchitis.

Wheatgerm Oil (*Triticum vulgare*)

Obtained from: The seed.

Best used for: 1.   Natural preservative
              2.   Eczema and other dry skin conditions
              3.   Inflammation

Wheatgerm oil contains essential fatty acids along with vitamins B and E. Cost of wheatgerm oil is fairly expensive, but well worth the investment as it is a natural anti-oxidant and can be added to any blend or carrier oil to stabilize it. Simply add 5-10% wheatgerm oil to naturally preserve any product that may be sitting on a shelf for a period of time.

Wheatgerm oil is a glorious deep brown colour and is a rich oil, good for dry skins. Wheatgerm is said to help remove cholesterol deposits from the arteries. One of its less favourable points is that wheatgerm oil tends to stain clothing.

FIXED OILS ARE ALL SOLUBLE IN:
ether, benzene, carbon disulphide, carbon tetrachloride, chloroform and petrol.
But, they are not soluble in alcohol or iso-propyl alcohol.

An Introduction to the Endocrine System

The endocrine or ductless glands pass their secretions or hormones directly into the blood stream. These hormone secreting glands are distributed throughout the body and include:

1. the pituitary
2. the thyroid
3. the parathyroids
4. the thymus
5. the supra-renal glands or adrenals
6. part of the pancreas
7. parts of the ovaries and testes

Although these glands are separate, it is certain that their function is closely related to each other because the health of the body is dependant upon the correctly balanced output from the various glands that form this system.

THE PITUITARY GLAND *(hypophysis)*

This gland has been described as the leader of the endocrine orchestra. It consists of two lobes, anterior and posterior.

The anterior lobe secretes many hormones including the growth promoting somatotropic hormone which controls the bones and muscles and in this way determines the overall size of the individual.

Over secretion of the hormone in children produces gigantism and under secretion creates *"dwarfism"*. The anterior lobe also produces gonadotropic hormones for both male and female gonad activity. Thyrotropic hormones regulate the thyroid and adrenocorticotropic hormones regulate the adrenal cortex. It also produces metabolic hormones.

The posterior lobe produces two hormones.

1. Oxytocin which causes the uterine muscles to contract. It also causes the ducts of the mammary glands to contract and, in this way, helps to express the milk which the gland has secreted into the ducts.

2. The second hormone it produces is vasopressin which is an antidiuretic hormone. This has a direct effect on the tubules of the kidneys and increases the amount of fluid they absorb so that less urine is excreted. It contracts blood vessels in the heart and lungs and so raises the blood pressure. It is not certain whether these two hormones are actually manufactured in the posterior lobe or whether they are produced in the hypothalamus itself and passed down the stalk of the pituitary gland to be stored in the posterior lobe and liberated from there into the circulation.

THE THYROID

The right and left lobes of this gland lies on either side of the trachea united by the isthmus. Average size of each lobe is one and a half inches long and three-quarters of an inch across. However, these sizes may vary considerably. The secretion of this gland includes thyroxine and tri-iodothyronine. Thyroxine controls the general metabolism. Both hormones contain iodine but thyronine is more active than thyroxin.

Under secretion of thyroxine and tri-iodothyronine hormone in children produces "the cretin", that is a child who when grown up suffers from dwarfism and mental deficiency.

Under secretion in adults results in a low metabolic rate. Over secretion in adults gives rise to exophthalmic goitre. The metabolic rate is higher than usual. Such persons may eat well but burn up so much fuel that they remain thin, usually accompanied by a rapid pulse rate. This gland has a profound influence on both mental and physical activity.

<u>Diagram of glands of the body</u>

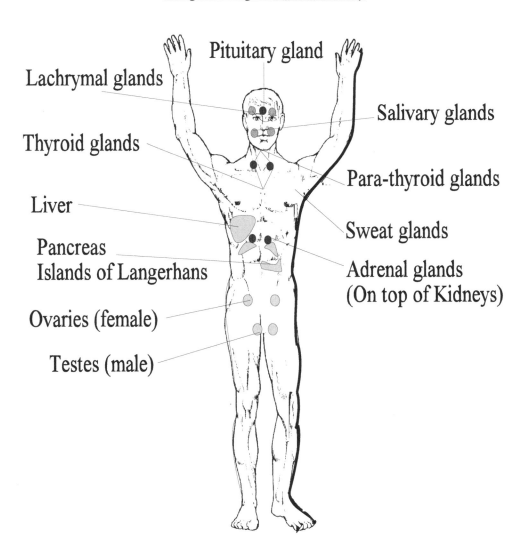

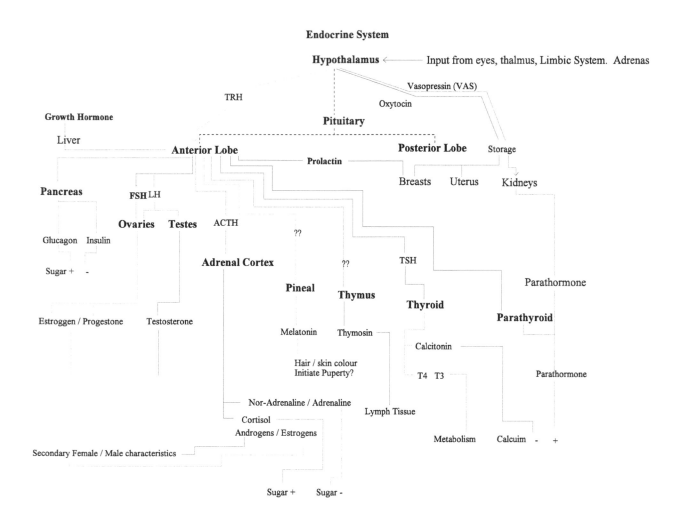

The Endocrine System diagram showing:

Endocrine System

Hypothalamus ← Input from eyes, thalmus, Limbic System. Adrenas

TRH

Vasopressin (VAS)

Oxytocin

Pituitary

Growth Hormone

Liver

Anterior Lobe

Prolactin

Posterior Lobe

Storage

Pancreas

FSH LH

Ovaries   Testes   ACTH

Breasts   Uterus   Kidneys

Glucagon   Insulin

Sugar +   -

??

Adrenal Cortex

??

TSH

Parathormone

Pineal

Thymus

Thyroid

Parathyroid

Estroggen / Progestone   Testosterone

Melatonin   Thymosin

Calcitonin

Hair / skin colour
Initiate Puperty?

T4 T3

Parathormone

Nor-Adrenaline / Adrenaline

Cortisol

Lymph Tissue

Androgens / Estrogens

Metabolism   Calcuim - +

Secondary Female / Male characteristics

Sugar +   Sugar -

THE PARATHYROID GLAND

There are four of these glands in total. Two are situated on either side of the thyroid with the two parathyroid glands lying behind it. Their secretion is parathormone.

The function of parathormone is to raise the blood calcium levels as well as maintain the balance of calcium and phosphorous in both the blood and bone structures. Under secretion gives rise to a condition known as tetany in which the muscles go into spasm. Over secretion causes calcium to be lost to the blood from the bones giving rise to softened bones, raised blood calcium and a marked depression of the nervous system.

THE THYMUS GLAND

This gland lies in the lower part of the neck and attains a maximum size of about two and a half inches long. After puberty the thymus begins to atrophy so by the time we reach adulthood, only fibrous remnants are found. Its secretion is thought to act as a brake on the development of sex organs so that as the thymus atrophies, the sex organs develop.

THE ADRENAL GLANDS

These are two adrenal glands, triangular in shape and yellow in colour. Each gland lies over each kidney. They are divided, like the kidney into two parts:

1. The cortex
2. The medulla

The cortex is the outer part of the gland and produces a number of hormones called cortico-steroids. Their function is to control sodium and potassium balance, stimulate the storage of glucose, and produces a sex hormone similar to that secreted by the testes.

The medulla or inner layer produces the hormone epinephrine, also called adrenaline. This is a powerful valvular constrictor. It can raise the blood pressure by constriction of smaller blood vessels, and increase the blood sugar levels by increasing the output of sugar from the liver.

The initial response to stress results in an increase in the amount of adrenaline that is produced. This prepares the body for a "fight or flight" response to a stressful situation. The purpose of adrenaline is to reduce the blood supply and the activities to specific organs (including the digestive system, the urinary tract and the sexual organs), in order to assist the more beneficial organs such as the heart, brain, muscles and lungs required for the anticipated reaction to the stressor. Once the "danger" passes, the body is meant to rest and recuperate, which unfortunately does not happen in this day and age. Chronic stress is another problem most people suffer from today. Ultimately, the adrenal glands are overworking and possible burnout resulting in fatigue, muscular aches and pains, heart disease, ulcers, digestive problems, coldness and infertility to name a few common symptoms.

The Gonads or Sex Glands

The sex glands are naturally different in men and women because they serve different, though, in many respects, complimentary functions. In the female the gonads are the ovaries and in the male the testes.

- ▸ Female sex hormones are estrogen and progesterone.
- ▸ The male sex hormone is testosterone.

Although each sex produces a specific sex hormone, each produces a small quantity of the opposite hormone. The female hormones are responsible for developing the rounded, feminine figure, breast growth, pubic and axillary hair and all the normal manifestations of femininity and reproduction.
Male hormone is responsible for voice changes, increased muscle mass, development of hair on the body and face and the usual development of manliness.

Pancreas

The Pancreas lies horizontally below and behind the stomach and consists of a head, neck and tail. The islets of langerhans is the part of the pancreas that produces Insulin. This substance regulates the sugar level in the blood and the conversion of sugar into heat and energy.

Insufficient insulin production results in a disease known as diabetes mellitus. This is a disease which normally occurs before the age of 25. It is considered juvenile onset. Diabetes can occur during middle age and this is caused by an insufficient amount of insulin, or the bodys inability to absorb that which is produced. It is a very common disease.

It is known that some half million people in the United Kingdom suffer from diabetes sufficiently to require treatment, but it has been estimated that there are many more people in whom the disease exists but at a sub-treatment level.

Drs. Banting and Best, discovered insulin and succeeded in 1922 in keeping a diabetic dog alive in a Canadian laboratory. Since then, by injection and, more recently, surgery, it has been possible to control this disease although the supplement of insulin is really a support treatment rather than a cure.

Common Diseases or Disorders

Disease or Disorder	HYPERTHYROIDISM
Description	Hyperthyroidism is a disorder in which the thyroid gland is overactive, resulting in an overproduction of thyroid hormone. Causes of this disease include; 1) thyroiditis - an inflammation of the thyroid 2) Graves disease - an immunologic reaction 3) toxic thyroid adenoma or toxic multi nodular goiter (Plummers disease) - presence of abnormal tissue growth within the thyroid gland. Common symptoms of an overactive thyroid gland include swollen bulging eyes, tachycardia, fatigue, increased appetite, weight loss, frequent bowel movements and/or diarrhea and nervousness.
Possible Allopathic Treatment	Anti-thyroid drugs may be prescribed to decrease the thyroid glands production of hormones. Propylthiouracil and methimazole are commonly used pharmaceuticals. Other options include surgical remove of the thyroid gland or treatment with radioactive iodine. Radioactive iodine destroys the thyroid gland. Doctors attempt to adjust the dosage to only partially destroy enough of the gland in hopes of regulation. However, in most cases, this treatment results in complete destruction leading to hypothyroidism which in turn requires its own therapy.
Possible Holistic Aromatherapy Treatment	There are no specific essential oils that can be used in place of allopathic medicine. Treatment may include Anti-depressant essential oil; *Basil, Bergamot, Lemon grass, Clary Sage, Geranium, Jasmine, Lavender, Melissa, Orange Blossom, Patchouli, Rose, Sandalwood and Ylang Ylang.* Auto-immune enhancers; *Cinnamon leaf, Clove bud, Frankincense.*

Disease or Disorder	HYPOTHYROIDISM
Description	Hypothyroidism is a deficiency in the production of thyroid hormone due to underactivity of the thyroid gland. The most common form of hypothyroidism is called primary hypothyroidism. It is thought to be an auto-immune disorder, resulting from a condition called Hashimoto's thyroiditis. It often begins with an enlarged thyroid and later in the disease process results in a shrunken fibrotic thyroid gland. Although rarely seen these days, a chronic lack of iodine in the diet produces an enlarged underactive thyroid gland. Salt manufacturers in many countries have virtually wiped out this problem by adding iodine to table salt. Early symptoms of hypothyroidism include slow speech, hoarseness, intolerance to cold temperatures, dull facial expression, weight gain and constipation. Symptoms of this disease can occasionally be mistaken for depression.
Possible Allopathic Treatment	Hypothyroidism is treated by replacing the deficient hormone. A synthetic T4 hormone is prescribed. There is a dried form of the hormone available. It is obtained from the thyroid gland of animals. The dried form is not used as frequently due to the difficulty in adjusting the dose to acquire a standardized amount. Regardless of the form of hormone given, small doses are initially prescribed and increased until the appropriate blood levels are restored to normal.
Possible Holistic Aromatherapy Treatment	There are no specific essential oils that can be used in place of the prescribed hormones. Treatment can include Anti-depressant essential oil; *Basil, Bergamot, Lemon grass, Clary Sage, Geranium, Jasmine, Lavender, Melissa, Orange Blossom, Patchouli, Rose, Sandalwood and Ylang Ylang.* Auto-immune enhancers; *Cinnamon leaf, Clove bud, Frankincense.*

Disease or Disorder	DIABETES MELLITUS
Description	A disorder of the pancreas resulting in an insufficient amount of insulin being produced, or the body's inability to use the insulin that the pancreas supplies. Insulin is a hormone that is responsible for maintaining blood sugar levels. Diabetes mellitus is classified into 2 different types: Type I - Insulin Dependent Diabetes (IDD) Generally develops before the age of 30. The cause is thought to be from either a viral infection or a nutritional factor in early childhood or early adulthood. The immune system destroys the insulin producing cells located in the pancreas resulting in diabetes. Up to 90% of the cells can be permanently destroyed. Type II - Non-insulin dependent diabetes (NIDD) This form of diabetes normally occurs after 30 years of age. The pancreas still manufactures insulin, sometimes at higher than normal rates. However, the body is unable to utilize it and develops a resistance to its effects. Obesity can increase the risk of developing NIDD. Symptoms include high blood glucose levels. Due to the body's attempt at releasing these excess sugars, the kidneys will pass additional water to dilute the glucose resulting in frequent urination. Abnormal thirst, weight loss (except in NIDD), nausea, fatigue, blurred vision and drowsiness may follow.
Possible Allopathic Treatment	Maintaining constant normal blood sugar levels is the most important aspect in the treatment of diabetes. Fluctuating blood sugar levels can lead to long term serious complications including stroke, heart disease, vision loss, neurological difficulties, poor healing, and susceptibility to infection. Maintenance of these glucose levels can be done as follows: Type I - Insulin is replaced through daily injections varying in frequency from 1 - 4 injection per day. Nutritional guidelines should be closely monitored avoiding refined sugar and related products. Regular exercise is important. Type II - Diet and exercise play an important part in NIDD and as with IDD, refined sugars and the related products should be avoided. There are some individuals who are able to regulate their blood sugar levels by diet and exercise alone. If this is not successful, then oral hypoglycemic drugs can be prescribed to help lower blood sugar levels while increasing the effectiveness of the insulin being produced. Some of these drugs include; Glimepiride, Glipizide, Glyburide, Chloropropamide, Acetohexamide and Tolazamide.
Possible Holistic Aromatherapy Treatment	There are no essential oils that will replace the effects of insulin or oral hypoglycemic drugs. You can help reduce the stress levels which can directly effect blood sugar levels. Other treatment options include the following; Immune enhancers Anti-depressant essential oil; *Basil, Bergamot, Lemon grass, Clary Sage, Geranium, Jasmine, Lavender, Melissa, Orange Blossom, Patchouli, Rose, Sandalwood and Ylang Ylang.* Auto-immune enhancers; *Cinnamon leaf, Clove bud, Frankincense.*

Essential Oils

GERANIUM

Latin name: *pelargonium graveolens*   Botanical family: *Geraniaceae*
              pelargonium adorantissimum

The three main areas where this oil can help are:

1.   Diuretic disorders
2.   Hormonal balancer
3.   Eczema and skin care

Properties	Uses
Diuretic	Urinary tract problems, water retention
Antiseptic	Skin care, sores, burns, sore throat
Cicatrisant/ Haemostatic	Wounds, aged skin, dermatitis, eczema, ulcers, cuts
Antidepressant	Depression, grief, sadness, anxiety
Tonic	Nervous system, liver, spleen, pancreas, kidney

Place of Origin
Geranium is a plant that can grow to the height of two foot. The leaves are serrated and pointed with a small pink flower. The whole plant carries the aromatic essence and it grows readily in the wild. The oil is often obtained from Europe specifically Spain, Morocco, Italy, and France as well as Russia and Egypt.

Method of Extraction
The essential oil of geranium is obtained by steam distillation of the leaves, flowers and stalks. This oil is clear to light green in colour with a floral scent. The principal chemical constituents are: geraniol, citronella, linalol, terpineol and alcohols.

Traditional Uses
Use of this plant include it as a vulnerary and styptic that healed wounds, ulcers and even fractures. Introduced in the 17thC, little historical reference has been made about this plant. In 1819 a French chemist by the name of Recluz was one of the first recorded people to distil the leaves.

Herbal Medicine

Known as early as the 1600's, pelargoniums were popularly used in the European countries for their astringent properties for wounds, as well as used as aromatic teas. Some herbalists have used them in the treatment of dysentery and ulcers of the stomach and upper intestines.

Aromatherapy

"Balancing" is the first word that comes to mind when utilizing the therapeutic properties of geranium. This essential oil is very versatile due to its balancing properties. This action arises because geranium is an adrenal cortex stimulant. The adrenal cortex secretes regulating hormones governing the balance of hormones secreted by other organs, including male and female sex hormones. Any disorders resulting from hormonal imbalance will benefit greatly from the use of geranium. PMS, menopause, irregular periods, heavy periods are problems that indicate use. The action on the adrenal cortex also allows this essence to assist in problems that stem from nervous tension.

Skin care problems, especially those that are due to hormonal fluctuations and/or imbalance improve with geranium. This essential oil has the ability to regulate the sebum (oil) production of the sebaceous glands. Many skin problems are a result of either excess sebum production (oily skin) or an inadequate production (dry skin).

Along with the cicatrisant (wound healing) properties other disorders that would benefit are wounds, cuts, burns, shingles, ulcers, dermatitis, and dry eczema. It has a haemostatic, cleansing action on the skin.

For those who have children that suffer from lice, geranium, lavender and eucalyptus combined and applied into the scalp after the hair has been freshly washed should see positive results. This may be used preventatively for school aged children during breakouts.

A diuretic, geranium will help for urinary tract infections as well as kidney stones and gallstones. It may relieve symptoms that occur from premenstrual tension and help relieve the excess fluid retention problems.

It is a tonic to the liver, kidney, spleen and pancreas. It has been used in the treatment of diabetes. This tonic action helps rid the body of built up toxins. This is an important action today, when you consider the overload of wastes that the liver has to filter. The added stimulating action on the lymphatic system boosts immunity and assists the body in the fight against infection.

Analgesic and antiseptic this oil is indicated in throat and gum infections, mouth ulcers or sore throats. A gargle is the most productive way in achieving results.

Geranium is indicated where there is heat or inflammation present. Diarrhea, gastroenteritis or peptic ulcers can be treated with a topical application over the abdomen. (Rub in a clockwise direction)

LEMONGRASS

Latin name: *cymbopogon citratus*   Botanical family: *Gramineae*
              cymbopogon flexuosus

The three main areas where this oil can help are:

1.   Insect repellant
2.   Auto-immune stimulant
3.   Headaches

Properties   Uses

Deodorant	Skin care
Stimulant	Nervous exhaustion, lethargy, fatigue, headaches
Digestive	Gastroenteritis, indigestion, colic, appetite stimulant, sluggish digestion
Antiseptic	Laryngitis, infections, sore throats

Place of Origin
Lemongrass is a native of India, but is also cultivated in other tropical areas, like Brazil, Sri Lanka and parts of Central Africa.   Cymbopogon citratus is from West India while cymbopogon flexuosus is from East India The grass grows to a height of three to four feet tall, and two or more crops may be harvested in one year.

Method of Extraction
Essential oil of lemongrass is obtained from the grass. Once harvested, this grass is finely chopped to facilitate the extraction of the essential oil by steam distillation. The main constituents of lemongrass oil is citral, which accounts for 70%-85% of its volume. Also, geraniol, farnesol, nerol, citrinellal and myrcene, with a number of aldehydes. The oil ranges in colour from yellow to a reddish-brown and has a strong lemony perfume.

Traditional Uses
Lemongrass has a very long history of its use in traditional Indian medicine, particularly against infectious illnesses and fevers. It is a very powerful antiseptic and bactericide, and a large number of laboratory trials have given scientific confirmation of its traditional uses. It has a powerful tonic and stimulating effect on the whole organism, and this too is of great value when treating feverish illness. It has been known as "Indian Verbena" or "Indian Melissa Oil".

Herbal Medicine

Lemongrass has been used as a remedy to reduce stress, especially when accompanied by headaches and dizziness. It appears to have an astringent effect on body tissue to help stop or slow the discharge of mucous.

Aromatherapy

Antiseptic and antibacterial in nature, lemongrass is wise to utilize in cases of infectious diseases. It is an immuno-stimulant and achieves this through increasing the action of the white blood cells. Lemongrass has been shown to be more effective against the bacteria staphylococcus aureus then penicillin.

It appears to have a positive effect on the nervous system. It helps to regulate the parasympathetic system. Combined with the antidepressant properties this oil would benefit those under stress, or suffering from burnout.

The crisp, clean scent can revive mental fatigue or lethargy. It also serves as an insecticide and deodorant. Skin care problems like acne, oily skin, congested skin will benefit from the tonifying and astringent effects. Do not use neat applications of this essence as it may irritate the skin.

Fungal infections and athletes foot respond to the use of lemongrass. Foot baths can ease odour problems and it is also wise to use the deodorant abilities in bath products.

Lemongrass has a positive effect on the digestive system. It is a stomachic stimulant and useful for colitis, gastroenteritis, indigestion and appears to increase the appetite. It will help tonify a sluggish digestive system that many people seem to suffer from today.

This essential oil is able to reduce lactic acid build up. Arthritis, rheumatism, gout and general aches that occur after a good workout would ease with the analgesic properties. The added astringent and stimulant effects would help varicose veins and reduce swelling, while stimulating the circulation.

Warning: *May irritate sensitive skin*

Mandarin

Latin name: *citrus reticulata*   Botanical family: *Rutaceae*
                   citrus madrurensis

The three main areas where this oil can help are:

1.   Balances metabolism
2.   Depression
3.   Digestive problems

Properties   Uses

Digestive	Appetite stimulant, flatulence, cramps, constipation, nausea
Antidepressant	Depression, sadness, grief, anxiety
Detoxifier	Cellulite, water retention
Astringent	Skin care, stretch marks

Place of Origin
A fruit bearing tree that prefers hot humid climates. Mandarin was originally cultivated in the Far East and China, and is now mainly produced in the countries that border the Mediterranean.

Method of Extraction
Essential oil of mandarin is expressed from the ripe fruit peel.   It is a light orange or amber in colour. Its main chemical constituents include: geraniol, citral, citronella, methyl anthranilate, and limonene.

Traditional Uses
The mandarin tree, originally found in the eastern countries was introduced to Europe in the early 19th century. The fruit was originally offered out of respect to the Chinese Mandarins. Obviously this is the origin of the name.

Herbal Medicine
There is no specific herbal reference to the medicinal use of mandarin in herbal medicine that the author is aware of. Although in France, the fruit has been used for treatment of digestive problems .

Aromatherapy

Mandarin has a clear, refreshing citrus scent that dispels anxiety, nervous tension or sadness. Its uplifting qualities settle the spirit and will help relieve depressive states. It is very similar in properties to sweet orange.

The main action of this essential oil is on the digestive system and can stimulate the appetite, while providing relief from cramps, flatulence, constipation and nausea. It will increase peristalsis, so any disorder resulting from slow digestion, such as dyspepsia, will show improvement with the use of this essence. It will assist the liver in the production of bile and will help break down the fats.

A very safe oil to use, mandarin is often used to treat children. It's soothing properties may prove useful to treat hyperactivity or apprehension in children.

Like other citrus oils, stretch marks, cellulite and the related body toxins can be reduced. Topical applications are the most useful application methods, bu remember, this must be done daily over a long period of time. Water intake, exercise and nutritional lifestyle changes are necessary to combat this predominantly female problem. After weight loss, mandarin can assist with the toning of the skin.

Skin care problems like acne, oily skin and congested pores will benefit from the toning and stimulant effects of mandarin.

Tangerine and mandarin essential oil are almost identical. The mandarin tree was renamed tangerine after it was taken to the United States. The tangerine fruit is slightly larger and has a stronger scent that mandarin.

Warning: *Possible skin irritant*
            Possible photo toxic -- avoid the sun after use.

SAGE

Latin name: *salvia officinalis*   Botanical name: *Labiatae*
                    salvia lavandufolia

The three main areas where this oil can help are:

1.   As a muscle relaxant
2.   Mouth and throat infections
3.   Menopausal problems

Properties	Uses
Digestive/Antispasmodic	Loss of appetite, constipation, indigestion, dyspepsia, weak digestion
Tonic	Liver, kidneys, reproductive system, nervous system
Stimulant	Rheumatism, arthritis, aches and pains, lymphatic system
Astringent	Bacterial infections, gingivitis, sore throats, bleeding gums, mouth ulcers

Place of Origin
Common sage "salvia officinalis" originated in the Mediterranean, but hardy enough to grow almost all over the world, both wild and as a garden plant. The main production of this essence is Yugoslavia, Dalmatia, France and Southern Europe. The Romans called it "herba sacra" or sacred herb. The Latin name is derived from the word of "salvation". The plant usually has purple green leaves and blue flowers. It grows to a height of 2 feet.

Method of Extraction
Essential oil of sage is steam distilled from the flowers and the leaves of the herb. It is a pale yellow-green with a distinctive clear scent. The main chemical constituents include:- borneol, salviol, cineol, thujone and phellandrene.

*** The high level of thujone makes this a potentially toxic essential oil and should be used with extreme care and caution. Spanish sage, "salvia lavandufolia" is not as high in thujone as common sage and would be a better choice for therapies.*

Traditional Uses
The Arabians associated sage with immortality and longevity while the Chinese found it more prized as a tea than their well respected green tea.

Sage has been used in cooking to enhance food and is used in male fragrances and toiletries.

Herbal Medicine
Herbal medicine uses sage for treatment of excess mucous discharges. Fresh leaves have been chewed to treat mouth and throat infections. Styptic in nature, it has been used to stop bleeding in cuts and wounds.

Aromatherapy

When dealing with sage (salvia officinalis) or common sage, caution should be exercised. The essential oil contains age amount of thujone. Thujone is toxic to the nervous system and can provoke epileptic seizures, muscle spasms, uterine spasm and is capable of inducing paralysis. Clary sage is similar in properties and is considered a safe alternative.

In extremely small doses (similar to the principal of homeopathy) sage can have a calming effect on the nerves, by soothing the parasympathetic system, stress, anxiety, tiredness and debility can be eased through this action. It is able to build stamina for those who have suffered from a convalescence. The stimulant properties will assist rheumatism, arthritis, and aches and pain. It is a warm, penetrating oil that "softens" the muscle.

Sage has been used to boost the lymphatic system and reduce swollen glands while increasing immunity.

Essential oil of sage seems to imitate estrogen and will help regulate the menstrual cycle and its related problems. Hot flashes, excess perspiration and menopausal symptoms improve. Do not use during pregnancy (due to the potential of creating uterine contractions) and after delivery it may reduce the flow of breast milk.

A tonic to the digestive system it will increase appetite. The kidneys will benefit in cases of edema and water retention. Styptic in nature, it will stop bleeding in cuts and wounds.

Warning: *Do not use during pregnancy*
                Use with extreme caution - high in thujone

MELISSA (LEMONBALM)

Latin name: *melissa officinalis*   Botanical family: *Labiatae*

The three main areas where this oil can help are:

1.   Depression
2.   Immuno-stimulant
3.   Anti-spasmodic

Properties   Uses

Antidepressant	Depression, grief, sadness
Nervine	Anxiety, nervous tension, stress, neuralgia, hysteria, shock
Antispasmodic	High blood pressure, heart palpitations, colic, flatulence
Digestive/Stomachic	Nausea, indigestion, vomiting
Antiviral	Herpes, influenza, smallpox, mumps

Place of Origin
Melissa (or sometimes known as lemonbalm), is found in Europe, Middle Asia, North America and England. The leaves are small and serrated and the flowers are white or yellow.

Method of Extraction
Steam distillation of the herb, leaves and flowers produces the oil. All parts of the plant yield essential oil which has a very strong scent of lemon, although they are of totally different botanical families. Main chemical constituents include; citronellol, citronellic, linalool, geraniol, and geranyl acetate.

Due to the high cost of the true melissa officinalis and the small amount of oil that is derived from the plant, blends of melissa essential oil are sold. Very often these blends are a mixture of lemongrass and citronella with naturally derived chemicals that are similar to the real constituents found in true melissa.*

Traditional Uses
Avicenna in his 11th C materia medica stated that melissa "maketh the heart merry and joyful and strengthen the vital spirit". It has been used since ancient times in cases of nervous disorders and cardiac problems. It has been used to treat cancer of the gums and for the pain resulting from stomach cancer.

Herbal Medicine
In past centuries melissa was used as a mild sedative. Nicholas Culpepper stated in the 17th Century that it "causes the mind and heart to become merry.....and driveth all troublesome cares and thoughts out of the mind, arising from melancholy".

A study has shown that the herb has a sedative effect on the central nervous system in mice.

Aromatherapy

True melissa is a very expensive, albeit useful essential oil. One of melissa's main action appears to be on the nervous system and is indicated for use in disorders that arise from nervous states. Common disorders that are associated with stress or burnout such as anxiety and nervousness show improvement. It may also prove useful in cases of neuralgia.

It is through this nervine action that it proves useful for hypertension or heart problems such as tachycardia, palpitations or panic attacks. Combined with the antispasmodic properties that melissa has, it imparts a calming action on the heart. Use where there is overstimulation or an overworked state present.

The antispasmodic properties make this essential oil helpful in the cases of colic, flatulence or painful periods. This same property will effect smooth muscle, to slow breathing and pulse.

Melissa possesses a "cooling" effect. With use during a fever, it appears to induce mild perspiration and help maintain homeostasis. Apply to the chest or diffuse through a sick room during colds and flu. Use is indicated in cases of asthma and bronchitis.

Also a digestive and stomachic, disorders like nausea, vomiting or indigestion and dyspepsia improve with the use of this oil.

Depression, grief, melancholy or sadness improve due to the uplifting and antidepressant properties of melissa as well as its calming abilities. It seems to have an affinity for the female reproductive system. Through a mild emmenagogic action, it helps to balance the system to restore function in its normal rhythm while removing tension and stress. It is of use for women suffering from menstrual irregularity and female infertility.

The antiviral effects of this essential oil have been put to use in Germany for the treatment of both acute and chronic oral herpes. 3 topical applications per day (undiluted, being careful not to touch the unaffected area to reduce skin irritation) is needed. Results have been seen in 24 hours.
Melissa, diluted in jojoba oil can be placed in a spritzer, and sprayed on for the treatment of chickenpox or even shingles.

Traditionally this plant has been used in the treatment of cancer. This may be an ideal oil to choose in aromatherapy. Three of the major constituents of this oil have been found to have an anti-tumoral effect to some degree.

Warning: *Mild emmenagogic - Avoid during pregnancy for safety.*
             Possible skin irritant

Question and Answer Sheets

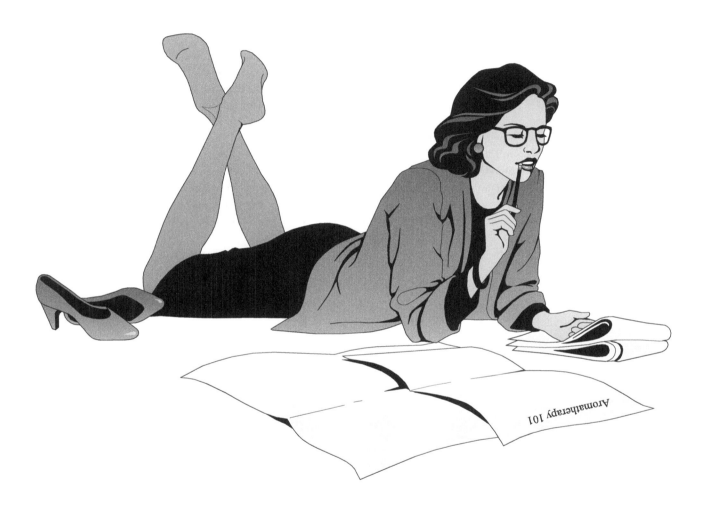

Please keep the questions for review.
Circle the correct answer/s on the Answer Sheets at the back of the book and
<u>return these sheets only</u> to your instructor.

Questions - Lesson #7

1. List the seven ductless glands which secrete hormones into the blood stream.
a. the axillary   b. the pituitary
c. the thyroid   d. the parathyroid
e. the gonadotropic   f. the thymus
g. the eccrine   h. the adrenals
i. part of the pancreas   j. parts of the ovaries and testes

2. Which gland is described as "the leader of the endocrine orchestra"?
a. the thyroid   b. the pituitary   c. the thymus

3. How many lobes does the pituitary gland have?
a. two   b. three   c. four

4. What is the name of the growth promoting hormone which controls the bones & muscles?
a. adrenocorticotropic   b. somatropic
c. thyrotropic   d. metabolic

5. If this hormone is over secreted in childhood, what condition occurs?
a. dwarfism   b. cretinism   c. gigantism

6. If this hormone is under secreted in childhood, what condition occurs?
a. dwarfism   b. cretinism   c. gigantism

7. Which lobe within the pituitary gland produces gonadotropic hormone?
a. the posterior lobe
b. the anterior lobe
c. the middle lobe

8. Which hormone regulates the thyroid?
a. adrenocorticotropic
b. somatropic
c. thyrotropic
d. gonadotropic

9. What two things does adrenocorticotropic hormone regulate?
a. the adrenal cortex and the metabolic hormones
b. the adrenal cortex and the kidneys
c. the metabolic hormones and the circulatory system

10. The posterior lobe of the pituitary gland produces two hormones, name them.
a. thyroxin and oxytocin

b. oxytocin and insulin
c. oxytocin and vasopressin

11. What is the function of the hormone oxytocin?
a. causes contraction of the diaphragm
b. causes contraction of the uterine muscle and mammary glands
c. causes contraction of the blood vessels in the heart and lungs

12. What are the functions of the hormone vasopressin?
a. increases the amount of fluid the kidneys absorb
b. contracts the diaphragm in the breathing process
c. contracts the blood vessels in the heart and lungs increasing the blood pressure
d. contracts the uterine muscles and mammary glands

13. Where in the body is the thyroid gland situated?
a. in the frontal lobe of the brain
b. on either side of the trachea
c. on top of both kidneys

14. What two hormones does the thyroid gland secrete?
a. thyroxine and tri-iodothyronine
b. thyroxine and cortico-steroids
c. cortico-steroids and tri-iodothyronine

15. What is the function of the hormone thyroxine?
a. it controls the sodium/potassium balance
b. it controls the general metabolism
c. it controls the fluid level in the cells

16. If this hormone is under secreted in childhood, what condition occurs?
a. dwarfism   b. cretinism   c. gigantism

17. If thyroxine is under secreted in adulthood, what condition occurs?
a. high metabolic rate
b. diabetes
c. low metabolic rate

18. How many parathyroid glands are there, and where are they positioned in the body?
a. four, two on each side of the thyroid
b. two, one on each side of the kidney
c. two, one on each side of the pituitary

19. Name the hormone that the parathyroid gland secretes.
a. tri-iodothyrnonine
b. parathormone
c. paratetany

20. Under secretion of this hormone causes something called tetany, what is that?
a. muscles go into spasm
b. calcium to be lost to the blood from the bones
c. softened bones and depression

21. Where in the body is the thymus gland positioned?
a. in the lower abdomen
b. in the frontal lobe of the brain
c. in the lower part of the neck

22. What is the function of the thymus gland?
a. to control the metabolic rate
b. control the development of the sex organs
c. to control growth

23. How many adrenal glands are there, and where are they positioned in the body?
a. there are two, one on top of each kidney
b. there are four, two on each side of the thyroid
c. there are two, one on each side of the pituitary

24. The adrenal glands are divided into two parts, they are?
a. the cortex and the medulla oblongata
b. the medulla and the cerebrum
c. the cortex and the medulla

25. What is the name of the hormones produced by the cortex part of the adrenal gland?
a. cortico-steroids
b. adrenalin
c. noradrenaline

26. What is the function of cortico-steroids?
a. control sodium/potassium balance and stimulate the storage of glucose
b. control the blood pressure by constricting the smaller blood vessels
c. controls the output of sugar from the liver

27. What part of the adrenal gland produces adrenaline?
a. the medulla oblongata
b. the cortex
c. the medulla

28. Describe the two functions of the hormone adrenaline.
a. control sodium/potassium balance and stimulate the storage of glucose
b. controls the output of sugar from the liver
c. controls the blood pressure by constricting smaller blood vessels
d. supplements the production of sex hormones

29. How is the amount of adrenaline secreted, affected?
a. in response to excitement, fear or anger
b. in response to exercise
c. in response to a large meal

30. The female gonads and hormones are called?
a. ovaries with oestrogen and progesterone
b. ovaries with oestrogen and testosterone
c. testes with testosterone and oestrogen

31. The male gonads and hormones are called?
a. ovaries with oestrogen and testosterone
b. testes with testosterone
c. testes with testosterone and progesterone

32. Where are the "Islets of Langerhans" found?
a. the pituitary gland   b. the thyroid gland
c. the adrenal gland   d.   the pancreas

33. What hormone is produced by the "Islets of Langerhans?"
a. insulin   b.   thyroxine   c. vasopressin

34. What is the function of this hormone?
a. controls blood pressure
b. controls the blood sugar level
c. controls growth

35. If too little of this hormone is produced, what disease occurs?
a. high blood pressure   b. diabetes mellitus
c. cretinism

36.   What is Addison's syndrome?
a. adrenal-cortical insufficiency characterised by hypotension, wasting, vomiting and muscular weakness
b. adrenal-cortical insufficiency characterised by hypertension, bloating and dizziness
c. adrenal-cortical excess characterised by moon face hypertension and muscular weakness

37.   What is meant by the term Amenorrhoea?
a. absence of menstruation   b. absence of appetite
c. absence of muscle tone

38.   What is Cushing's syndrome?
a. adrenal-cortical insufficiency characterised by hypotension, wasting, vomiting and muscular weakness
b. adrenal-cortical excess characterised by hypertension, bloating and dizziness
c. adrenal-cortical excess characterised by moon face, hypertension and muscular weakness

39.   What is hyperthyroidism?
a. increased metabolic rate
b. decreased metabolic rate
c. alteration of function of thyroid

40.   What is meant by the term menopause?
a. cessation of menses at the end of reproduction cycle
b. absence of menses
c. absence of male influence and hormones

41.   What is premenstrual tension or syndrome?
a. an imbalance of hormones
b. a syndrome of depression, irritability and bloating occurring about a week before the onset of menstruation
c. a syndrome of depression and irritability occurring a short time before the onset of labour

42.   What is a steroid?
a. a generic name given to various compounds of internal secretions
b. a hormone used to increase muscle size
c. a hormone used to counter inflammation of muscles and joints

43.   Label the diagram of the glands.
(SEE ANSWER SHEET FOR DIAGRAM)

44. What is a fixed oil?
a. a stabilized oil of either plant or animal origin
b. a non-essential oil
c. an oil to be used on humans not vehicles
d. an carrier oil that does not evaporate when warmed or in contact with air

45. What happens to a carrier oil that is exposed to the air for long periods?
a. they go sticky and unusable
b. they go rancid
c. they discolour
d. they change chemical constituency

46. What is the main difference between sweet and bitter almond oil?
a. sweet almond oil is used for cooking and bitter almond is used in massage
b. sweet almond oil is used for dry skins and bitter almond is used for oily skins
c. bitter almond contains prussic acid when crushed with water
d. bitter almond is crushed using heat and sweet almond is cold pressed

47. For which skin condition would you use almond oil?
a. psoriasis
b. chapped and cracked skin
c. acne
d. relieving itching caused by eczema

48. Which types of avocado should not be used for Aromatherapy?
a. bleached oil   b. heat pressed
c. cold pressed   d. solvent processed

49. What properties and vitamins are in avocado oil?
a. A, B, C, D, E, and F
b. Lecithin and vitamins A, B, and D
c. Lecithin and vitamins A and F
d. linoleic acid and vitamins A, E and F

50 What are the main constituents of Borage seed oil?
a. Fatty acids, Vitamins D, and F
b. Rich in Gamma-linolenic Acid, (GLA) vitamins and minerals
c. Lecithin and vitamin K
d. Glycerol and fatty acids

51 Calendula oil is also known as?

a. sunflower oil   b. extra virgin Olive-oil

c. marigold oil   d. canola oil

52 For which skin problem is calendula oil used?

a. psoriasis   b. chapped and cracked skin

c. eczema   d. acne

53. Which vitamins are found in carrot oil?

a. A, B, C, D, E, and F

b. lecithin and vitamins A, B, and D

c. lecithin and vitamins A and F

d. linoleic acid and vitamins A, E and F

54. Which carrier oil is good in assisting tanning (sun tan)?

a. calendula oil because of its golden colour

b. avocado oil because of its high content of vitamin A

c. coconut oil because it does not filter the sun's rays

d. sunflower oil because of its golden colour

55. For what conditions would you used evening primrose oil?

a. menstrual, pre-menstrual problems

b. most skin diseases including cancer

c. dry, itchy skins due to allergies

d. all of the above

56. Which carrier oil is most used by aromatherapists?

a. borage, its cheaper than the other oils

b. coconut oil, its easy to obtain

c. grapeseed, its odourless, and will not effect the aroma of the blend

d. almond oil, you can buy it in large quantities

57. For which condition would you use hazelnut oil?

a. eczema   b. psoriasis

c. chapped skin   d. acne

58. For which condition would you used jojoba oil and why?

a. eczema, it protects from bacteria

b. psoriasis, it heals the infection

c. acne, it protects from bacteria

d. acne, it dissolves sebum

59. Which condition would you use St. Johns Wort?

a. M.S. Wounds and bruises, inflammation and burns

b. Acne, high blood pressure and dry skin

c. Psoriasis, eczema and M.S.

d. Weight loss and oedema

60. What is the main constituent in Macadamia oil?

a. Palmitoleic acid   b. Noradrenaline

c. Ascorbic acid   d. Nitric acid

61. When olive oil is first pressed, what is the resulting oil called?

a. virgin oil   b. extra virgin oil

c. first pressing   d. florence oil

62. What are the problems of using olive oil as a massage oil?

a.   no guarantee as to what the quality is

b.   it's prone to be thick unless heated

c.   it has a very characteristic odour that is not always acceptable (too smelly)

d.   it is processed with solvent

63. Which oil is the same as peach kernel oil?

a. apricot oil   b. avocado oil

c. grapeseed oil   d. almond oil

64. What is Rose Hip oil best used for?

a. For tea

b. Burns and scars, nourishes the skin

c. Sprains and bruises

d. Antidepressant

65. What would you use Sunflower oil for?

a. Heart disease   b. Eczema, dry or mature skin

c. Antispasmodic   d. Burns and wounds

66. Which oil can be used as a cheap substitute for almond oil?

a. apricot oil   b. grapeseed oil

c. peanut oil   d. avocado oil

67. What are the problems with using peanut oil for massage?

a. distinctive odour and too "oily"

b. distinctive odour and dries too fast

c. too "oily" and price

d. distinctive odour and too calming

68. Sesame seed oil is rich in which vitamins?

a. A, B, C, D, E and F

b. A, and E

c. lecithin and vitamins A, E and F

d. A, E and linoleic acid

69.   Sesame seed oil is used by aromatherapist in Scandinavia to help what problems?

a. psoriasis   b. dry eczema

c. acne   d. excessively oily skins

70. What is the principal use of wheatgerm oil?

a. to stabilize grapeseed oil in blends

b. to balance the adrenal system in a client

c. to balance the oil production on skin

d. to increase the vitamin content of the massage oil

71. What are the problems involved with using wheatgerm oil?

a. the smell

b. people's allergies to wheat

c. tends to stain clothing

d. the consistency

72. List as many carrier oils as you can that are mentioned in the course.

73. What part of the plant is used to obtain essential oil of geranium?

a. the seeds of the plant

b. the leaves, stem and flowering tops

c. the grass

d. the fruit or berries of the plant

e. the whole plant

74. What three main areas will geranium help most?

a. hormonal balancing properties

b. insect repellant

c. regulates blood pressure

d. heals skin disorders

e. diuretic/detoxifying

75. What part of the plant is used to obtain essential oil of lemongrass?

a. the seeds of the plant

b. the leaves, stem and flowering tops

c. the grass

d. the fruit or berries of the plant

e. the whole plant

76. What three main areas will lemongrass help most?

a. digestive properties

b. insect repellant

c. autoimmune enhancer

d. heals skin disorders

e. analgesic for headaches

77. What do you have to be careful of when using lemongrass?

a. pregnancy   b. skin irritant

c. epilepsy   d. toxic

e. no contra-indications

78. What three main areas will mandarin help most?

a. digestive properties

b. depression

c. balances metabolism

d. helps skin tone

e. respiratory tract infections

79. What do you have to be careful of when using mandarin?

a. pregnancy

b. skin irritant

c. photosensitivity

d. low blood pressure

e. no contra-indications

80. What part of the plant is used to obtain essential oil of melissa?

a. the seeds of the plant

b. the leaves, stem and flowering tops

c. the grass

d. the fruit or berries of the plant

e. the whole plant

80. What do you have to be careful of when using melissa?

a. pregnancy

b. skin irritant

c. photosensitivity

d. low blood pressure

e. no contra-indications

81. What three main areas will melissa help most?

a. anti-depressant

b. immuno-stimulant

c. antispasmodic

d. analgesic

e. calms nervous system

82   What three main areas will sage help most?

a. anti-depressant

b   muscle relaxant

c. skin healer

d. mouth/throat infections

e. urinary tract infections

f. menopausal problems

83. What do you have to be careful of when using sage?

a. large amounts are toxic to the nervous system

b. can provoke epileptic fits

c. capable of inducing paralysis

d. all of the above

Answer Sheet - Lesson #7

(Keep the questions for review. Circle the correct answer/s and return these sheets only to your instructor.)

1   A   B   C   D   E   F   G   H   I

2.   A   B   C

3.   A   B   C

4.   A   B   C   D

5.   A   B   C

6.   A   B   C

7.   A   B   C

8.   A   B   C   D

9.   A   B   C

10.   A   B   C

11.   A   B   C

12.   A   B   C   D

13.   A   B   C

14.   A   B   C

15.   A   B   C

16.   A   B   C

17.   A   B   C

18.   A   B   C

19.   A   B   C

20.   A   B   C

21.   A   B   C

22.   A   B   C

23.   A   B   C

24. A   B   C

25. A   B   C

26. A   B   C

27. A   B   C

28. A   B   C   D

29. A   B   C

30. A   B   C

31. A   B   C

32. A   B   C   D

33. A   B   C

34. A   B   C

35. A   B   C

36. A   B   C

37. A   B   C

38. A   B   C

39. A   B   C

40. A   B   C

41. A   B   C

42. A   B   C

43.   Label the following diagram

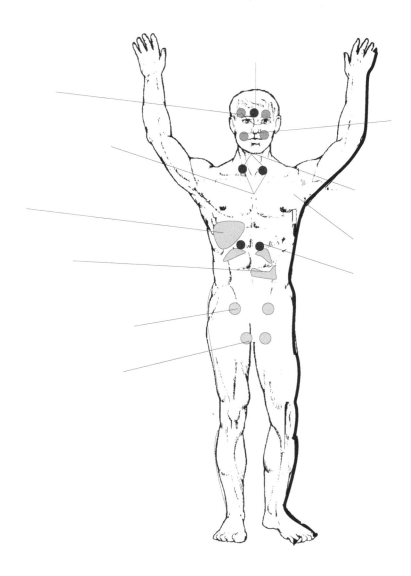

44.   A   B   C   D

45.   A   B   C   D

46.   A   B   C   D

47.   A   B   C   D

48.   A   B   C   D

49.   A   B   C   D

50. A   B   C   D

51. A   B   C   D

52. A   B   C   D

53. A   B   C   D

54. A   B   C   D

55. A   B   C   D

56. A   B   C   D

57. A   B   C   D

58. A   B   C   D

59. A   B   C   D

60. A   B   C   D

61. A   B   C   D

62. A   B   C   D

63. A   B   C   D

64. A   B   C   D

65. A   B   C   D

66. A   B   C   D

67. A   B   C   D

68. A   B   C   D

69. A   B   C   D

70. A   B   C   D

71. A   B   C   D

72. List as many carrier oils as possible

_____

_____

_____

73. A   B   C   D   E

74. A   B   C   D   E

75. A   B   C   D   E

76. A   B   C   D   E

77. A   B   C   D   E

78. A   B   C   D   E

79. A   B   C   D   E

80. A   B   C   D   E

81. A   B   C   D   E

82. A   B   C   D   E   F

83. A   B   C   D

LESSON
EIGHT

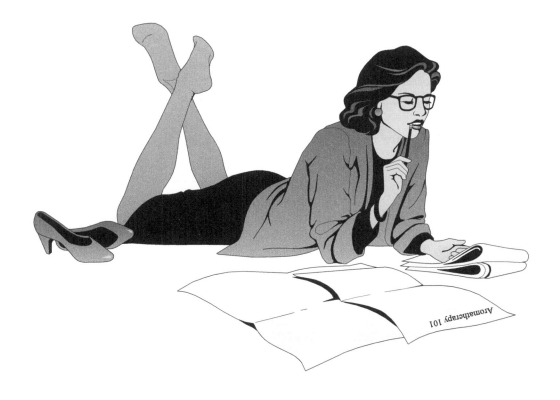

Lesson #8

Table of Contents

The Respiratory System

The respiratory system is responsible for taking in oxygen and giving off carbon dioxide and some water. It normally divides into the upper respiratory tract and the lower respiratory tract. The process of taking in air into the body is normally referred to as inspiration and getting rid of air from the body expiration.

DIAGRAM OF THE RESPIRATORY SYSTEM

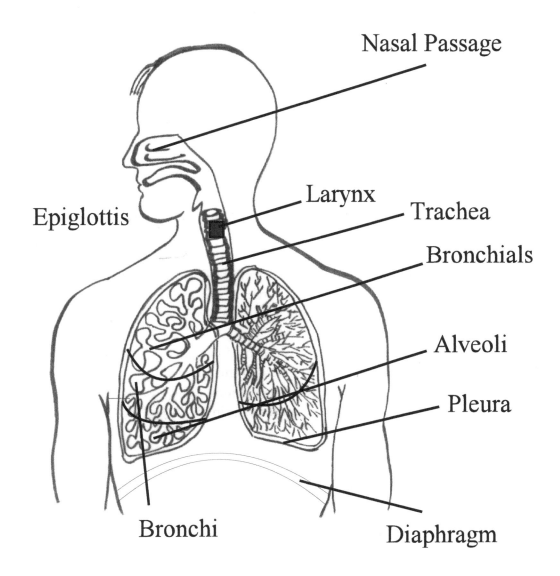

Nasal Passage

Epiglottis

Larynx

Trachea

Bronchials

Alveoli

Pleura

Bronchi

Diaphragm

The respiratory system consists of:

- ▸ The upper respiratory tract including the nose, the mouth, the throat, the larynx and numerous sinus cavities in the head. Any air that is brought in through the nose is filtered and warmed before passing down a tract into the lungs.

- ▸ The lower respiratory tract includes the trachea (or windpipe), the bronchi and the lungs themselves which contain bronchial tubes bronchioles and alveoli or air sacs.

The two lungs which are the principal organs of the respiratory system, and are situated in the upper part of the thoracic cage. They are inert organs, which means, they do not work by themselves but they work by a variation of atmospheric pressure which is achieved by a muscular wall known as the diaphragm.

The contraction and relaxation of the diaphragm results in an alteration of atmospheric pressure within the lungs themselves. Expiration occurs when the pressure is increased and the air in the lungs rushes out. When the pressure is decreased, the air rushes in. This causes *inspiration*.

The inspired air, which contains oxygen, passes down into the billions of minute air chambers or air cells known as alveoli which have very thin walls. Around these walls are the capillaries of the pulmonary system. It is at this point that the blood becomes oxygenated and the lungs remove the carbon dioxide from the blood which is then expelled with the expired air.

An average adult breathes approximately 13,500 litres of air a day. This is not only the body's largest intake of any substance, but it is the most urgently important to the life process. It is possible to live without food for many days, without water a few days but without air only for a very few minutes.

The trachea or windpipe measures about four and a half inches in length and is approximately one inch in diameter. It passes through the neck in front of the oesophagus branching into two bronchi, the right bronchus being an inch long and the left bronchus two inches long. The bronchi branch into smaller and smaller tubes ending in the bronchioles which have no cartilage in their walls and have clusters of the thin walled air sacs or alveoli.

The lungs are greyish in colour and are spongy in appearance. The right lung has three lobes divided into the, upper, middle and lower, and the left lung has two lobes divided into the upper and lower portions, because it must leave room for the heart.

DIAGRAM OF THE RESPIRATORY PASSAGES

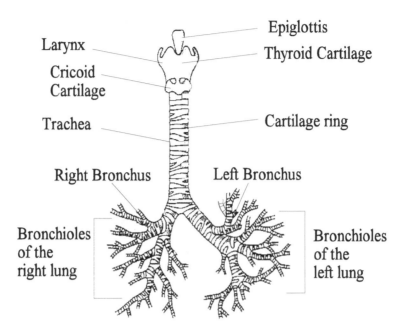

The pleura is the serous membrane which covers the lungs.

The visceral layer is in close contact with the lung tissue and the parietal layer lines the chest wall, between these layers being the pleural cavity. In health it is a natural cavity because the two membranes are fluid lubricated on their opposing surfaces and slide easily over each other as the lungs expand and contract. Air going into the lungs follows the same throat passageway as food for a short distance but there is a ingenious trapdoor called the epiglottis which permits the passage of air to the lungs, but closes it when liquids are swallowed.

With each quiet breath cycle of an adult about one pint (.568 litres) of air flows in and out of the lungs. This is known as tidal air. If one continues to inhale at the end of a quiet inspiration almost an additional half pint (.284 litres) of complemental air can be forced into the lungs. Equally, if one continues to exhale at the end of exhalation, almost a pint and a half (.852 litres) of supplemental air can be forced out of the lungs. There always remains in the lungs about one and a half pints (.852 litres) of air which is known as residual air and this cannot be forced out. The normal rate of inspiration and exhalation is about sixteen times a minute.

Common Diseases or Disorders

Disease or Disorder	BRONCHITIS
Description	Bronchitis is an inflammation of the bronchi that is generally caused by an infection either bacterial or viral in nature. It is more commonly found in individuals who; 1) have lung disorders 2) are smokers or those who live in a smoke filled environment Bronchitis can appear in either one of two forms Acute bronchitis - the symptoms may include cough, fever, back pain, sore throat and chills Chronic bronchitis - normally produces an excess of mucous and coughs, lasting for a minimum of three months. It appears to be related to cigarette smoking, chronic infections and other irritants.
Possible Allopathic Treatment	Medical treatment usually includes bed rest until the fever subsides. Antibiotics may then be prescribed. These may include tetracycline, ampicillin or amoxicillin. Aspirin or acetaminophen are advised to help reduce fever or pain symptoms.
Possible Holistic Aromatherapy Treatment	Expectorant essential oils like; *Basil, Bergamot, Cedarwood, Eucalyptus, Fennel, Ginger, Hyssop, Immortelle, Marjoram, Myrrh, Peppermint, Pine, Sandalwood, Tea tree, Yarrow* Anti-inflammatory oils; *Caraway, Tea tree, Camphor, Chamomile, Fennel, Geranium, Jasmine, Peppermint, Benzoin, Frankincense, Myrrh, and Patchouli* Analgesic oils like; *Bergamot, Cajeput, Coriander, Eucalyptus, Lemongrass, Niaouli, Black pepper, Camphor, Cypress, Fennel, Geranium, Hyssop, Juniper, Lavender, Marjoram, Pine, Rosemary and Ginger* Antiseptic oils like; *Bay, Benzoin, Basil, Black pepper, Camphor, Cedarwood, Citronella, Clary Sage, Cypress, Eucalyptus, Fennel, Frankincense, Geranium, Hyssop, Jasmine, Juniper, Lavender, Lemon, Lemongrass, Marjoram, Myrrh, Neroli, Niaouli, Patchouli, Rose, Rosemary, Sandalwood, Tea Tree, Yarrow, Ylang ylang*

**An effective and simple way of dealing with any respiratory disturbance is through the use of steam inhalations using the appropriate indicated essential oil(s) to help clear the condition. Prepare a bowl of hot steaming water and place 1-2 drops of essential oils into it. A towel is placed over the head while the face is placed within a close but safe distance from the bowl. Deep breathing is encourage. The oils will penetrate into the air passages and throughout the body, helping to clear congestion, and assist with fighting the infection.

Disease or Disorder	ASTHMA
Description	A respiratory disorder that results in a narrowing of the airways due to hyper reactivity to certain stimuli which produces inflammation. Stimuli may include stress, allergies, perfumes, pollutants, infection, excess exercise and/or smoke. During an asthma attack, the smooth muscles of the bronchi go into spasm, the tissue that lines the airways swell from inflammation and secrete mucous into the airway. Breathing becomes difficult.
Possible Allopathic Treatment	In allopathic treatment, the trigger factors should be determined and avoided. Drug treatment is recommended. This could include corticosteroid inhalants used to block the inflammatory response. Beta-Adrenergic Receptor Agonist (B-Agonists) drugs are bronchodilators prescribed to relax the smooth muscle of the bronchioles. Commonly used B-Agonist drugs may include albuterol, theophylline and epinephrine. Other prescriptions may include anticholinergic drugs like atropine an ipratropium bromide to reduce the amount of mucous
Possible Holistic Aromatherapy Treatment	Expectorant essential oils like; *Basil, Bergamot, Cedarwood, Eucalyptus, Fennel, Ginger, Hyssop, Immortelle, Marjoram, Myrrh, Peppermint, Pine, Sandalwood, Tea tree, Yarrow* Anti-inflammatory oils; *Caraway, Tea tree, Camphor, Chamomile, Fennel, Geranium, Jasmine, Peppermint, Benzoin, Frankincense, Myrrh, and Patchouli* Antispasmodic essential oils; *Aniseed, Basil, Bergamot, Black Pepper, Cajeput, Chamomile, Clary-Sage, Coriander, Cypress, Fennel, Ginger, Hyssop, Jasmine, Juniper, Lavender, Marjoram, Melissa, Orange, Peppermint, Patchouli, Petitgrain, Rosemary, Thyme*

Disease or Disorder	SINUSITIS
Description	Sinusitis is an inflammation of one or more sinuses. It is caused by an allergic reaction or, a bacterial, fungal or viral infection. Sinusitis can be either acute or chronic in nature. Acute sinusitis can be caused by streptococci, pneumococci or staphylococci and usually develops after a viral infection in the respiratory tract. Chronic sinusitis in the maxillary sinus cavity stems from a dental infection. Both acute and chronic sinusitis produce similar symptoms. These include pain, tenderness and swelling over the affected sinus area. Maxillary sinusitis can produce pain below the eyes, on the cheeks, toothache and headache. Frontal sinusitis produces headache in the forehead in the frontal area, while ethmoid sinusitis causes pain behind and between the eyes along with a frontal headache.
Possible Allopathic Treatment	Allopathic treatment encourages draining of the sinus cavity. This helps improve the sinus congestion and helps to heal the infection. Steam inhalations can be used to facilitate the drainage. Antibiotic treatment for a ten to twelve day period is used for acute sinusitis. Chronic infections are treated with antibiotics for a six to eight week period to clear the problem. If sinusitis is not responsive to antibiotic therapy, then surgical intervention may be suggested to improve ventilation and drainage.
Possible Holistic Aromatherapy Treatment	Expectorant essential oils like; *Basil, Bergamot, Cedarwood, Eucalyptus, Fennel, Ginger, Hyssop, Immortelle, Marjoram, Myrrh, Peppermint, Pine, Sandalwood, Tea tree, Yarrow* Anti-inflammatory oils; *Caraway, Tea tree, Camphor, Chamomile, Fennel, Geranium, Jasmine, Peppermint, Benzoin, Frankincense, Myrrh, and Patchouli* Analgesic oils like; *Bergamot, Cajeput, Coriander, Eucalyptus, Lemongrass, Niaouli, Black pepper, Camphor, Cypress, Fennel, Geranium, Hyssop, Juniper, Lavender, Marjoram, Pine, Rosemary and Ginger* Antiseptic oils like; *Bay, Benzoin, Basil, Black pepper, Camphor, Cedarwood, Citronella, Clary Sage, Cypress, Eucalyptus, Fennel, Frankincense, Geranium, Hyssop, Jasmine, Juniper, Lavender, Lemon, Lemongrass, Marjoram, Myrrh, Neroli, Niaouli, Patchouli, Rose, Rosemary, Sandalwood, Tea Tree, Yarrow, Ylang ylang*

Disease or Disorder	PNEUMONIA
Description	Pneumonia is an infection of the lungs. It affects both the alveoli (the small air sacs) and the tissue surrounding the lungs. It can affect the whole lobe or just an area of one. A virus may cause pneumonia although bacteria appears to be the main cause of the infection. It can be transmitted through inhalation of the organism. Occasionally the infection may be carried to lungs via the bloodstream. Other times it could migrate to the lungs from another infected area. High risk individuals include young children, the elderly, cigarette smokers, diabetics, or those suffering from heart failure, alcoholism, or suppressed immune disorders/problems. Symptoms include cough, chills, fever, the presence of sputum and chest pain either on its or pain with breathing.
Possible Allopathic Treatment	Antibiotic therapy is prescribe in the treatment of this disease. Penicillin is the most commonly prescribed drug. However, in 25% of the cases, the infecting bacteria is resistant to this drug. Furthermore, in many cases of these strains that are resistant to penicillin, the bacteria is also resistant to other antibiotics. In these cases, replacement drugs may include cefotaxime, ceftriaxone, levofloxacin, sparfoxacin, trovafloxacin, erythromicin or clindamycin. Analgesics are recommended for any associated pain.
Possible Holistic Aromatherapy Treatment	Expectorant essential oils like; *Basil, Bergamot, Cedarwood, Eucalyptus, Fennel, Ginger, Hyssop, Immortelle, Marjoram, Myrrh, Peppermint, Pine, Sandalwood, Tea tree, Yarrow* Analgesic oils like; *Bergamot, Cajeput, Coriander, Eucalyptus, Lemongrass, Niaouli, Black pepper, Camphor, Cypress, Fennel, Geranium, Hyssop, Juniper, Lavender, Marjoram, Pine, Rosemary and Ginger* Antiseptic oils like; *Bay, Benzoin, Basil, Black pepper, Camphor, Cedarwood, Citronella, Clary Sage, Cypress, Eucalyptus, Fennel, Frankincense, Geranium, Hyssop, Jasmine, Juniper, Lavender, Lemon, Lemongrass, Marjoram, Myrrh, Neroli, Niaouli, Patchouli, Rose, Rosemary, Sandalwood, Tea Tree, Yarrow, Ylang ylang*

Essential Oils to Restore Health and Vitality

Today, more and more people are looking for more "natural" alternatives from health care to cosmetics. This is an area to be utilized to a professionals advantage. Not only is it less expensive to incorporate the use of natural products into health and skin care, but the results are generally better, if not equal. Exploring the effects of plant and plant products is a great opportunity which every aromatherapist should do. The extent to which it is done is dependant on each individual therapist. From the simple act of adding a few drops of a high quality essential oil into an existing skin care product, to making your own line of products for home or client use is all up to each and every one of us.

METHODS OF APPLICATION

Diffuser blends

Vapourizing is a easy way to obtain benefits from essential oils. Not only does it affect moods, but this method of use is very effective in killing any airborne bacteria or viruses that may be present. An aromatic diffuser which disperses essential oils into the air without altering or heating them is available. Even a small inexpensive potpourri filled with water and a few drops of essential oils with a lit candle underneath will heat the water and allow the oils to evaporate into the air. This method can be used to enhance moods, aid in relaxation and even promote sleep, help allergies and/or sinus congestion, and deodorize a room, to name but a few uses.

The use of aromatic diffusion is very ancient. Priests and healers of all traditions have used it extensively in their ceremonies and various rituals.

Ancient Egyptians burned perfumes in the streets and inside the temples. Each deity was represented by a different scent.

More than 2,000 years ago, *Hippocrates, the father of Western medicine*, successfully struggled against the epidemic of plague in Athens.

In the 14th Century, the *Bubonic plague* was warded off through the burning of pine and frankincense. It was a fact that through the ages, *perfumers were known to be resistant to diseases*.

The Catholic church was and is still known for their diffusion of *frankincense* inside their churches to promote spirituality.

Diffuser blend recipes....

Calming and Uplifting 2 drops Lavender 1 drop Ylang Ylang 1 drop Rose	Antiseptic 1 drop Pine 2 drops Eucalyptus 1 drop Tea Tree	To Promote Sleep 1 drop Lavender 1 drop Chamomile 1 drop Clary Sage
Allergies/Sinus Congestion 3 drops Eucalyptus 1 drop Camphor	Meditation 1 drop Frankincense 1 drop Clary Sage 1 drop Hyssop	Stimulating 2 drops Rosemary 1 drop Basil 1 drop Grapefruit

Asthmatic blend 2 drops of Eucalyptus 1 drop of Chamomile	Antiseptic blend 4 drops of Ti-tree 1 drop of Lemon Mix into one teaspoon of Vodka Top-up with 125ml Distilled water	Morning Wake-Up Call 4 drops of Lemon 2 Drops of Rosemary 1 drop of Orange 1 drop of Rose

Specific usage...

Cuts Place 1-2 drops of Myrrh without diluting it or adding anything to it, directly onto the wound. Repeat two to three times a day	Burns Place a few drops of undiluted Lavender directly onto the burn, the pain will subside very soon	Fungus on nails Place one drop of Ti-tree directly on the nail and repeat twice a day until it is gone

Baths

An enjoyable and effective use of essential oils is in a bath. The aroma combined with the warmth of the water has definite beneficial effects through comfort and relaxation. The mind, through the inhalation of the scented oil, can be treated as effectively as the body through the absorption of these essences into the skin and eventually into the bloodstream. When using essential oils in the bath, it is important to remember to add the oils once you are in the bath because they evaporate so quickly. This obtains greater results due to the fact that the oils will evaporate during the filling process. Fill the tub, then place your essential oils into the water just prior to entering the bath. Do not use soaps, bubble bath or other products in the tub until you have soaked for 15 - 20 minutes.

It is wise to remember that essential oils lose their therapeutic property when mixed with soaps, although they will retain their fragrance. If an emulsifier is required it is best to purchase a specially formatted soubliser or bath dispersant from a professional supplier. This will allow the therapeutic value of the essential oils to be utilized to the fullest extent. Once finished soaking, then use your necessary personal grooming products.

Baths can be done to incorporate the full body, or just afflicted parts, ie, foot, hand and sitz baths. Baths can be used to treat a variety of complaints including *irritating skin conditions, muscular aches and pains, rheumatism and arthritis* as well as *emotional states* such as stress-related complaints like *anxiety, insomnia, irritability and fatigue.*

Another method to obtain the maximum therapeutic effects is to dilute the essential oils in a carrier oil and pour this into the bath. The carrier oils will counter any drying effects on the skin. *Dead sea salts* that have had essential oils added also create a more therapeutic effect on the skin.

Bath blend recipes...

Relaxing, Uplifting Bath 2 drops Lavender 2 drops Chamomile 1 drop Ylang Ylang 1 drop Patchouli	Stimulating Morning Bath 2 drops Peppermint 2 drops Rosemary 2 drops Juniper	Foot Bath for Tired Feet 1 drop Lavender 1 drop Peppermint 1 drop Lemon
Muscular Aches and Pains 2 drops Marjoram 2 drops Black Pepper 2 drops Lavender	Cellulite Bath 2 drops Grapefruit 2 drops Juniper 2 drops Cypress	Cleansing, Detoxifying Bath 2 drops Lemon 2 drops Juniper 2 drops Geranium

Creams

Hypo-allergenic cream bases derived from natural sources are the best medium to mix essential oils into. Carrier oils are just as effective. These creams or carrier oils can be customized to suit any problem from *headaches, sinus infections* or problems with skin care, aches and pains etc. These creams can then be applied to the affected area to help alleviate the existing problem.

Recipes...

Headache Cream 3 drops Peppermint 3 drops Lavender 30 ml Base Cream	Sinus Cream 2 drops Eucalyptus 2 drops Camphor 1 drop Peppermint 30 ml Base cream If an infection is present versus just congestion, then 2 drops of tea tree can be used as well.
Aches and Pains 3 drops Marjoram 2 drops Black Pepper 2 drops Lavender 30 ml Base Cream	Skin Care 3 drops Lavender 3 drops Geranium 3 drops Roman Chamomile (1 drop if using German Chamomile) In 30 ml Base Cream 10 drops oil of Evening Primrose

Undiluted oils

It is best to remember that the quality of the base will effect the efficacy of the essential oils. *Soaps, preservatives and chemical based ingredients* will hinder or potentially stop the therapeutic action of the oils. In most cases, essential oils should not be applied neat to the skin. There are certain circumstances where they can be used neat, but this is the exception and not the rule.

Massage is the most common form of application of essential oils when dealing with a professional aromatherapist. The type of massage used is normally very relaxing and gentle. It provides the therapeutic benefit of lymphatic drainage.

Lymphatic drainage helps the body assist in the elimination of toxins as well as building the immunities. This type of technique will only benefit the recipient of an aromatherapy treatment. There are benefits of receiving aromatherapy through massage. Touch plays a significant factor in contributing to good health.

Modern research has proven that animals and babies who are stroked or touched regularly have a better immunity to disease and are less subject to stress than those who are not. What better method of application than a massage performed by a qualified aromatherapist with a caring compassionate touch.

Essential oils in general...

UPLIFTING OILS	Grapefruit, Rose, Jasmine, Ylang-ylang, Neroli, Orange, Lime, Linden Blossom

ANXIETY	Basil, Bergamot, Cedarwood, Roman Chamomile, Geranium, Jasmine, Juniper, Lavender, Marjoram, Neroli, Petitgrain, Rose, Ylang-ylang.

DEPRESSION	Basil, Bergamot, Roman Chamomile, Clary sage, Frankincense, Geranium, Grapefruit, Jasmine, Lavender, Lemon, Mandarin, Neroli, Orange, Sandalwood, Ylang-ylang.

CALMING	Roman Chamomile, Cypress, Jasmine, Lavender, Marjoram, Ylang-ylang.

SEDATIVE	Basil, Roman Chamomile, Clary sage, Lavender, Mandarin, Marjoram, Neroli, Sandalwood, Ylang-ylang.

Poultices and Compresses

Compresses can draw out impurities from the skin, help soothe any irritation, pain and/or infection present. They are an old and very good method of applying oils to a specific area of the body. They can be done either hot or cold. A hot compress should be as hot as possible. These are used to reduce muscular and rheumatic pain, to draw out boils, splinters or infections, to relieve menstrual cramps, toothaches, etc. A cold compress may be used for sprains, swelling, headaches and to reduce fever. If a cold compress is called for, add ice cubes in the water to reduce the temperature further. Compresses can also be used to aid the absorption of essential oil applied with massage to the area of the body requiring treatment. For example, you could apply an expectorant chest rub, then a compress. This will work because the essences are absorbed into the skin even when the temperature of the compress changes.

To make a compress add approximately 4 drops of essential oil to about 1000 ml (1 litre) of water. Saturate the compress by dipping it close to the surface of the water so that much of the floating oil is absorbed into the compress. Squeeze out the excess water. For added effectiveness, an herbal infusion of the same plant can be used instead of water.

Abscesses/Boils
2 drops Tea Tree
2 drops Eucalyptus

Burns
Apply lavender neat onto the skin.
For a analgesic effect, apply a cool compress with
2 drops Lavender
2 drops Chamomile

Itching and Eczema
2 drops Chamomile
1 drop Lavender
1 drop Geranium

Insect Bites/Poison Ivy
2 drops Eucalyptus
1 drop Lavender
1 drop Tea Tree

ESSENTIAL OILS AND THE COMPATIBILITY WITH THE HUMAN BODY

Essential oils and human beings have a great deal in common. We are both alive, chemically, and electrically. Essential oils come from plants. They are considered the *"life force"* of these plants, and the finest that these organisms have to offer. We, as human beings rely totally on plants for our sustenance. We eat plants and animals which eat plants and breathe the air made possible by plants. Human beings and plants are related because all living organisms are descended from the same single-cell line. The chemical composition of DNA in plants and people is virtually the same. Because of these similarities, essential oils, derived form these plants seem to be in perfect harmony with the human organism.

Through natural human evolution, our genetic structure has experienced many of the natural compounds that effect our health and causes illness, but our genes or genetic memory has had little or no experience with the synthetics used extensively today.....

Through maternal and/or cytoplasmic inheritance, our immune systems have also experienced many of the natural compounds, but no one knows the long term effects of tomorrow's synthetics on our bodies.

Essential oils have an effect on the brain via two different routes.
One is olfaction while the other is essential oil absorption.

The olfactory bulb, which is just above the top of the nose, is actually part of the brain extending from the limbic system. The limbic system is a link between the voluntary and involuntary nervous centres and a link between left and right brain. Essential oils connect directly into this system through the olfactory bulb.

The second route is through cutaneous absorption. The excellent permeability of essential oils is usually attributed to their high lipophilicity. In other words, they are soluble in lipids, or fats. This makes a carrier oil an excellent medium for essential oils.

The skin also has a solubility factor when it comes to lipids. The membrane of a human cell is composed of an outer layer of protein, followed by a bi-lipid layer , and then another layer of protein. (More on this in chapter 10)

Two factors of solubility pertaining to the cell are:

1)   Size of molecule - the size of the molecule wanting to gain entrance into the cell will be a determining factor as to whether it will be allowed in or not. Large molecules will not be allowed in. *Essential oils are very small in their molecular make-up* and will gain entrance into the cell.

2)   Solubility in lipids - substances that are soluble in lipids will have a higher permeability factor as well. Due to the fact that essential oils are soluble in lipids and also the fact that the *cell membrane is high in lipid content* allows essential oils to penetrate into the cell.

Once through the epidermal layer of the skin, molecules are transported by the capillary blood and by interstitial fluid. *(Heat tends to favour their absorption. A warm room and a massage will enhance the absorption factor.)* When the essential oils enter the bloodstream, they will be transported around the body and eventually into the brain to benefit the recipient of aromatherapy.

In the circulatory system, there is a structure of systems that prevent large molecules from passing into the brain. This is called the blood-brain barrier. Again the small size of these molecules allow them to *pass this barrier and enter the brain, as do many chemical drugs.*
Having gained entrance into the circulatory system, the body will begin to reap the benefits.

The frequently asked question is how do essential oils work on the brain?
We really do not know. It is thought that because human beings rely so totally on plants for sustenance and well-being and because the chemistry of human and plants is so similar, they might be thought of as a set of keys for turning on the body's mechanisms.

There are many different ways that drugs can affect brain chemicals, they block the synthesis of a naturally occurring chemical, or block its transport down an axon of a nerve, its formation into vesicles, its release into the synapse, its attachment to the receptor and so on. Science does not often exactly understand which mechanisms are at work. *It seems unreasonable, therefore, to expect us to know exactly how essential oils work, but, many authors claim to know. These however are theories at this stage.*

PLANT EXPERIENCE
Natural medicines have evolved over thousands of years, time enough for people to come to know which natural products are good to eat, which are poisonous, which heal and which do not. It is upon this wealth of experience that aromatherapy draws, and indeed, upon which chemical companies draw as they search for medications to synthesize chemically in the lab.

The adverse side effects of chemical drugs are becoming more well known due to the efforts of the media and there are now several good books available to the public on that subject. It is ludicrous to criticize natural therapies on the basis of their potential toxicity when so very few toxic effects have been observed or reported.

At the same time, it is a well known fact that chemical drugs have many side effects and potential toxicity when used. In *the Journal of American Medical Association, Nov 27, 1987*, we read that one patient in every thousand admitted to the hospital will be killed by the medicine that they receive there, and according to the Chemical Marketing Reporter Jan. 2 1989, as a result of the 68 million prescriptions for non-steroidal anti-inflammatory drugs given to American sufferers of arthritis, 10,000 - 20,000 deaths occur each year while others suffer various side effects.

Natural medicines are often dismissed in the medical field as ineffective or placebos. However, essential oils do work. They, like anything else are not cure-all, but they do have many benefits. When a professional quality is used properly by a professional trained in their uses, they can enhance and benefit almost anyone.

BENEFITS OF AROMATHERAPY

The main benefits of aromatherapy are through relaxation. To alleviate stress and any anxiety that an individual may be suffering from. This in turn will positively affect the immune system. Aromatherapy is best used as a means of prevention to help stop the onset of disease. But prevention in any case is the best method.

Essential Oils

CAMPHOR

Latin name: *cinnamomum camphora*   Botanical family: *Lauraceae*

The three main areas where this oil can help are:

1.   Common cold
2.   Stimulant properties (circulatory and respiratory systems)
3.   Nervous system

Properties	Uses
Stimulant	Respiratory system, circulatory system; heart
Rubefacient	Sprains, aches and pains, rheumatism, gout, bruises
Antispasmodic	Diarrhea, constipation, colic, vomiting, gastroenteritis, flatulence
Antiseptic	Colds, cough, bronchitis, breathing difficulties, pneumonia

Place of Origin
Camphor is obtained from trees grown in Formosa, China and Japan. It has been cultivated in other sub-tropical countries such as India, Ceylon and Madagascar. The tree which is an evergreen may reach the height of 100 feet with a trunk roughly 10 feet in diameter. The leaves are small with serrated edges with clusters of small white flowers and dark red berries.

Method of Extraction
Essential oil of camphor is extracted from the branches by chipping the wood and then boiling it in water. The camphor then rises to the surface and becomes solid as the water cools. The oil is extracted by steam distillation. It is clear with an obvious medicinal camphorous smell, similar to that of Eucalyptus.

Traditional Uses
Camphor has been used to protect against influenza and other infectious disorders. It was worn around the neck in small bag for protection from these diseases.
The Chinese liked the fragrance of the camphor tree and would use the wood to build their ships.

Herbal Medicine
Camphor has been used in herbal medicine in creams and lotions to help relieve any pain or itching.

Aromatherapy

Only white camphor should be used in aromatherapy. Avoid the use of yellow or brown camphor.

Due to the antiseptic properties of camphor it has been known for its use in respiratory disturbances. Disorders like colds, bronchitis, or when there are breathing difficulties, an inhalation of camphor would ease the restriction. It is effective against the pneumococcus bacteria and is suitable for use in any "cold" conditions. Applied externally camphor can numb the peripheral nerve endings.

Constipation, diarrhea, vomiting, colic and gastric spasms will benefit from the calming, balancing action of this essential oil. It is also antispasmodic in nature.

Essential oil of camphor is a respiratory and circulatory stimulant. It is indicated for heart problems like low blood pressure, heart failure and even cardiac disease.

The use of camphor may be needed when other oils have been explored and have not been effective. Camphor gives more of a shock to the system and tends to produce better results in those harder cases.

Inflammatory problems will find a topical application of camphor beneficial. It appears to have a cooling action on the area. Use when heat is present.

Psychosomatic or nervous disorders (anxiety, stress, hysteria, shock, etc) find positive results with the use of this essence. This is probably due to its balancing action on the nervous system.

Warning;   *Avoid with pregnancy, asthma and epilepsy*
             High doses could cause convulsions

EUCALYPTUS

Latin name: *eucalyptus globulus*   Botanical family: *Myrtaceae*
                 eucalyptus radiata

The three main areas where this oil can help are:

1.   Respiratory disorders
2.   Viruses
3.   Analgesic and temperature reducing properties

Properties	Uses
Expectorant	Asthma, bronchitis, coughs, colds, emphysema, sinusitis, allergies, hay fever
Antiseptic	Viral infections, cystitis, fevers, leucorrhea, ulcers, wounds
Stimulant	Fatigue, debility, lack of concentration
Analgesic	Headaches, migraines, arthritis, rheumatism, aches and pains

Place of Origin
There are approximately 300 plus varieties of eucalyptus. The eucalyptus used in aromatherapy are traditionally either eucalyptus globulus or eucalyptus radiata. Eucalyptus globulus is traditionally distilled from the "Gum tree" in Australia, but there are roughly 15 other species that produce this oil.
The leaves of a mature tree are long, pointed and yellow-green.

Method of Extraction
The oil is distilled from the leaves. It is almost clear in colour with a very familiar crisp and refreshing scent. The main chemical constituents include: eucalyptol (80%), ethyl alcohol, various aldehydes, camphene, eudesmol, phellandrene, pinene and aromadendrene.

Traditional Uses
Australians have used eucalyptus in the treatment of wounds. Burning leaves were used as a form of fumigation in the treatment of infectious disorders and fever. The dried leaves have been rolled and smoked for respiratory problems. The tree was introduced in Europe in the 19 th century as an ornamental species, but has developed certain characteristics that do not appear in its native home. Eucalyptus has been known to secrete a specific substance that does not allow other plants to grow in the area.

Herbal Medicine
Herbalists use steam inhalations with the plant to help with respiratory ailments and to alleviate the symptoms of these problems. Infusions or baths are used to help relieve joint and muscular aches and pains.

Aromatherapy

Jean Valnet has given data on the bactericidal properties of this essential oil. A 2% dilution of eucalyptus in a spray form will kill 70% of the staphylococci in the air. It has been shown that the whole synergistic value of eucalyptus essential oil is more effective than the chemical constituent of eucalyptol on its own. Today the pharmaceutical industry uses just the main chemical constituent. The effectiveness of the oil seems to be due to the constituents of aromadendrene and phellandrenes. When these substances come into contact with the air, a chemical reaction occurs and they produce ozone. Bacteria is not able to live in this.

A powerful antiseptic and antiviral agent, it can be used to treat viral infections like herpes. Herpes remain dormant within the body and flairs in states of physical exhaustion or stress. The blisters will then appear on the area of skin that is over the affected nerve fibres. A combination of eucalyptus, bergamot and/or tea tree will fight off the virus.

Another "nerve" fibre problem is shingle. This will benefit from the application of the essential oil of eucalyptus. The inflamed and painful nerves will improve due to the analgesic action. Joint stiffness, rheumatism and arthritis would benefit from the rubefacient and analgesic abilities, especially when there is cold and damp weather conditions.

An excellent preventative measure in cases of colds, influenza or other contagious illnesses, vaporisation of this oil would kill the germs. If there is an allergy or hay fever sufferer in the house, they would also benefit from the use by way of topical application over the sinus areas as well as through diffusion or vaporisation.

The expectorant properties are highly known and can help ease mucous build up with respiratory ailments like colds, coughs, sinusitis, bronchitis and emphysema. It will assist in clearing the head that is desperately needed in these disorders.

Sores and burns could be bound in wraps with eucalyptus. The antiseptic and healing properties have been well utilized by the Australian aborigines. They bind serious wounds with eucalyptus leaves. Surgeons have used solutions with eucalyptus to wash out operation cavities and place dressings on them with the essence as well. Burns will benefit through the new tissue growth.

Urinary tract infections, cystitis, and gallstones clear with the use of this essential oil. However, *eucalyptus citradoria* seems to be slightly more beneficial in cases associated with the urinary tract. Beware that large doses may overtax the kidneys.

Warning: *Never take internally due to the toxicity.*
             Avoid on people suffering from high blood pressure or epilepsy.
             May antidote homeopathic preparations.

FRANKINCENSE

Latin name: *boswellia thurifera*   Botanical name: *Burseraceae*
               boswellia carteri

The three main areas where this oil can help, are:

1.   Respiratory disorders
2.   Nervous tension
3.   Skin care

Properties   Uses

Properties	Uses
Expectorant	Asthma, coughs, colds, laryngitis, catarrh, bronchitis
Digestive	Indigestion, dyspepsia
Cicatrisant	Wounds, ulcers, skin care
Sedative	Nervous tension, anxiety, stress
Astringent	Cystitis, haemorrhoids, haemorrhage

Place of Origin
Frankincense originates from the Land of Punt. It was imported by the Egyptians approximately 5,000 years ago. A small tree that was native to North Africa and Arabia. The gum nowadays comes from Arabia and Somaliland.

Method of Extraction
Essential oil is obtained from the resin of the bark through steam distillation. A deep incision is made into the trunk to encourage the production of resin. Over a period of weeks, a milky juice is excreted which hardens when in comes into contact with the air. The oil varies in colour from colourless to a pale yellow.

Its main chemical constituents include: phellandrene, l-pinene, dipentene, camphene, olibanol and various resins.

Traditional Uses
Frankincense was one of the most valuable commodities of the ancient world and this is why it was offered as a gift to Jesus. Both the Egyptians and the Hebrews spent excessive amount of money to import this precious product for their religious purposes. An alternative name for Frankincense is olibanum.

Herbal Medicine
No info found

Aromatherapy

For years, Frankincense has been dispersed as a fragrance in the Catholic church. It deepens breathing, calms and uplifts the mind and prepares the body for states of meditation or prayer.

The sedative action and its effects on the respiratory system make in an invaluable oil to use for states of anxiety, stress or nervous tension.

Combined with the expectorant properties, Frankincense can help with mucous build-up in cases of colds, cough, bronchitis as well as asthma and laryngitis.

Frankincense has been used for centuries for skin care purposes. The astringent properties appear to be somewhat anti-inflammatory, and help to slow down time and the appearance of wrinkles and other abominations of old age including lost facial tone. An expensive yet beneficial product for skin care. The cicatrisant effect will assist healing wounds and ulcers. It will reduce scar tissue.

The astringent properties carry over into the genito-urinary filed and treats cystitis, nephritis and haemorrhoids.

Menstrual problems like heavy flow or uterine haemorrhages ease with the use of this essential oil. Use in a bath or as a topical preparation. This is a safe oil to use during pregnancy and childbirth.

In China, it has been used in the treatment of scrofula, which is tuberculosis of the lymph glands and even leprosy.

It's calming and soothing effects on the mind as well as the respiratory changes it produces in breathing make it an invaluable oil in aromatherapy today. Many people are unable to relax and breathe appropriately due to the day to day demands and stress we place on our body. A delightful addition to a diffuser in any home or workplace.

PINE

Latin name: *pinus sylvestris*   Botanical name: *Pinaceae*

The three main areas where this oil can help are:

1.   Respiratory problems
2.   Genito-urinary problems
3.   Circulatory stimulant

Properties   Uses

Expectorant	Respiratory infections, asthma, bronchitis, colds, flu, pneumonia, tuberculosis, catarrh
Stimulant	Exhaustion, poor concentration, mental fatigue
Rubefacient	Strains, sprains, rheumatism, arthritis
Diuretic	Kidney problems, gallstones
Antiseptic	Urethritis, cystitis, urinary tract infections

Place of Origin
Pine essential oil is also known as Scotch pine . A tree with reddish bark and sharp pointed cones. It is found in the cold regions of Europe, Scandinavia and the USSR. The best quality tends to come from the trees that grow in the far northern regions.

Method of Extraction
This oil is produced by steam distillation of the needles, twigs, cones, resins and buds of the tree. An inferior oil can be made from the wood. The main chemical constituents include: borneol, bornyl acetate, terpinyl acetate, cadinene, camphene, dipentene, phellandrene, pinene, sylvestrene.

Traditional Uses
Avicenna used pine for lung infections and pneumonia due to its known effects on the respiratory system. American Indians used the needles to fill a mattress to sleep on and this is occasionally still used in the treatment of rheumatism in the Swiss Alps.
Today it is used as a disinfectant and deodorizer in many commercial preparations.

Herbal Medicine
Shavings off the tree have been used as an aid in the treatment of asthma. The shavings were used as a pillow.

Aromatherapy

Throughout history pine has been known for its effect on respiratory ailments that range from infections to bronchitis to pneumonia and tuberculosis. An effective means of treatment for these problems is to place 1-2 drops of pine essential oil in a steaming bowl of hot water and use it as an inhalation. Topical application would benefit as well to help ease breathing. It will assist in removing the mucous build up commonly found in respiratory infections. Use it in a diffuser to fight against any infectious diseases in the home or workplace.

The antiseptic properties of pine is apparent in its effectiveness against genito-urinary tract disorders like cystitis, urethritis, pyelitis and even hepatitis. It cleanses the kidneys and helps with gallstones.

Mental fatigue, lethargy and exhaustion improve from the stimulating properties of pine. It can be used in the bath, particularly after a tiring day. However, *pine may irritate sensitive skin*, so a low dilution should be used and it should be dissolved in some carrier base to dissipate the essence into the water.

Symptoms of arthritis, rheumatism, sprains or aches and pains would ease from a topical application or bath with pine. The rubefacient properties will increase circulation. It can also create a warming feeling that helps decrease the pain.

Scabies, lice and fleas do not appreciate the fresh scent of pine. Use preventatively when required.

Warning: *possible skin irritant*

The safest pine to use in the field of aromatherapy is "pinus sylvestris. There are other species of this oil available and one of them, "dwarf pine" or pinus pumilio is considered hazardous.

Ti-Tree (Tea Tree)

Latin name: *melaleuca alternifolia*   Botanical family: *Myrtaceae*

The three main areas where this oil can help are:

1.   Auto-immune system stimulant
2.   Colds, influenza, viral infections
3.   Strong anti-septic/anti-fungal for nails and skin care

Properties   Uses

Antiviral	Influenza, warts, herpes, cold sores
Antifungal	Candida, athlete's foot, thrush, yeast infections, fungal infections, genital warts
Antiseptic	Cystitis, urinary tract infections, skin care, boils, acne, mouth ulcers, gum infections
Immunostimulant	Infections, debility, infectious diseases

Place of Origin
This tree is primarily a native of Australia. It is a member of the Myrtacaceae family as eucalyptus and clove. It is a relative new comer to the Aromatherapy field, yet highly regarded for its diversified uses.

Method of Extraction
The essential oil of tea tree is distilled from the leaves of the plant. The main chemical constituents include:- terpineol with various alcohols and monoterpenes. The oil may be colourless to a pale yellow hue with a distinctive medicinal odour.

Traditional Uses
The Aborigines in Australia have used the plant to help heal wounds. It was introduced to the European countries in the late 1920's and was used in first aid kits by the military in World War 2. Today, many products are using tea tree in deodorants, toothpastes, skin care produces and more for its versatile nature.

Herbal Medicine
Tea tree has been used in dermatological conditions such as acne vulgaris

Aromatherapy

Tea tree has a wide range of uses in the aromatherapy field. This is due to the fact that it is antiviral, antifungal and antibacterial in nature.

It has been proven to be a very powerful immune system stimulant. It does this by activating the white blood cells to fight off any intruders (virus, bacteria and fungi). Glandular fevers, debility and other debilitating illnesses are indications for treatment with tea tree. It may possibly be effective for AIDS.

Viral infections from influenza to warts and herpes (both oral and genital) respond to this essential oil. Sprays can be made up to use in infected rooms. The spray is also safe to use in the case of herpes, or you may wish to apply a drop directly onto the affected area. Warts need an application a minimum of one per day. It may take a few weeks to see results, but it is an effective means of treatment.

Many people today suffer from candida and other yeast infections as well as fungal infections like athletes foot and thrush. Use tea tree for these problems, but it is important to continue the use of this essence for 1-2 months after the symptoms disappear. Sprays or douches are effective means for treating vaginal yeast infections.

Tea tree may induce perspiration when used to alleviate colds and flu. This is a good sign as it increases the immune response. Most naturopaths believe in allowing a fever to run its course without medication as long as it stays below 104 degrees F. This does not hold true in infants, young children, geriatrics and the chronically ill. It is important to seek the appropriate medical attention in these cases in order to maintain safety.

Essential oil of tea tree may be used as a gargle for the treatment of gum diseases. Bad breath or mouth ulcers. Do not swallow.

Question and Answer Sheets

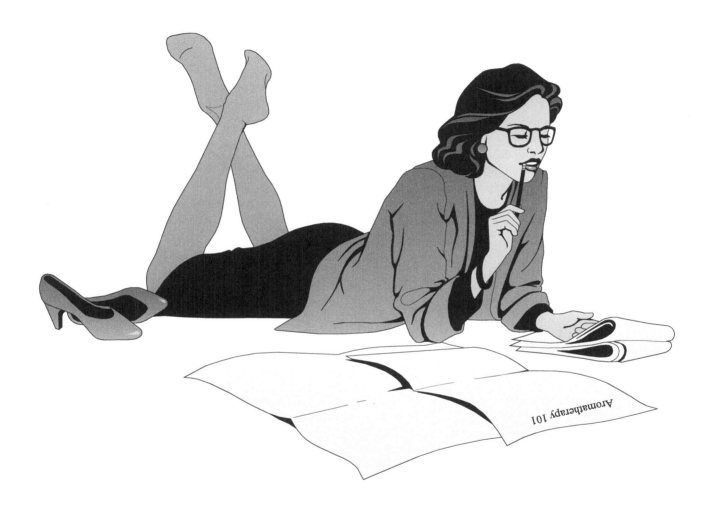

Please keep the questions for review.
Circle the correct answer/s on the Answer Sheets at the back of the book and
<u>return these sheets only</u> to your instructor.

Questions - Lesson #8

1. What are the main functions of the respiratory system?
a. to allow intake of air for breathing
b. to take in oxygen and give off carbon dioxide and water
c. to provide air for the sense of smell
d. movement of the upper and lower respiratory tracts.

2. What is the definition of "inspiration".
a. the process of breathing
b. getting rid of air from the lungs
c. coughing
d. the process of taking air into the lungs.

3. What is the definition of "expiration"?
a. the process of breathing in and out
b. the process of taking air into the lungs
c. The process of removing air from the lungs
d. the cause of death due to smoking cigarettes.

4. What are the two principal organs of the respiratory system?
a. the two lungs
b. the lungs and the diaphragm
c. the trachea and the lungs
d. the sphenoid sinus and the epiglottis.

5. How do lungs work?
a. at the normal rate of 16-20 breathes per minute, average
b. the diaphragm causes a change of atmospheric pressure to occur in the lungs
c. air is drawn in and out, causing the diaphragm to rise and fall
d. by unconscious control of the bronchioles enlarging and causing air to be drawn in and contracting causing air to be pushed out.

6. What is the name of the muscular wall involved in the process of breathing?
a. the diaphragm
b. the pleura
c. the visceral layer
d. the great wall of China.

7. What are the air chambers or cells in the lungs called?
a. the bronchi
b. the pleura
c. the blasts

d. the alveoli

8. How many litres of air does the average adult breath daily?
a. 852   b. 10
c. 1,350   d. 13,500

9. How many lobes does each lung have?
a. the right lung has two, the left has three
b. both lungs have three
c. the right lung has three, the left has two
d. the lungs don't have lobes, they have one big cavity each.

10. Name the serous membrane which covers the lungs.
a. the visceral layer
b. the pericardium
c. the parietal layer
d. the pleura.

11. What lies between the visceral layer and the parietal layer?
a. lung tissue
b. blood vessels
c. pleural cavity
d. residual air.

12. What is the epiglottis?
a. a "trap-door" which permits the passage of air into the lungs but closes when liquids are swallowed
b. the rings of cartilage around the trachea
c. the tubes leading into the lungs
d. the valve at the base of the oesophagus responsible for the "gag-reflex" when choking.

13. What is meant by the term "tidal air"?
a. the rate of inspiration/expiration
b. the contraction and relaxation of the diaphragm
c. the quiet flow of air into and out of the lungs
d. the mixture of salt water and air when choking while swimming in the ocean.

14. What is meant by the term "residual air"?
a. the remaining air coughed out when choking
b. air breathed in that is tainted with toxic air-born chemicals
c. the term given to air that is in the lungs due to inspiration
d. a reservoir of air amounting to .852 litres which constantly remains in the lungs.

15. What is asthma?
a. wheezy sounding breathing
b. breathing difficulty due to allergies
c. difficulty in breathing due to narrowing of the airways
d. infection in the lungs.

16. What is bronchitis?
a. inflammation of the bronchioles
b. inflammation of the pleura
c. removal of the bronchi
d. an infection of the bronchi.

17. Name the two forms of bronchitis.
a. acute and chronic bronchitis
b. right and left bronchitis
c. normal and abnormal bronchitis
d. acute and infectious bronchitis.

18. Describe in your own words the difference between the two forms of bronchitis mentioned above.

19. What is sinusitis?
a. a viral infection affecting the nose and ears
b. an inflammation of the mucous lining of the sinuses
c. an inflammation of the eustachian tube between the nose and the ears

20. What is pneumonia?
a. a viral or bacterial infection of the bronchi
b. a viral or bacterial infection of the lungs
c. an inflammation of the lungs

21. Label the diagram of the respiratory system.
(SEE ANSWER SHEET FOR DIAGRAM)

22. Label the diagram of the respiratory passages.
(SEE ANSWER SHEET FOR DIAGRAM)

23. Name four different methods of using essential oils, other than massage.

24. The benefit(s) of using vapourizers include;
a. pain relief
b. changes mood
c. kills viruses/bacteria
d. does nothing

25. Soap enhances the therapeutic effects of essential oils.
a. true
b. false

26. Which of the following effects does lymphatic massage have?
a. builds immunities
b. relaxes the client
c. eliminates toxins
d. all of the above

27. Essential oils effect the brain via two different routes. Name these two.

28. What part of the plant is used to obtain essential oil of eucalyptus?
a. the flowering tops
b. the rind of the fruit
c. the leaves
d. the wood

29. What three main areas will eucalyptus help the most?
a. Decongestant and anti-viral
b. Digestive problems
c. Analgesic
d. Temperature reducing
e. Hypotensive

30. What do you have to be careful of when using eucalyptus?
a. internal toxicity
b. will antidote homeopathic remedies
c. high blood pressure
d. epilepsy
e. all of the above

31. What part of the plant is used to obtain essential oil of tea tree?
a. the flowering tops
b. the rind of the fruit
c. the leaves
d. the wood

32. What three main areas will tea tree help the most?
a. bacterial infections
b. respiratory infections/problems
c. fungal infections
d. headaches
e. stimulates white blood cells

33. What do you have to be careful of when using ti-tree?
a. internal toxicity
b. during pregnancy
c. high blood pressure
d. epilepsy
e. none of the above

34. What part of the plant is used to obtain essential oil of camphor?
a. the flowering tops
b. the rind of the fruit
c. the leaves
d. the wood
e. the berries/fruit

35. How is essential oil of camphor obtained?
a. distillation
b. pressing
c. maceration
d. enfleurage

36. What three main areas will camphor help the most?
a. respiratory infections
b. anti-spasmodic
c. circulatory stimulant
d. balances nervous system
e. helps addictions

37. What do you have to be careful of when using camphor?
a. asthma
b. during pregnancy
c. high blood pressure
d. epilepsy
e. none of the above

38. What part of the plant is used to obtain essential oil of pine?
a. the needles, twigs and cones
b. the rind of the fruit
c. the leaves
d. the wood
e. the berries/fruit

39. What part of the plant can be used to obtain an inferior quality essential oil?
a. the needles, twigs and cones
b. the rind of the fruit
c. the leaves
d. the wood
e. the berries/fruit

40. What three main areas will pine help the most?
a. respiratory infections
b. anti-spasmodic
c. circulatory stimulant
d. balances nervous system
e. Genito-urinary problems

41. What do you have to be careful of when using pine?
a. asthma
b. during pregnancy
c. high blood pressure
d. epilepsy
e. none of the above

42. Where does essential oil of frankincense originate?
A. Land of Punt, Somaliland, Arabia
b. Nairobi, India, Virgin Islands
c. Eygpt, Somaliland, India
d. Eygpt, Canada, England

43. How is essential oil of frankincense obtained?
a. distillation
b. pressing
c. maceration
d. enfleurage

44. What three main areas will frankincense help the most?
a. respiratory infections
b. anti-spasmodic
c. circulatory stimulant
d. balances nervous system
e. skin care

Answer Sheet - Lesson #8

(Keep the questions for review. Circle the correct answer/s and return these sheets only to your instructor.)

1.   A   B   C   D

2.   A   B   C   D

3.   A   B   C   D

4.   A   B   C   D

5.   A   B   C   D

6.   A   B   C   D

7.   A   B   C   D

8.   A   B   C   D

9.   A   B   C   D

10. A   B   C   D

11. A   B   C   D

12. A   B   C   D

13. A   B   C   D

14. A   B   C   D

15. A   B   C   D

16. A   B   C   D

17. A   B   C   D

18. The difference between the two types of bronchitis is

_____

_____

_____

19. A   B   C

20. A   B   C

21.   Label the following diagram.

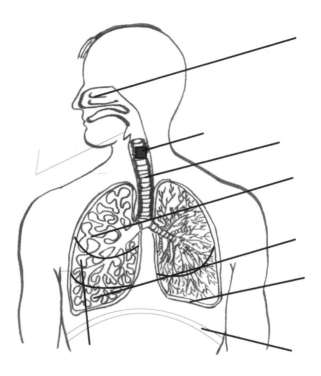

22.   Label the following diagram.

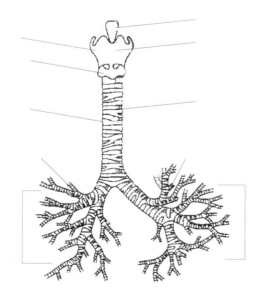

23. Four different methods of using aromatherapy include
    1.
    2.
    3.
    4.

24. A   B   C   D

25. A   B

26. A   B   C   D

27. The two different routes that essential oils effect the brain are:

    1._____

    2._____

28. A   B   C   D

29. A   B   C   D   E

30. A   B   C   D   E

31. A   B   C   D

32. A   B   C   D   E

33. A   B   C   D   E

34. A   B   C   D   E

35. A   B   C   D

36. A   B   C   D   E

37. A   B   C   D   E

38. A   B   C   D   E

39. A   B   C   D   E

40. A   B   C   D   E

41. A   B   C   D   E

42. A   B   C   D

43. A   B   C   D

44. A   B   C   D   E

LESSON NINE

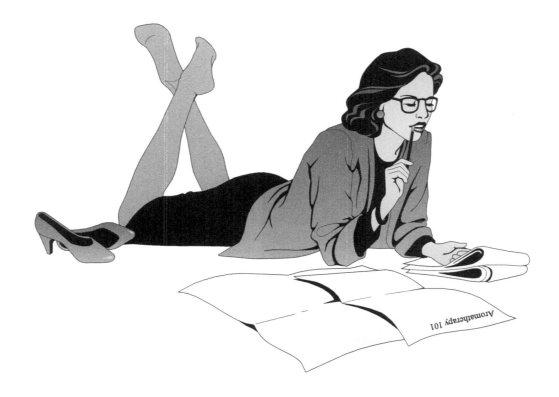

Lesson #9
Table of Contents

Bibliography:

The Simon & Schuster, Anatomy & Physiology by Dr. James Bevan.
Aromatherapy A to Z by Patricia Davis.
Aromatherapy Workbook by Shirley Price
A Textbook of Holistic Aromatherapy by Arnould-Taylor

An Introduction to the Genito-Urinary and Kidney System and the Reproductive System

THE GENITO-URINARY SYSTEM

Many anatomical textbooks divide the genito-urinary systems into:
- the reproductive system; and
- the excretive system.

But because a number of the organs involved are common to both systems, for the purpose of this course we will treat them under this one heading.

The principal organs involved in this dual system are;
- ovaries, fallopian tubes, uterus, testes, urethra, ureter and the urinary bladder.

There are a number of smaller accessory organs involved and these will be dealt with appropriately in due course.

Diagram of the section of:
<u>The female pelvic cavity</u>   Diagram of the section of:
<u>The male pelvic cavity</u>

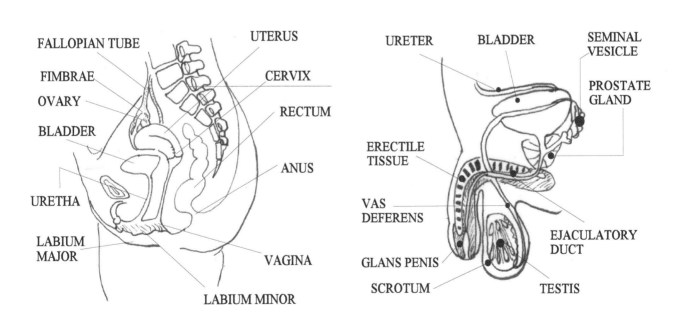

First we have the right and left ovaries in the female anatomy. These are quite small and are about the size of an almond.

They consist of masses of very small sacs known as the "ovarian follicles" and each follicle contains an "ovum".

The ovaries have two principal functions:

1. To develop the ova and expel one at approximately twenty-eight day intervals during the reproductive life.

2. To produce hormones *(oestrogen and progesterone)* which influence secondary sex characteristics and control changes in the uterus during the menstrual cycle.

The fallopian tubes - Sometimes referred to as the uterine tubes, are about four inches long and their function is to transport the ova from the ovaries to the uterus.

The uterus is a muscular organ approximately pearshaped, about three inches long by two inches wide and inch thick. It is positioned in the centre of the pelvis with the bladder in front and the rectum behind.

For the purpose of description, it is normally divided into three parts:

1. The fundus being the broad, upper end.
2. The body is the central Part.
3. The cervix is about an inch long and is the neck which projects into the vagina.

The vagina is the muscular canal which connects the above organs to the external body at the point collectively known as the vulva which includes the clitoris which is a small, sensitive organ containing erectile tissue corresponding to the male penis.

The male genital organs are comparatively simple in comparison to the female genital organs. The principal organs are the testes or testicles which are the essential male reproduction glands.

The scrotum which is a pouch-like organ containing the testes and the penis which is suspended in front of the scrotum.

The kidneys are two bean shaped organs, approximately four inches long, two inches wide and one inch thick. They are positioned against the posterior wall at or above the normal waistline. quite often the right kidney is slightly lower than the left kidney.

The kidneys consist of three principal parts:

1. The cortex or outer layer which is light brown in colour.
2. The middle portion which is inside and is dark brown in colour.
3. The pelvis which is the hollow, inner portion from which the Ureters open.

The function of the kidneys is to separate certain waste products from the blood and this renal function helps maintain the blood at a constant level of composition despite the great variation in diet and fluid intake.

Diagram of section of kidney

As blood circulates in the kidneys a large quantity of water, salts, urea and glucose are filtered into the capsules of bowman and from there into the convoluted tubules. From here all the glucose, most of the water and salts and some of the urea are returned to the blood vessels.

The remainder passes via the calyces into the kidney pelvis as urine. It is estimated that 33-40 gallons (150-181 litres) of fluid are processed by the kidneys each day but only about 2 and half pints (1.42 litres) of this leave the body as urine.

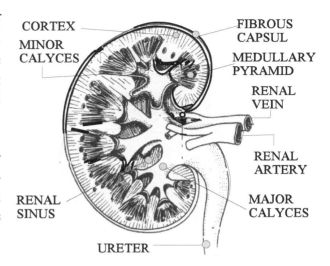

Diagram of internal kidney structure

Did you know?
It is estimated that up to 40 gallons or 181 Litres of fluids are processed by the Kidneys each day, but only about 2 ½ pints or 1.42 litres leaves the body as urine.

The average composition of urine is 96% water, 4% solids and of the 4%, 2% represents urea.

The ureters are two fine muscular tubes, ten to twelve inches long, which carry the urine from the kidney pelvis to the bladder. This is a very elastic muscular sac lying immediately behind the symphysis pubis.

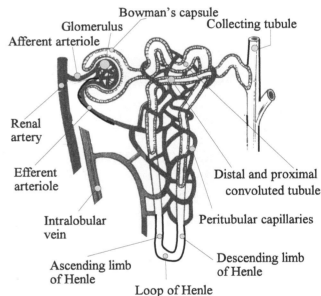

The urethra is a narrow muscular tube passing from the bladder to the exterior of the body. The female urethra is 1 to 1 ½ inches long and the male urethra 6 -8 inches long.

In the male, the urethra is the common passage for both urine and the semen or reproductive fluid. Also, in the male, it passes through a gland known as the prostate gland which is about the size and shape of a chestnut. It surrounds the neck of the bladder and tends to enlarge after middle life when it may, by projecting into the bladder produce urine retention.

DIAGRAM OF THE EXCRETORY SYSTEM

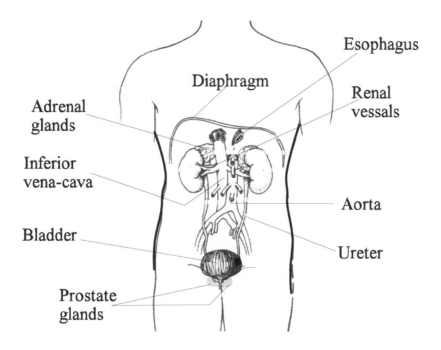

Additional notes on the functions of the genito-urinary system

The 2% urea compares with 0.04% urea in blood plasma so it will be seen that concentration has been increased some fifty times by the work of the kidneys.

The salts consist mostly of sodium chloride, phosphates and sulphates produced partly from the presence of these salts in protein foods. These salts have either to be reabsorbed or got rid of by the kidneys in sufficient quantities to keep the blood at its normal reaction and balance.

The urine also contains traces of a number of other substances, all of which combine to produce, in the urine, a reasonable pattern of the state of the body itself.

Its analysis indicates a number of physiological states including the amount of alcohol in the body, whether a female is pregnant or not and whether a person has diabetes.

It is estimated that, at birth, there are some thirty thousand ova or eggs in a female child. No fresh ova are formed after birth but, during the reproductive female life, That is commencing between ten and sixteen years of age and concluding between 45 and 55 years of age, these ova develop within the follicles or sacs in which they are embedded and progressively come nearer to the surface of the ovary where they mature and increase in size.

Then, about every 28 days, one of these follicles bursts and the ovum it contains, together with the fluid surrounding it, is expelled into the fallopian tubes and then into the uterus where it may or may not be fertilised.

If the ovum is fertilised by a male Reproductive cell or spermatozoon it then attaches itself to the uterine wall and there develops. If the ovum does not become fertilised within a few days it is cast off and the process termed menstruation is initiated.

The spermatozoa which are responsible for fertilisation are contained in a substance known as seminal fluid. An average ejection of seminal fluid contains several hundred million of these mobile units which look rather like a miniature elongated tadpole, and 1/500th of an inch in light.

It consists of a headpiece, a middle piece and a long whip-like tail which gives the spermatozoon its mobility. The single fertilized ovum soon becomes many cells which develop in a bag of membranes which soon fill the uterine cavity. At one part of this sac, at the point where the ovum first embedded itself in the uterine wall, the placenta or afterbirth develops.

The umbilical cord contains blood vessels and runs from the navel of the foetus to the placenta. The placenta receives the mother's blood from the wall of the uterus and the infant's blood via the umbilical cord so that, at no stage, does the mother's blood pass directly into the child. It is through the placenta that the child's blood is able to absorb food, oxygen and water from the mother and, in turn, give off its waste products.

The skin is, of course, an organ very closely connected with the excretatory system but, as it is a multipurpose organ, it is dealt with later on in the course.

Terminology

Cervicitis: This is an infection of the cervix that is, the neck of the uterus, and is reasonable common. It may be due to gonorrhoea, syphilis or a specific infection.

Kidney stones: Stones in the kidney are quite common and precipitate out of the urine, which has already been explained as a complex solution of many substances. Surgical operations for the removal of stones have a very long history. The Greek Doctor Hippocrates, admonished fellow physicians not to cut out stones but to leave it to the specialist. Whilst, nearer to our time, Samuel Pepys describes his own operation for the cutting of stone on march 26th 1658. He notes in his diary that he spent twenty four shillings *"for a case to keep my stone that I was cut of"*.

Nephritis or Bright's disease: This was first described by Dr. Richard Bright of London, England, in 1827. The single disease which he diagnosed has now been subdivided into a number of conditions which may, in a broader way, be called nephritis; An inflammation of the kidney not resulting from infection in the kidney.

Calculus: Stone e.g. Renal calculus; Stone in the kidney

Catheter: A hollow tube for introduction into a cavity through a narrow canal for the purpose of discharging fluid from a cavity. For instance, passing water from the bladder for the relief of urinary retention.

Ectopic: Gestation development of the ovum in a fallopian tube instead of the uterus

Enuresis: The involuntary discharge of urine.

Foetus: The unborn child dating from the end of the third month until birth

Intra-uterine: Within the uterus. Relating to conditions which occurred before birth

Menopause: Also called climacteric. The physiological cessation of menstruation.

Micturition: The act of passing urine.

Common Diseases or Disorders

Disease or Disorder	ENDOMETRIOSIS
Description	The cause of endometriosis is unknown. This disorders results from endometrial tissue that normally lines the uterus, spreads and grows in other sites like the fallopian tubes, ovaries and occasionally to the bladder, small or large intestines. Because this tissue responds to the same hormonal influence as the uterus, it can bleed during menstruation, causing pain, irritation, cramps and even scar tissue. Endometriosis can occur in 10 to 15% of menstruating women between the ages of 25-45. It can be a main cause of infertility. Symptoms may include pain in the lower back, abdomen, and/or pelvic area prior to and during menstruation, nausea, vomiting, constipation.
Possible Allopathic Treatment	Normally some form of "anti-estrogen" medication is used to reduce the estrogen within the body. This is used because the growth of the endometrial tissue is dependent on this hormone. Blocking the production of estrogen is suppose to shrink the patches of growth. Analgesics such as aspirin and acetaminophen are used for pain relief. Surgery may be required in more extreme cases.
Possible Holistic Aromatherapy Treatment	Analgesic essential oils like; *Bergamot, Cajeput, Coriander, Eucalyptus, Lemongrass, Niaouli, Black-pepper, Chamomile, Jasmine, Lavender, Marjoram, Peppermint, Rosemary and Ginger.* Hormonal essential oils like; *Geranium, Rose* Anti-depressant essential oils; *Basil, Bergamot, Lemongrass, Clary Sage, Geranium, Jasmine, :Lavender, Melissa, Neroli, Patchouli, Rose, Sandalwood and Ylang ylang*

Disease or Disorder	DYSMENORRHEA
Description	Dysmenorrhea is painful or difficult menstruation. It normally occurs as abdominal pain stemming from uterine cramps during menstruation. This disorder affects more than 50% of women with severe symptoms occurring in about 10% of the cases. When this occurs in younger women, it may be due to the uterus not having reached full maturity. Other reasons may include the ovulation cycle. As well, the production of certain prostaglandins can cause painful uterine contractions.
Possible Allopathic Treatment	NSAIDS (non-steroidal anti-inflammatory drugs) such as ibuprofen, naproxen and mefenamicacid are used as may be drugs that block prostaglandin production like low dose oral contraceptives that have estrogen and progesterone. In more extreme cases, artificial dilation of the cervix is performed. This relieves the pain for several months. Pregnancy is also been known to alleviate cramps after the first delivery due to the stretching of the cervix during delivery.
Possible Holistic Aromatherapy Treatment	Reproductive oils like *Rose, Neroli, Jasmine, etc.* Analgesic essential oils like: *Bergamot, Cajeput, Coriander, Eucalyptus, Lemongrass, Niaouli, Black-pepper, Camphor, Cypress, Fennel, Geranium, Hyssop, Juniper, Lavender, Marjoram, Pine, Rosemary and Ginger.* Anti-depressant essential oils; *Basil, Bergamot, Lemongrass, Clary Sage, Geranium, Jasmine, Lavender, Melissa, Neroli, Patchouli, Rose, Sandalwood and Ylang ylang* Evening Primrose oil would help as either a topical carrier oil or as an internal supplement. It contains GLA (gamma-linoleic acid) which is a precursor of beneficial prostaglandins.

Disease or Disorder	CYSTITIS
Description	Cystitis is an inflammation of the bladder. It is ten times more commonly found in females then males due to the smaller urethra in women. Due to the short length of the female urethra, bacteria enters the bladder easily and can cause infection and inflammation. Symptoms include increased urination with greater urgency and pain. The urine is often cloudy with a strong odour. There could be blood present in the urine. Nearly 85 % of urinary tract infections are caused by the bacteria "Escherichia coli". Chlamydia may also be a cause of bladder problems. If bladder infections are left untreated, they can lead to kidney infections.
Possible Allopathic Treatment	Traditionally antibiotics are used in order to kill the bacteria. For people suffering from recurrent infections (3 or more per year), long term doses of antibiotics are given as treatment. Atropine may be given to relieve the muscle spasms often associated with cystitis and phenazopyridine is prescribed for pain reduction and to soothe the inflamed tissue
Possible Holistic Aromatherapy Treatment	Anti-inflammatory oils; *Caraway, Tea tree, Camphor, Chamomile, Fennel, Geranium, Jasmine, Peppermint, Benzoin, Frankincense, Myrrh, and Patchouli* Analgesic essential oils; *Bergamot, Cajeput, Coriander, Eucalyptus, Lemongrass, Niaouli, Black-pepper, Camphor, Cypress, Fennel, Geranium, Hyssop, Juniper, Lavender, Marjoram, Pine, Rosemary and Ginger.* Antispasmodic essential oils; *Aniseed, Basil, Bergamot, Black Pepper, Cajeput, Chamomile, Clary-Sage, Coriander, Cypress, Fennel, Ginger, Hyssop, Jasmine, Juniper, Lavender, Marjoram, Melissa, Orange, Peppermint, Patchouli, Petitgrain, Rosemary, Thyme.* Antibacterial essential oils; *all essential oils possess some form of anti-bacterial property.*

Disease or Disorder	YEAST INFECTIONS
Description	Yeast infections normally stem from an overgrowth of yeast such as candida albicans. This fungus infects the vagina and causes a form of vaginitis. Itching, local irritation, burning accompanied by an abnormal discharge are signs of yeast infections in females. In males, there may be a slight discharge from the penis and the end of it may be red with small crusted blisters or sores present. The cause of yeast infections stem from oral contraceptives, pregnancy (due to the altered pH state and sugar content of vaginal secretions), diabetes (due to the high sugar content - yeast thrives in this type of environment), IUD's, antibiotic therapy and corticosteroid therapy.
Possible Allopathic Treatment	Antifungal preparations such as clotrimazole (Canesten), miconazole (Monistat) and nystatin are some commonly used products for people suffering from yeast infections. They can be prescribed for either local or systemic applications Discontinuation of oral contraceptives may be requested for several months to reduce the severity of the infection.
Possible Holistic Aromatherapy Treatment	Antifungal essential oils such as; *Tea tree, Myrrh, Cedarwood, Immortelle, Lavender, Lemongrass, and Patchouli*

Disease or Disorder	HERPES SIMPLEX VIRUS (HSV)
Description	Herpes is a virus that has an affinity for the skin and the nervous system. There are two types HSV 1 - this is oral herpes, normally found around the mouth and nose HSV 2 - this is genital herpes, which is a sexually transmitted disease caused by the herpes simplex virus. Herpes generally appear on the vulva, vagina or penis after contact. Initial symptoms begin with tingling, itching or discomfort followed by the appearance of small vesicles filled with clear fluid. The vesicles can vary in size from .5 to 1.5 cm. After the vesicles have appeared, they begin to dry out and form a yellow crust/scab. Complete clearing of the lesions normally takes place between 8-12 days. Herpes can remain dormant for a period of time and recur due to stress (either emotional or physical), after illness or immunosuppression and even overexposure to sunlight.
Possible Allopathic Treatment	Antibiotics are prescribed to be used topically on the affected area. These drugs may include acyclovir, valacyclovir, and famciclovir. If severe infection is present, the medications may be given orally to facilitate a systemic treatment. **Herpes are extremely contagious and should not be touched under any circumstances.
Possible Holistic Aromatherapy Treatment	Antiviral essential oils like; *Tea tree, Eucalyptus, Manuka, Immortelle, Lavender, Lime and Palmerosa* Analgesic oils like; *Bergamot, Cajeput, Coriander, Eucalyptus, Lemongrass, Niaouli, Black Pepper, Camphor, Cypress, Fennel, Geranium, Hyssop, Juniper, Lavender, Marjoram, Pine, Rosemary and Ginger.* Anti-depressant essential oils; *Basil, Bergamot, Lemongrass, Clary Sage, Geranium, Jasmine, :Lavender, Melissa, Neroli, Patchouli, Rose, Sandalwood and Ylang ylang*

Disease or Disorder	URINARY TRACT INFECTIONS
Description	This is an infection of one or more structures in the urinary tract. Urinary tract infections (UTI) can be caused by bacteria, fungus or parasites. The most common cause of infection is bacteria. UTI's are found more frequently in women than men. The condition may be asymptomatic or may produce pain or burning during urination. There may be the presence of pus and/or feeling the constant need to urinate with no success.
Possible Allopathic Treatment	Antibiotics are prescribed to eradicate the cause of the infection. If there is pain present, analgesics like NSAIDS (non-steroidal anti-inflammatory drugs) may be suggested
Possible Holistic Aromatherapy Treatment	Antiseptic oils like; *Bay, Benzoin, Basil, Black pepper, Camphor, Cedarwood, Citronella, Clary Sage, Cypress, Eucalyptus, Fennel, Frankincense, Geranium, Hyssop, Jasmine, Juniper, Lavender, Lemon, Lemongrass, Marjoram, Myrrh, Neroli, Niaouli, Patchouli, Rose, Rosemary, Sandalwood, Tea Tree, Yarrow, Ylang ylang* Analgesic oils like; *Bergamot, Cajeput, Coriander, Eucalyptus, Lemongrass, Niaouli, Black pepper, Camphor, Cypress, Fennel, Geranium, Hyssop, Juniper, Lavender, Marjoram, Pine, Rosemary and Ginger.* Antibacterial essential oils; *all essential oils possess some form of anti-bacterial property.*

Aromatherapy with Pregnancy and Treating Babies

INTRODUCTION

The mammary glands or breast

These are accessories to the female reproductive organs and secrete milk during the period of lactation. They enlarge at puberty, increase in size during pregnancy and atrophy in old age. The breast consists of mammary gland substance or alveolar tissue arranged in lobes and separated by connective and fatty tissues. Each lobule consists of a cluster of alveoli opening into lactiferous ducts which unite with other ducts to form large ducts which terminate in the excretory ducts. As these ducts near the nipple expand they create a reservoir for the milk, thus being called the lactiferous sinuses.

The breast also contains a considerable quantity of fat which lies in the tissues of the breast and also in between the lobes. It also contains numerous lymphatic vessels which commence as tiny plexuses which unite to form larger vessels which eventually pass mainly to the lymph node in the axilla. The nipple is surrounded by a darker coloured area known as the mammary areola.

The breasts are very greatly influenced by hormone activity. Hyper-secretion of the thyroid can lead to atrophy of the breasts whilst hypo-secretion can be the cause of too greatly developed breasts. Both the ovarian hormones influence the condition and appearance of the breast whilst the pituitary hormone prolactin starts lactation at the end of pregnancy.

When considering the use of aromatherapy during pregnancy, you should first become aware that there are a small group of essential oils which should never be used in the first few months of pregnancy, partly because of the risk of toxicity with certain oils and also because of the possible harm to the growing foetus or because they involve some risk of miscarriage.

Provided these oils are carefully avoided, aromatherapy techniques can be used very safely and beneficially to maintain the general health of the expectant mother, and to help minimise the various discomforts of pregnancy, such as nausea, backache, swollen legs and ankles.

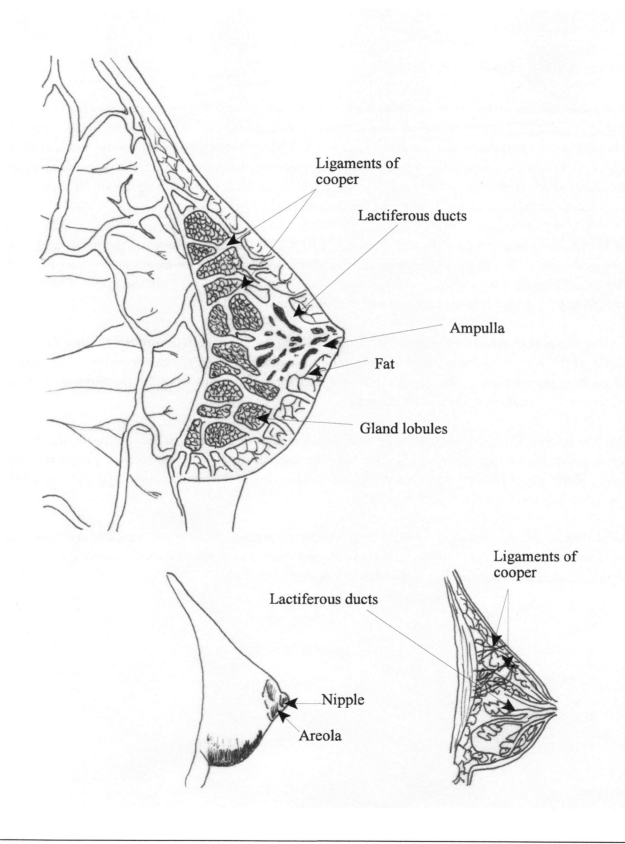

Ligaments of cooper

Lactiferous ducts

Ampulla

Fat

Gland lobules

Lactiferous ducts

Ligaments of cooper

Nipple

Areola

AROMATHERAPY WITH PREGNANCY

When considering the use of aromatherapy during pregnancy, you should first become aware that there are a small group of essential oils which should never be used in the first few months of pregnancy. There is the risk of toxicity with certain oils, as well as the possibility of harming the growing fetus or increasing the risk of miscarriage.

Provided these oils are carefully avoided, aromatherapy techniques can be used very safely and beneficially to maintain the general health of the expectant mother, and to help minimise the various discomforts of pregnancy, such as nausea, backache, swollen legs and ankles.

The oils which must be avoided during the first three or four months of pregnancy include:

1. Those which are described as "emmenagogue", which means that they will induce menstrual flow.
2. Those which are recommended for use during labour to strengthen contraction and,
3. Essential oils that are considered to be toxic, which could harm both the mother and the foetus

The oils that should NOT be used at this time are:

Aniseed,	Armoise (mugwort),	Arnica,	Basil,
Clary-sage,	Cypress,	Fennel,	Hyssop,
Jasmine,	Juniper,	Marjoram,	Myrrh,
Origanum,	Pennyroyal,	Peppermint,	Rose,
Rosemary,	Sage,	Thyme,	Wintergreen.

Plus any other oil described as toxic.

Camomile and lavender are also described as emmenagogue, but can be used with care and in small amounts or low dilutions, except where the mother has reason to fear a possible miscarriage. For instance, if she has previously miscarried, or if there is a history in the family of miscarriages, or if there has been any abnormal bleeding and of course if her doctor has informed her that there is some risk.

Later in pregnancy (after six months) lavender and rosemary has proved beneficial in relieving backache, and of course rosemary and geranium are useful for oedema of the legs which sometimes occurs in later months, use firm strokes moving away from the feet and towards the thighs.

For the nausea which often accompanies the first few months, fennel tea is a safe and effective remedy (please note that fennel oil is to be avoided).

A great many women experience some low back pain as their pregnancy advances, due not only to the increased weight of the baby, but to the changing shape of their own bodies, and the way this increases the lumbar curve of the spine. Gentle exercise could prove beneficial, however, massage with essential oils will give a tremendous amount of relief from pain and help to tone the muscles which are carrying the increased load. Obviously, as the baby grows, it will not be possible to lie the mother on her tummy to be massaged.

It is possible to give back massage with the woman lying on her side, or if she wants to sit up, I have found it easier for both the giver and the receiver this way. The lower (lumbar) area of the back should only be massaged lightly during the first four months, by the time the back starts to become a problem around the six month period the pressure can be safely massaged with good firm strokes by this time.

The same comments apply to massage of the abdomen. Work very lightly in this area for the first four to six months, after this period, massage will not only be beneficial but most enjoyable. Very often, the developing child responds to the massage given to its mother. A lively baby which may be causing its mother some discomfort, will be still for quite a while when its mother has been massaged with a soothing, calming oil and babies whose mothers have received regular massage throughout their pregnancy are generally very peaceful when they are born.

As well as receiving regular treatments from you the therapist, she should also massage oil into her own tummy and hips each day from about the fifth month onwards, to prevent stretch marks. Neroli or mandarin might be a good choice.

Aromatic baths can be enjoyed right throughout pregnancy, and can in fact be one of the expectant mother's greatest luxuries and forms of relaxation. Once again, simply avoid the risky oils and also avoid over-hot bath water.

When using pure essential oils yourself, on their own or undiluted, please refer to the following lists/guidelines

List "A"

Oils that in my opinion may be used with safety during the whole of pregnancy, provided that you do not massage the abdomen and there is no history of misscarrage or related problems:
Use only Quinessence Essential oils at low dilution (1/2 measures)

Cedarwood (Cedrus atlantica)
Ginger (Zingiber officinale)
Neroli (Citrus aurantium amara)
Petitgrain (Citrus aurantium amara)
Rose Otto (Rosa centifolia)
Rosewood (Aniba rosaeodora)
Sandalwood (Santalum album)
Tea Tree (Melaleuca alternifolia)
Ylang Ylang (Cananga odorata)

List "B"

Oils which have a very mild diuretic or emmenagogic properties but are nevertheless considered almost as safe to use as list "A" after the first trimester pregnancy. provided that you do not massage the abdomen and there is no history of misscarrage or related problems:
Use only Quinessence Essential oils at low dilution (1/2 measures)

Bergamot *(Citrus bergamia)*
Bitter Orange *(Citrus aurantium amara)*
Chamomile German *(Matricaria chamomilla)*
Chamomile Roman *(Anthemis nobilis)*
Chamomile Moroccan *(Ormenis mixta)*
Geranium *(Pelargonium graveolens)*
Grapefruit *(Citrus Paradis)*
Lavender *(Lavendula angustifolia)*
Lemon *(Citrus Limon)*
Mandarin *(Citrus reticulata)*
Marjoram sweet *(Origanum majorana)*
Sweet Orange *(Citrus aurantium sinensis)*

Unless recommended by an Aromatherapists, it is best during pregnancy not to use any unknown oils or any not mentioned in list "A" or "B" or "C".

The following oils contain Ketones or phenols and although, they have not been proved to be dangerous at low levels, they are best used only by trained (completed the Advanced Course) therapists and treated with great respect.

List "C"

Basil *(Ocimum basilicum)*
Camphor *(Cinnamomum camphora)*
Clove *(Eugenia caryophyllata)*
Cinnamon *(Cinnamomum zedylanicum)*
Hyssop *(Hyssopus officinalis)*
Lemongrass *(Cymbopogon citratius)*
Origanum *(Origanum vulgare)*
Sage *(Salvia officinalis)*
Savory *(Satureia montana)*
Tarragon *(Artemisia dracunculus)*
Thyme *(Thymus vulgaris)*

TREATING BABIES

There are one or two additional factors to be considered when treating babies, as opposed to treating children.

Babies often suck there thumbs, or hands, and rub their fists into their eyes. Essential oils can find there way into the babies eyes or mouth with dangerous consequences. What could be just unpleasant with an adult, could cause permanent damage to the eyes of babies.

Before adding essential oil to a bath for babies (not new born babies), first mix the essential oil (maximum one drop) to a carrier oil. A single drop of camomile or lavender will be sufficient in a bath to ease minor discomforts and to promote sleep. Regular additions of the oils to the bath is a good preventive measure against nappy-rash, as almost all essential oils will prevent bacteria developing on the skin for some time.

If nappy-rash does become a problem, creams containing oil of calendula or camomile are very healing, and benzoin or myrrh might be added for cracked or slow to heal skin.

A very safe and effective method of administering essential oils is via inhalation. A drop of the appropriate oil on the sheet in the cot (not near the head), a better method would be a vaporiser in the same room.

If the baby is suffering from colic, he or she can be comforted and the pain reduced by very gentle massage on the tummy and lower back, making sure that the baby doesn't try to get the oils on his or her hands. Dress the baby as soon as you have finished, this will protect baby from ingesting the oil or rubbing it into his or her eyes.

During teething for older babies, rub a very diluted camomile over the cheeks and side of the face, remembering to wipe away any excess oil to prevent contamination into the eyes or mouth.

RECIPES

Constipation	3 drops Orange, 3 drops Chamomile, 3 drops Black pepper applied twice daily onto the small of the back and lower abdomen
Heartburn	3 drops Chamomile, 3 drops Petitgrain, 3 drops Sandalwood
Bath treatment for backache	2 drops chamomile, 2 drops Lavender
Stretch marks	3 drops Lavender, 3 drops Chamomile, 3 drops Frankincense
Varicose veins	3 drops lemon, 3 drops Cypress, 3 drops Lavender
Haemorrhoids	3 drops cypress, 3 drops Lemon, 3 drops Sandalwood
Labour lotion	3 drops Lavender, 3 drops Mandarin, 3 drops Sandalwood
To promote lactation	3 drops Fennel
To stop lactation	3 drops Cypress, 3 drops Geranium
General baby mix	1 drop Lavender, 1 drop Mandarin

To keep baby calm, put one drop of essential oil on a tissue out of reach of the baby but near the child whilst feeding. They soon learn to associate the smell with warmth, comfort, etc.

When leaving the baby with a baby-sitter, simply give her a tissue too. For children that are restless during the night, use the same oil on a tissue besides them, or on their night clothes, but not near the face, it's calming effect will get back to sleep.

Since Aromatherapy was introduced in this country, mothers-to-be have used essential oils during early pregnancy including many of the so-called *"forbidden"* oils (under the direction and guidance of a qualified Aromatherapist. To-date, no ill effects have been reported, possibly because most people use common sence and when in doubt, they leave the oil out. Many of the oils contain a chemical that is deemed un-safe or toxic, and if this chemical was to be used on its own, it would be unsafe. However, when used in its natural state, *(not singled out)* the damaging effect is not evident.

Many of the books talk about contra-indications and toxic levels etc. Not without cause, their advise should always to taken into consideration and you are advised to err on the side of caution. There are several oils that should not be used on a regular basis during the first five months of pregnancy. ie. emmenagogue oils. Many of the essential oils on the *"best to avoid list"* can still be used safely in room diffusers

Inhalations and baths are very useful for helping *"morning sickness"*/nausea. Pregnant women have a heightened sense of smell and this can contribute to the feeling of sickness, especially during cooking or being in the company of a smoker. However, Petitgrain and sweet Orange essential oils, when used in a vaporiser, can be a great help towards preventing nausea.

LABOUR

Inhalation is an effective method of using essential oils while in labour, to help contractual pains. During contractions place a few drops each of lavender and clary sage onto a cotton wool ball and inhale as required, or use a room vaporiser.

Preparation for labour

Towards the end of pregnancy, ie. the last 6 weeks, oils can be used to prepare the uterus for labour. Adding 1 drop of, rose Otto, Lavender, Chamomile and Frankincense to 25ml of carrier oil, helps the uterus to regain tone.

Commencement of labour

If you are not taken unawares, mix 2 drops each of chamomile Mandarin and Sandalwood to 25ml of carrier oil and apply to the lower back and tummy.

Post natal/after birth

Bath containing Cypress and Lavender to deal with bruising or excess bleeding.

Oils for childhood conditions

Chicken pox	Lemon and Lavender
Measles	Eucalyptus and Lavender
Colds & coughs	Tea-Tree and Eucalyptus
Colic	Orange and Chamomile
Insomnia	Sandalwood and Lavender
Calming	Lavender and Chamomile

Mechanical Methods of Contraception

1. The natural or rhythm method
which requires restricting intercourse to the non-fertile period of the woman which only lasts a few days after ovulation. Taking the body temperature assists in determining the exact date of ovulation.

2. Birth control pill taken orally contains a mixture of oestrogen and progesterone-like hormones which fool the body into thinking it is already pregnant via the endocrine system.

3. Surgical intervention involves a vasectomy for men and tubal ligation for women. This is where the reproductive tubes are simply cut and tied.

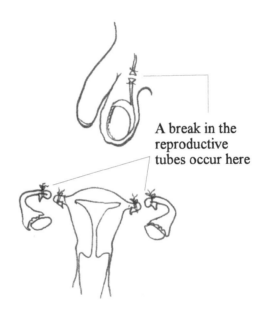

A break in the reproductive tubes occur here

Essential Oils

ANISEED

Areas that this oil can help:

1. Calm digestive or menstrual pain.
2. Respiratory tract infections.
3. Anti-parasitic in treating lice.

Properties   Uses

Narcotic	Anti-spasmodic	Slows down circulation
Addictive	Carminative	Calm digestive pain
Galactagogue		Calm menstrual pain

Place of Origin
Aniseed *(pimpinella anisum).*
Is a native of most Mediterranean countries, where it grows wild.

Method of Extraction
The oil is extracted from the seed of the plant. Obtained by Steam distillation.
It was particularly favoured by the Romans, who used the seeds to sweeten breath and as an aphrodisiac. Today the essential oil of aniseed is seldom used, because of its relatively high toxicity. Also when used in high doses, or taken over a long period of time, it acts as a narcotic which slows the circulation, damages the brain and is addictive *(the addiction to absinthe which was common in the 19th century France).* Theoretically, it can be used to calm digestive or menstrual pain, stimulate the flow of breast milk, or treat heart and lung disease, but as there are other safe essential oils with the same properties, it is better to leave this one well alone.

It is used to flavour medicines, confectionary and dental preparations, it is also thought to help alleviate the effects of a hangover. It is stimulating to the respiratory tract, and is helpful for asthma, coughs, colds and sore throats. The antispasmodic effect also helps relieve period pains. Galactagogue means that it is a useful post-natally to help stimulate milk flow.
Being anti-parasitic it has proved useful in the treatment of lice and scabies.

Note: aniseed has been avoided by many therapists due to suspected side effects. The cheap alcoholic drink *"absinthe",* contained alcohol distilled from wormwood, which had a very bitter taste. The aniseed was used to conceal the taste. It was not however, the cause of the side effects. It must be emphasized that it was the wormwood which resulted in the high toxic effects of brain damage and addiction not the aniseed.

BENZOIN

The three main areas where this oil can help are:

1. Urinary tract problems like cystitis, etc.
2. Respiratory disorders like colds and flu. Asthma and bronchitis.
3. Skin problems, where there is redness, irritation, cracked or dry skin and even for   wounds.

Properties   Uses

Antiseptic	Carminative	Arthritis	Asthma
Cordial	Deodorant	Bronchitis	Colic
Diuretic	Expectorant	Coughs	Gout
Sedative	Vulnerary	Laryngitis	Wounds
		Skin irritations	
		Spermatorrhoea	

Place of Origin
Benzoin *"styrax benzoin"*. Used to be known as *"gum benjamin"*. The Benzoin tree is cultivated in Java, Sumatra, and Thailand. Benzoin has been imported for centuries by the Chinese, and a similar product to our modern Benzoin absolute is mentioned by Li Shih-Chen.

The granulated gum called, *"gum benjamin"* in old herbals, is a dark reddish-brown, and is often used as a fixative in pot pourris, but the form in which Benzoin is probably best known is as, *"friar's balsam"*, or compound tincture of Benzoin.

Method of Extraction
Gum from the tree is not naturally produced, but forms when a deep incision is made in the trunk. This produces a slow exudation, which is collected from the tree when it has sufficiently hardened.
The gum is a greyish colour with dark red streaks in it. These red parts contains most of the aromatic material. A resinoid, or absolute is produced from the gum. It is a beautiful reddish-brown colour, and has the consistency of a fatty oil.

Benzoin is not a true essential oil, as pure Benzoin is a resin and has to be melted by heating over hot water before it can be used. When you buy Benzoin from an essential oil supplier it is usually dissolved in ethyl glycol, but this method is not very satisfactory from the point of view of a natural therapy using plant products, so it is worth finding a supplier who dissolves the Benzoin resin in wood alcohol, or buying it in the solid state and melting it when needed.

The active constituents of pure benzoin include benzoic acid, bemzoresinal, siaresinotannol and vanillin, which gives it its characteristic *"ice cream"* aroma.

Benzoin has been used for thousands of years as an ingredient of incense, and to drive out evil spirits. It is very warming, soothing and stimulating, and this makes it particularly helpful for colds, flu, coughs and sore throats.

It use in the form of *"friar's balsam",* as an inhalation for sore throats and loss of voice, is probably it's best known virtue. Because of its ability to stimulate at the same time as sooths, it seems to get things moving in the body, whether it is clearing mucus, stimulating the circulation, expelling gas or increasing the flow of urine. It is very comforting for griping pains in the stomach, and for urinary tract infections.

Benzoin is used for healing many kinds of skin lesions, from cracked and chapped hands to chilblains. Friar's balsam has long been used by ballet dancers to heal cracked toes and prevent further cracking. It would be a good idea to put benzoin into hand creams for older people who work out side in the open.

On the psychological plane, as with many essential oils, we find a parallel with its physical properties. People respond to the use of Benzoin who are sad or depressed.

JASMINE

The three main areas where this oil can help are:
1. emotional problems
2. has an affinity for the female reproductive system
3. skin care.

Properties		Uses	
Antidepressant	Antiseptic	Anxiety	Cough
Antispasmodic	Aphrodisiac	Depression	Dysmenorrhoea
Galactagogue	Parurient	Frigidity	Impotence
Sedative		Nervous chills	
Tonic (especially uterine)		Skin care	Uterine disorders

Place of Origin

The Jasmine plant is a creeper, with white or yellow flowers. It is cultivated in Algeria, Morocco, France, China, Egypt, Italy and Turkey; the French oil is the most expensive. The oil is a deep reddish-brown colour and contains the chemical constituents, methyl anthranilaye, indol, benzyl acetate, linalol and linalyl acetate.

Method of Extraction

Jasmine Oil is very costly, because of the enormous quantity of flowers needed to produce a relatively small amount of oil, and because it is extracted by the labour-intensive method of enfleurage. In the case of Jasmine, the labour costs are further increased by the need to gather the flowers at night, for the odour of Jasmine is more powerful after dark, due to changes in the plant's internal chemistry. The flower continues to release essential oil for several days after being picked, so are left on the cotton cloths soaked in olive oil until all possible oil has been extracted. The olive oil is afterwards extracted with spirits, leaving the true Jasmine essence. A cheaper grade of Jasmine oil is made by extracting directly from the petals with petroleum spirits, this does not produce the quality or intensity of odour, as the spirit kills the flower instantly. This grade of Jasmine is of little use in Aromatherapy, and remember *"bargains"* in Jasmine oil will be avoided by caring therapists.

Two varieties of Jasmine are used in making the essential oil: Jasminium officinal and Jasmine grandiflorum.

Jasmine oil works primarily on the emotional level and has been found to have a significant effect on psychological and psychosomatic problems. Although it does have physiological effects, its use is especially indicated when these are linked to an emotional problem. It is a good oil to use when someone lacks confidence, self esteem, and has been described by many noted Aromatherapists as uplifting. It is these properties which make Jasmine an excellent anti-depressant, and very useful when treating impotence or frigidity resulting from anxiety and tension.

Jasmine has a strong affinity for the female reproductive system and is noted for being a uterine tonic. It is valuable in relieving menstrual pain both in the abdomen and lower back.

Jasmine is also particularly effective in giving relief from premenstrual syndrome, whether on its own or as part of a synergistic blend. It is also effective in helping women who are going through the menopause.

Jasmine is valuable in helping women in childbirth, as it relieves the pain and helps strengthen contractions, when massaged into the lower back. It will also aid in the expulsion of the placenta. Post-natally, it promotes the flow of breast milk, and is valuable in helping relieve post-natal depression.

Jasmine is a wonderful oil to use for skin care, especially hot, dry and sensitive skins. It will help relieve redness and itching and so is useful in treating dermatitis especially if accompanied by a psychological problem such as depression. It is delightful to use as a facial oil due to its lovely aroma. But only a small amount is needed, as it is concentrated and therefore, a fairly powerful oil and too much can have an opposite effect to what is needed.

Rose

The four main areas where rose oil can help are:

1. The female reproductive system. Uterus disorders, excessive menstrual flow, irregular menstruation.
2. Skin care. Acts as a skin astringent, tonic, helps eczema, wounds and cuts, bruises, dry and inflamed skin, skin allergies.
3. Treats depression, sadness, grief and p.m.s.
4. As an aphrodisiac.

Properties   Uses

Antidepressant	Antipholistic	Cholecystitis	Conjunctivitis	Stomachic
Antiseptic	Antispasmodic	Constipation	Depression	Nausea
Aphrodisiac	Astringent	Frigidity	Haemorrhage	
Choleretic	Depurative	Headache	Hepatic congestion	
Emmenagogue	Haemostatic	Impotence	Insomnia	
Hepatic	Laxative	Irregular menstruation		Sterility
Sedative	Splenetic	Leucorrhoea	Menorrhagia	
		Tonic (heart, liver, stomach, & uterus)		
		Cell and skin rejuvenation		Skin care
		Nervous tension	Ophalmia	
		Uterine disorders	Vomiting	

Place of Origin

Roses have been used for their appearance, their scent, and their therapeutic properties from time immemorial. They were used extensively by the Romans for garlands, perfumes, and scented baths, just to name a few.

Today the finest and most expensive Rose oil comes from Bulgaria and is known as Bulgarian Rose Otto. It is extracted from the Damask Rose, from this plant it takes about 30 roses to make one drop of Bulgarian Rose Otto, and 60,000 roses to make one ounce.

Three varieties of rose are used commercially for the production of oil of Rose:

1. Rosa centifolia.
2. Rosa damascena.
3. Rosa gallica.

A slight variation of aroma and colour will be found in the oils made from the different varieties, from a greenish-orange to a deep browny-red.

Rose de mai (rosa centiflora) is cultivated in the grasse region of southern France, but it is only used for the production of an absolute, not an Otto. The finest Rose oil, and the most costly, is Bulgarian Attar of Roses, but excellent oil is also produced in the area around Grasse, a slightly cheaper oil comes from North Africa. The French and Bulgarian oils are produced by Enfleurage, while the North African is now generally obtained by the organic solvent method, which is considerably cheaper but less refined than the oils made according to traditional methods.

Method of Extraction
The major production of essential oil of Rose is not by distillation, which yields only a very small amount of essential oil as a secondary product during the extraction of rosewater *(Otto)*. Today, Rose oil is extracted by the Enfleurage method. The very high price of rose oil is due to the huge quantity of rose petals needed to extract a tiny amount of oil, and also because of the labour costs involved in this method of extraction.

However the *"Otto of roses"* extracted in this way is so concentrated that only a tiny amount is required For each treatment. The *"Otto"* is actually solid in the bottle at room temperatures, only turning into a thick oil when the bottle is warmed in the hands. The oil itself is a deep-reddish brown colour, and has been traditionally thought of as the queen of essential oils.

Rose oil takes preference in aromatherapy, when treating disorders of the female reproductive system. It has a powerful effect on the uterus, being cleansing, purifying, regulating and a tonic. It can be used to help regulate the menstrual cycle, and reduce excessive loss. Rose oil tones the vascular and digestive system by purging or cleansing, rather than stimulating. It has a soothing action on the nerves, which may induce sleep, although it is not a strong sedative.

As a well known aphrodisiac, it is used in the Hindu pharmacopoeia reinforced with Sandalwood. Aromatherapists have experienced a considerable influence with regard to the female sexual organs and Rose Oil. Not by stimulus, but on the contrary, by cleansing and regulating their functions.

Rose oil is used for regulating menstrual functions, it is a gentle emmenagogue, and cleanses the womb of impurities. It may be used for most disorders of the genito-urinary systems. Its action on the vascular system is manifold; it promotes the circulation, cleanses the blood, relieves cardiac congestion, regulates the action of the spleen and heart, and tones the capillaries. Its action on the digestive system is almost as important, it strengthens the stomach, promotes the flow of bile, and the elimination of faeces. It is also useful for nausea, vomiting and coughing.

The triple action of rose on the vascular, digestive, and nervous systems, and more especially the nature of its action, render it particularly suitable for the conditions of stress which are becoming more and more common today; nervous tension, peptic ulcers, heart disease and so on.

Rose oil, is perhaps surprisingly, one of the most antiseptic essence. This, combined with its slightly tonic and soothing essences, together with its slightly tonic action on the capillaries, makes it useful for virtually all types of skin. It is particularly good for mature, dry or sensitive skin, and for any kind of redness or inflammation. Rose is the least toxic of all essences. For most therapeutic purposes.

Note: *This expensive absolute oil should not be taken internally.*

Sandalwood

The three main areas where this oil can help are:

1. Urinary antiseptic.
2. Inhalation for coughs and throat infections.
3. Will help many skin problems.

Properties   Uses

Antidepressant	Acne	Nausea
Antiphlogistic	Blennorrhoea	Nervous antiseptic
Tonic	Bronchitis	Skin care
Antispasmodic	Catarrh	Tuberculosis
Aphrodisiac	Cough	Vomiting
Astringent	Cystitis	Tension
Carminative	Depression	
Diuretic	Diarrhoea	
Expectorant	Hiccough	
Sedative	Insomnia	
	Laryngitis	

Place of Origin
Sandalwood is a small evergreen, parasitic tree, which obtains its nourishment by attaching suckers to the roots of other trees. The variety *"santalum album"* grows in India and various Islands of the Indian Ocean, with the best quality being found in the province of Mysore. Santalum spicatum grows in Australia and yields a somewhat inferior oil.

Method of Extraction
The trees are very slow-growing, and only very mature trees, which are nearing the end of their life, are cut. The trunks are left to lie in the forests until the outer wood has been eaten away by ants, and *only the heartwood, which the insects will not attack,* is then used for building, furniture making, incense and the extraction of essential oil by steam distillation.

The oil contains santalol, fusanol, santalic acid, terasantalic acid and carbides, and varies from yellowish to a deep brown. It is extremely thick and viscous, the odour although not initially strong, develops when applied to the skin, and is amazingly persistent.

The taste is bitter in the extreme, which makes it very unpalatable for use as a gargle.

Sandalwood has been used in India for many centuries, both in traditional Ayur-Vedic Medicine, and as a perfume and incense. Its most important medicinal use is as a powerful urinary antiseptic. It has been used for at least two and a half thousand years for the treatment of various infections of the urinary tract, such as cystitis. It is also a very good pulmonary antiseptic, and has proved useful for dry, persistent and irritating coughs, for it is also very sedative. It is one of the best essential oils to use in the treatment of chronic bronchitis, and can also be used for soothing sore throats. The best methods of use are inhalations and external application to the chest and throat.

As a cosmetic ingredient, Sandalwood is far more than a perfume, for it is beneficial to many different skin types and problems. It can be used for dry and dehydrated skins, especially in the form of a warm compress, but at the opposite end of the scale it is helpful for oily skins and acne, as it is slightly astringent and a powerful antiseptic. It is one of the perfumes that seems to be as popular for use by men as it is with women.

Question and Answer Sheets

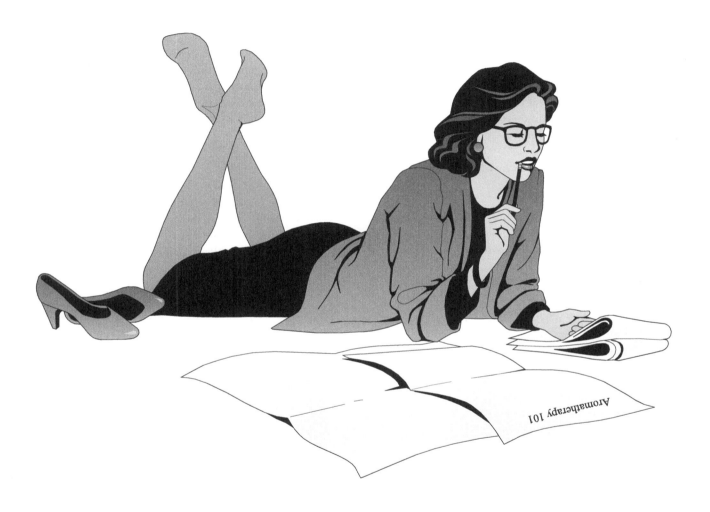

Please keep the questions for review.
Circle the correct answer/s on the Answer Sheets at the back of the book and
<u>return these sheets only</u> to your instructor.

Questions - Lesson #9

1. What is the difference between sexual and asexual reproduction?
a. nothing
b. asexual only occurs in mammals
c. sexual reproduction requires two individuals, male and female, while asexual requires just one   organism
d. asexual reproduction requires two individuals,   male and female, while sexual requires just one organism

2. Gonads form specialized sex cells that are called?
a. gametes   b. ovaries
c. testes   d. sex cells

3. What is the function of the uterus?
a. it connects all sex organs together
b. supplies blood to the ovaries
c. transports the ova
d. its an organ that provides an environment for a developing fetus

4. What are the two principal functions of the ovaries?
a. to develop the ova & expel/to produce hormones
b. to develop the hormones/to distribute through the body
c. to develop the ova/to expel one at approx. 28-day cycles
d. to attach fertilized egg to uterine lining/to aid in fetal development.

5. What is the function of the fallopian tubes?
a. provide passage of urine
b. allow for passage of sperm to unite with the ova
c. to transport the ova from the ovaries to the uterus
d. it doesn't serve any useful purpose.

6. Where is the uterus positioned?
a. in the back of the rectum and up under the kidneys
b. in the front of the bladder just beneath the navel
c. in the centre of the body
d. in the centre of the pelvis with the bladder in front and the vagina below.

7. The uterus is divided into three main parts; name them:
a. the fondue, the body and the cerebellum
b. the fundus, the body and the cervix
c. the body, the cervix and the canal
d. the cerebellum the clavicle and the femur.

8. What is the name of the muscular canal that connects the above organ to the external body?
a. the vagina   b. the rectum
c. the pharynx   d. the Nile

9. Name two of the principle male reproductive glands?
a. the urethra   b. the bladder
c. the ureter   d. the testes

10. Where are the kidneys positioned?
a. against the posterior abdominal wall, along either side of the gluteus maximus
b. against the posterior abdominal wall, at the normal waistline on either side of the body
c. against the anterior abdominal wall, under the rib cage
d. in the direct centre of the body, protected by all the other organs.

11. What is the function of the kidneys?
a. to separate waste products from the blood and remove them from the body
b. to circulate large quantities of water throughout the body
c. to add water to the blood and also to remove salts
d. to maintain constant levels of glucose found in the blood.

12. When the blood circulates through the kidneys, what substances are filtered into the Bowmans capsule?
a. water
b. blood, water and vitamins
c. coffee
d. water, urea, glucose and salts.

13. The excess products are removed from the body,
a. through bile   b. through urine
c. are not removed   d. thru sweating

14. Blood is supplied to the kidneys via the,
a. Bowmans artery   b. renal vein
c. renal artery   d. Bowmans vein

15. What is the function of the ureters?
a. to carry urine from the bladder to the outside of   the body
b. to provide passage for the male's reproductive   fluid
c. to retain water
d. to carry urine from the kidney pelvis to the bladder.

16. What is the urethra?

a. the passage for urine to pass from the bladder to   t h e outside of the body

b. to provide passage for the male's reproductive   fluid

c. to retain water

d. to carry urine from the kidney pelvis to the bladder.

17. What is the function of the urinary bladder?

a. to produce urea

b. to store urine from the kidneys

c. filters waste

d. has no purpose

18. What is the difference between the male urethra, and the female urethra?

a. nothing, they are quite similar

b. the male urethra is the passage for both semen and urine

c. the male urethra is the passage for both semen and urine, as well as differing in dimensions, being 6-8 in. long

d. the male urethra contains the prostate gland, which females don't have.

19. Where is the prostate gland positioned?

a. it encircles the urethra

b. at the top of the ureters

c. inside of the bladder

d. behind the left knee.

20. What common problem occurs with the prostate gland in middle aged men?

a. it shrinks, causing uncontrolled release of urine

b. it shrinks, causing urine retention

c. it enlarges, causing uncontrolled release of urine

d. it enlarges, causing urine retention.

21. What is endometriosis?

a. inflammation of the endometriosis

b. growth of endometrial tissue that has spread to   other sites

c. a form of uterine cancer

d. heavy bleeding with menstruation

22. What is cystitis?

a. a growth in or on the skin called a cyst

b. an infection of the cervix , (neck of the uterus)

c. inflammation of the bladder

d. a shortened urethra.

23. What is a yeast infection?

a. infection of the cervix

b. an overgrowth of yeast infecting the vaginal area

c. infection of the ureter

d. infection of the vagina.

24. What is a urinary tract infection?

a. kidney inflammation

b. inflammation of the cervix

c. inflammation of the ovaries

d. an infection of one or more structures in the urinary tract

25. What is herpes simplex caused by?

a. bacteria   b. fungus

c. virus   d. parasite

26. Herpes simplex is not considered contagious.

a. true

b. false

27. The rule of thumb when treating babies and young children is to use;

a. 2 drops of essential oils per year in age

b. 3 drops of essential oils per year in age

c. 1 drop of essential oils per year in age

d. ½ drop of essential oils per year in age

28. Where does the finest essential oil of rose originate?

a. Rose Otto from Bulgaria

b. Rose centifolia from Yugoslavia

c. Rose centifolia from China

d. Rose gallica from Canada

29. How is the finer quality of rose extracted?

a. steam distillation of the petals

b. steam distillation of the leaves

c. enfleurage of the petals

d. maceration of the petals

30. What are the three main areas that rose can help?

a. female reproductive system

b. tonic to the body

c. headaches

d. fungal infections

e. uplifter, treats depression, grief, etc.

31. Where does essential oil of jasmine originate?

a. Algeria, Morocco, Egypt

b. France, China, Italy

c. Turkey, England, Germany

d. Algeria, Morocco, France, Egypt, China, Italy Turkey

32. How is jasmine extracted?
a. enfleurage of the flowers
b. pressing of the flowers
c. steam distillation of the flowers
d. maceration of the flowers

33. What are the three main areas that jasmine can help?
a. female reproductive system
b. tonic to the body
c. skin care
d. fungal infections
e. uplifter, treats depression, grief, etc.

34. When should you avoid using jasmine?
a. high blood pressure
b. its a skin irritant
c. pregnancy
d. low blood pressure

35. How is essential oil of sandalwood extracted?
a. steam distillation of the leaves
b. enfleurage of the whole tree
c. pressing of the tree bark
d. steam distillation of the mature heartwood of the tree

36. What are the three main area that sandalwood can help?
a. skin problems   b. high blood pressure
c. urinary tract problems d. respiratory problems
e. nervous disorders

37. When should you avoid using sandalwood?
a. no known contra-indications
b. its a skin irritant
c. pregnancy
d. low blood pressure

38. Where does essential oil of benzoin originate?
a. Guave, Java and Sumatra
b. China, Japan, and India
c. Canada, United Kingdom and Iraq
d. Java, Sumatra and Thailand

39. How is benzoin extracted?
a. a resinoid or absolute produced from the gum of the tree
b. a resinoid or absolute produced from the flowers of the tree
c. a distillation from the leaves and the twigs of the tree
d. a resinoid dissolved in ethyl glycol

40. What are the three areas where benzoin can help?
a. skin problems   b. high blood pressure
c. urinary tract problems d. respiratory problems
e. nervous disorders

41. When should you avoid using benzoin?
a. no known contra-indications
b. its a skin irritant
c. pregnancy
d. low blood pressure

42. Which type(s) of essential oils should   NEVER be used during the first 3 - 4 months of pregnancy?
a. emmenagogue
b. anti-spasmodic
c. toxic
d. muscle relaxant
e. those that strengthen contraction
f. diuretics

43. Chamomile and lavender should NEVER   be used during pregnancy.
a. true
b. false

44. Which essential oils should not be used during pregnancy?
a. aniseed   b. armoise
c. arnicad   d. basil
e. black pepper   f. bergamot
g. clary sage   h. coriander
i. cypress   j. dill
k. eucalyptus   l. fennel
m. frankincense   n. geranium
o. hyssop   p. jasmine
q. juniper   r. marjoram
s. melissa   t. manuka
u. myrrh   v. origanum
w. pennyroyal   x. peppermint
y. rosemary   z. rosewood
aa. rose   bb. sage
cc. sandalwood   dd. tea tree
ee. thyme   ff. wintergreen

Answer Sheet - Lesson #9

(Keep the questions for review. Circle the correct answer/s and return these sheets only to your instructor.)

1. A   B   C   D

2. A   B   C   D

3. A   B   C   D

4. A   B   C   D

5. A   B   C   D

6. A   B   C   D

7. A   B   C   D

8. A   B   C   D

9. A   B   C   D

10. A   B   C   D

11. A   B   C   D

12. A   B   C   D

13. A   B   C   D

14. A   B   C   D

15. A   B   C   D

16. A   B   C   D

17. A   B   C   D

18. A   B   C   D

19. A   B   C   D

20. A   B   C   D

21. A   B   C   D

22. A   B   C   D

23. A   B   C   D

24. A   B   C   D

25. A   B   C   D

26. a. true   b. false

27. A   B   C   D

28. A   B   C   D

29. A   B   C   D

30. A   B   C   D   E

31. A   B   C   D

32. A   B   C   D

33. A   B   C   D   E

34. A   B   C   D

35. A   B   C   D

36. A   B   C   D   E

37. A   B   C   D

38. A   B   C   D

39. A   B   C   D

40. A   B   C   D   E

41. A   B   C   D

42. A   B   C   D   E   F

43. a. true   b. false

44.
a.   b.   c.   d.
e.   f.   g.   h.
i.   j.   k.   l.
a.   n.   o.   p.
q.   r.   s.   t.
u.   v.   w.   x.
y.   z.   aa.   bb.
cc.   dd.   ee.   ff.

LESSON
TEN

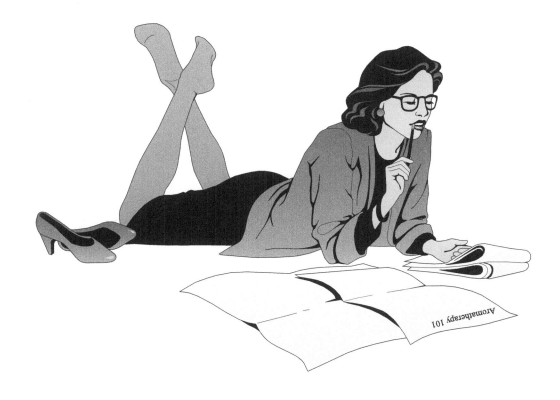

Lesson #10

Table of Contents

Bibliography:
The Simon & Schuster, Anatomy & Physiology by Dr. James Bevan.
Aromatherapy A to Z by Patricia Davis.
Aromatherapy Workbook by Shirley price
A textbook of Holistic Aromatherapy by Arnould-Taylor

An Introduction to the Skin

THE CELL

Our bodies are composed of cells, tissues organs and systems. Each of these could not exist without the other, as they depend upon one another on an interactive level for health and communication. The levels of organization are as follows:

Cells build tissues
Tissues form organs
Organs create a body system
Body systems form an organism ie. humanity.

The cell is the smallest, basic structural unit of the skin, yet it is responsible for the body's metabolism and reproduction. It is the fundamental basic unit of all living matter. Although every part of the body is made up of cells, each cell is different in size, shape and structure, according to its function. Therefore, each cell is specialized to allow the body to carry out its vital functions. For example, blood cells transport oxygen through the blood vessels and remove carbon dioxide. Nerve cells communicate and co-ordinate the body systems, muscle cells provide movement of the limbs, and bone cells support the body.

Function of the cell
1. To create and repair all parts of the body.
2. To help blood circulation by carrying food to the blood and waste matter away from the blood.
3. To control all body functions.
4. Certain cells are capable of reproduction.
5. The cell is capable of metabolism (*absorbing and consuming nutrients to form energy*)

Structure of the cell
It is estimated that the human body consists of over 75 trillion cells. The individual size of a person is not determined by the cell size, but rather the number of cells an individual possesses. The cell has three main components:
1) Cell (*plasma*) Membrane - this forms the outer boundary
2) Cytoplasm -this is found inside the cell membrane and surrounds the nucleus and other organelles.
3) Organelles - these are specialized structures within the cell that carry out specific functions

1. Cell Membrane
This is a very thin porous skin that is composed of several layers of molecules. The inner and outer layers are composed of protein molecules. Between this is a double layer of fat molecules (*lipids*). These lipids provide a barrier between water soluble materials both inside and outside the cell and protects the cell from the external environment.

2. Cytoplasm

   Is the living liquid matter that is found between the cell membrane and the nucleus. It contains 75 - 90% water plus organic and inorganic compounds. Its consistency is slightly thicker than water which holds the organelles in suspension.

3. Organelles

   These are specialized structures that perform specific cellular functions. Some of these include:

   Centrosomes   which are important in cell reproduction.

   Mitochondria which contain enzymes that provide the cell with energy and also is responsible for cell respiration.

   Vacuoles   are fluid filled bubbles found in the cytoplasm that contain food material or waste supplies

   Ribosomes   make proteins for the cells use.

   Lysosomes   manufacture digestive enzymes that break down large molecules into smaller ones, so these products can be converted into other necessary chemicals and substances.

4. Nucleus   Is found in the centre of the cell.
   - It is enclosed by a nuclear membrane, which is a thin porous layer of tissue.
   - It is responsible for cell reproduction and cell metabolism.
   - It contains one or more small bodies called nucleoli which float freely inside the nucleus, which are responsible for the synthesis of RNA.

The nucleus is the largest organelle of the cell. It is the control centre of the cell because it is responsible for all metabolic functions and plays an important part in cell reproduction.

Both RNA and DNA (*ribonucleic acid and deoxyribonucleic acid*) are found within the nucleus.

DNA is a long spiral-shaped molecule (*similar in appearance to a twisted ladder*) that has the ability to duplicate itself, therefore passing on all necessary information to any new cells, DNA is also the building blocks of chromosomes. The DNA contains genes, these genes contain an individuals' hereditary information or genetic code.

Each human chromosome (*there is 46 in total*) contains 20,000 genes. It is very easy to understand why no two people in the world are identical, taking into consideration the vast number of possible genetic combinations.

Cell Metabolism

METABOLISM   Is the chemical change that absorbed foods undergo in the body cells.

There are two forms of metabolism.

1.	ANABOLISM	The building up of cellular tissues. During anabolism, the cells absorb water, food, and oxygen for growth, reproduction and repair. This is considered the constructive part of metabolism.
2.	CATABOLISM	Breaks down cellular tissue. During catabolism, the cells consume what they have absorbed to perform specialized functions, such as muscular effort, secretion, or digestion. This is considered the destructive part of metabolism.

Metabolism goes on continually inside the cell.
A simpler example of metabolism is that people require nutrients and food for growth, repair and maintenance of a healthy body - this is anabolism because we are feeding the body to build up cellular tissue.

Then, during physical activity catabolism takes place because the cells are consuming or using up the nutrients they have absorbed by breaking down cellular tissue.

Cell Reproduction

Cells reproduce by division called mitosis. This enables growth and repair of tissue. It is the replication of a cell, into two daughter cells, resulting in both of these newly formed cells being identical to the original cell. Mitosis assures that any newly formed cells contain the same number and composition of chromosomes.

Mitosis is generally a process that is controlled. Therefore, the replication process will be dormant when there is no need for additional cells to be produced. Occasionally, the control is lost and the cells continuously undergo division, which lead to the formation of tumours. Tumours are either benign (*do not spread*) or malignant (*cancerous and do spread throughout the body*).

Cell Permeability

All materials that enter or exit the cell (*ie: food, water, oxygen, etc.*) must pass through this cell membrane.   Only certain molecules are allowed to enter and exit.   This is called selectively permeable.

The permeability of the cell will depend on four different things:

1) Size of molecules - water and amino acids are allowed easy access in and out of the cell, while larger protein molecules are restricted due to their size. (Essential oils are very minute in their molecular structure.)

---

2)   Solubility in lipids - the cell membrane is composed of 50% of lipids.   Therefore the natural path of penetration of the skin is through lipids. If the substance is soluble in lipids, entrance to the cell will be gained. (Essential oils are soluble in lipids.)

3)   Presence of a carrier molecule - there are specialized molecules that are "carriers". Their sole purpose is to carry certain substances into the cell. Glucose requires a carrier in order to gain entry into a cell.

4)   Charge of an ion - the skin is capable of ionization. In other words, if the charge of an ion (substance) is an opposite charge to that of the cell membrane, then the ion will be attracted into the cell. Similar charges will result in a "repelling" of each other.

TISSUES

Definition - tissues are made up of similar constructed cells carrying out the same functions. The cell shape, size and arrangement determine the structure of the tissue.

There are five types of tissue.
1. Epithelial tissue
2. Connective tissue
3. Muscular tissue
4. Nerve tissue
5. Liquid tissue

We are going to discuss the first two:
Epithelial tissue covers the surface of the body, lines the internal organs, respiratory and digestive tract. Epithelial tissue is packed tightly together with little intercellular material between them.

The surface or top layer is always free and is exposed, as it is not attached to any other tissue. It contains no blood vessels and is nourished by the underlying tissue, it regenerates rapidly, as large amounts are destroyed and replaced or sloughed-off.

There are two types of epithelial tissue:
a. Simple
b. Stratified

Simple Epithelial tissue -consists of one layer of cells. These cells are renewed by minor mitosis and are nourished by the underlying tissues as there are no blood vessels in this area. This type of tissue is found internally - it lines the body's inner organs such as blood vessels, the small intestines and the lungs.

This type of tissue can be squamous, cuboidal or columnar.

Stratified Epithelial tissue - consists of more than one layer of cells, one on top of the other. Its main purpose is to protect the underlying tissue and the area of the body that are subject to considerable surface friction. It protect the mouth, oesophagus and makes up the outer layer of the skin.

Note: *Most common types of cancer arise from the epithelial tissue. One reason for this may be due to the frequent exposure that these cells have with carcinogens (cancer causing agents).*

Connective tissue - supports, protects and binds together the organs and other tissues of the body. Some example of connective tissue are:

Cartilage: gives strength, support.

Bone: protects the body

Tendons: connects bone to muscles

Ligaments: attach one bone to another

Adipose tissue: this type of tissue contains fat cells. Fat is stored in the cell pushing the cytoplasm and nucleus towards the cell membrane. This fatty tissue is found under the skin. It protects and supports and is a reserve source of energy and is used when the body runs out of carbohydrates.

Most cells found within connective tissue are fibroblasts which are long irregularly shaped cells. These cells produce two different types of fibres;

Collagen fibres - Gives strength and flexibility to the connective tissue. It is the main constituent of connective tissue. These are white fibres, formed from protein, that are very tough and resistant to a pulling force, but are somewhat flexible.

Elastin fibres - contain the protein elastin which allows the ligament to be stretched. These fibres give an elastic quality to the expandable tissue such as the arteries, vocal cords and the loose connective tissue under the skin. These are smaller than collagenous fibres but also provide strength and have great elasticity.

Fibroblast production decreases as we age. There is less collagen and elastin fibres being produced, resulting in loss of elasticity, sagging and ageing the skin.

DIAGRAM OF THE SKIN

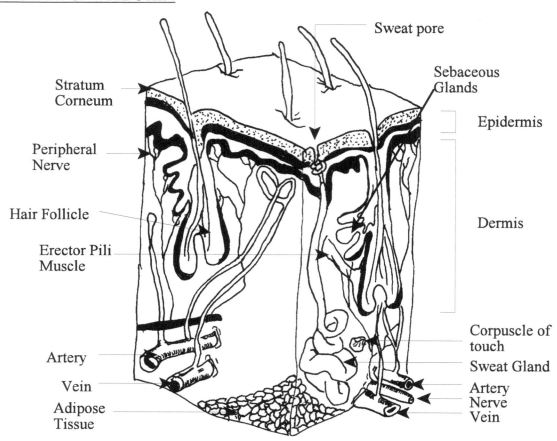

Sweat pore

Stratum Corneum

Sebaceous Glands

Epidermis

Peripheral Nerve

Hair Follicle

Dermis

Erector Pili Muscle

Artery

Corpuscle of touch

Sweat Gland

Vein

Artery
Nerve
Vein

Adipose Tissue

The skin and its derivatives (hair, glands and nails) constitute the integumentary system. It is the largest organ of the body. It makes up 15% of our total body weight. The skin is constantly shedding and replacing itself through new cells from below. It varies in thickness in different areas of the body. The thickest areas are the palms of the hands and the soles of the feet while the thinnest areas are the eyelids and the lips.

The skin provides a protective barrier that helps prevent damage occurring to internal organs from traumas as well as substances like chemicals, pollution, bacterial invasion, microorganisms and ultraviolet radiation.

Vitamin D is metabolized in the skin. This is an important ingredient in the formation of bone.

The skin is able to absorb and excrete. It can move substances such as chemicals and drugs into the skin. This is the premise in which aromatherapy essential oils work. Not only are they able to gain easy access into the skin (refer to the factors of permeability), but they are further absorbed into the bloodstream and carried throughout the body to assist in healing.

Temperature regulation of the skin occurs through specialized receptor cells called thermoreceptors. They will react to heat by inducing sweating, or in cold situations, they will create shivering to induce warmth.

Touch receptors called Meissners corpuscles are located all over the skin.

The Epidermis
The epidermis is the outermost part of the skin that is composed of different layers. It is devoid of blood vessels, and nerves.

The top layer is known as the stratum corneum and is composed of tightly packed dead cells call keratin. This is the layer that is visible to us. These cells are rubbed off during the normal wear and tear of the skin.

Beneath the stratum corneum lies the stratum germinativum or granular layer. Then we have the squamous cell layer. This layer contains the most abundant cells of the skin. Then finally we have the stratum germinativum or the basal cell layer. This is the lowest layer of of the epidermis and it sits upon the dermal layer. It contains specialized cells called melanocytes which produce a pigment called melanin, which is responsible for the colouring of the skin. The more active the cells, the greater the quantity of melanin produced, hence the varied colours in different races of people. Melanin protects the skin from sun damage and the darker your natural skin colour is, the greater protection you have from the sun. Sun tans do not protect your skin, remember to use a sunscreen for protection.

New cellular growth begins in the basal layer. As this growth takes place, the cells move upwards towards to stratum corneum and gradually keratinize (die) during this process. Once they have reached the upper layer, they have died. This cycle takes approximately 28 days for completion. The cells spend approximately 2 weeks moving towards the stratum corneum and then another 2 weeks before they are shed.

The keratinization process is the change in the epidermal cells within their compositional structure as they are created in the basal layer and pass upwards into the uppermost layer of the epidermis known as the stratum corneum. From living metabolically functioning cells, that gradually change into flat lifeless cells composed of the complex protein substance called keratin. It is the unique properties of keratin that gives the skin its protective properties.

Keratin serves as a barrier to physical and chemical injury and provides a protective covering membrane that helps maintain the body's internal homeostasis.

Dermis
The dermis, varies in thickness from 1-4mm, is composed of dense fibrous tissue that provides for strength, extensibility and elasticity. The dermis is the underlying, or inner layer of the skin. It is a highly vascular and sensitive layer of connective tissue, that is made up of three types of fibres. These are called collagen, elastin and reticulum.

The dermis contains blood vessels, lymph vessels, nerves, sweat and oil glands, hair follicles, erector pili muscles and papillae.

The nerve endings in the skin are responsible for the feelings of sensation. For the therapist it is the hands which are the most important communicating role. Touch is fundamental to the development of a healthy human being, and touch deprivation in the early stages of life is known to inhibit the emotional and physical growth of a child. It is important to remember that the need to be touched in a caring way does not stop in childhood. The power of a caring touch and its ability to heal, share empathy and to comfort is vital in the holistic field. Touch can be remarkably effective in the reduction of pain, lowering of blood pressure, and control of nervous irritability.

The main objective of touch is to soothe and to provide a comforting connection that is calming and allows the powerful healing mechanisms of the body to function.

Collagen and elastin fibres are abundant in the dermis. Collagen makes up about 70% of the dermis. It gives structure and support for cells and blood vessels, allows for stretching and contraction of the skin, provides strength and aids in the healing of wounds. Reticulum fibres help link bundles of collagen together while the protein called elastin, gives elasticity and pliability to the dermis..

Moisture is important in keeping this network supple. It is the skins collagen condition and not the facial muscles that causes the lines and the wrinkles. Cells within the dermis called fibroblasts are responsible for producing the collagen and elastin fibres. As we age, the fibroblasts decrease their production ability.

Subcutaneous Tissue
This is a fatty layer found below the dermis, also referred to as adipose tissue. It attaches the skin to the underlying tissue and organs. It is thicker than the dermis but is absent in areas such as the eyelids, nipples, and shins. It serves as a heat insulator and stores fats for use as energy, all while acting as a shock absorber to protect the internal organs from trauma. It varies in thickness according to age and health of the individual. It gives smoothness and contour to the body and is distributed differently in males and females.

Epidermis - this is the outermost layer of the skin. It forms the protective covering of the skin of the body. It contains no blood vessels, but has many small nerve endings the epidermis is approximately 0.5 mm thick on the eyelids to about 6mm on the soles of the feet, and contain the following layers:

Stratum germinativum (Basal layer)
This single layer contains cells from which new epidermal cells are constantly being produced. It is found resting on the papillae of the dermis. The cells are closely packed together and are conical in shape. As they multiply, the previously formed cells are pushed towards the surface.

This cellular multiplication is known as "cellular regeneration" and it may be increased or decreased by a number of factors from old age to health states. Melanocyte cells are responsible foe producing the pigment melanin and are found withing this basal layer. Melanin determines the colour of skin.

Aromatherapy For Holistic Therapists - Lesson Ten

Stratum spinosum (Stratum malpighii)
This layer is composed of several layers (5-10) of nucleated cells which vary in size and shape. It is the upper portion of this layer which is called the prickle cell layer. This is because the cells are linked by fine threads and their projections give a prickly or spiky appearance. These cells have tonofilaments (tiny fibres, similar to rope) that crisscross the cytoplasm attaching to other prickle cells. Their function is to hold the cells together, giving stability and holding the epidermis intact.

Stratum Granulosum (Granular layer)
This has between one and four layers of flattened cells that contain a nucleus. As the cells from the layer beneath ascends to the surface they become progressively larger and accumulate granules containing a substance called "keratohyalin" which is involved in the first step of keratin formation on the skin.

Stratum Lucidum
This layer contains a narrow transparent layer of cells that are almost at the end of their life span. The cells are becoming dehydrated, and filled with a substance called "eleidin", which is produced from keratohyalin, and will eventually form keratin. This layer forms a barrier, an electro-physical barrier that prevents the penetration of water and other substances into the deeper layers. It holds in moisture and is found on the palms and soles of the feet.

Stratum Corneum (Horny layer)
This is the external layer of the skin and is composed of some 15-20 layers of flattened irregular shaped cells that are sometimes referred to as "corneocytes". They assume this flattened form from evaporation of fluid contents. There is only 10-15% water in this layer, as compared to 70% in deeper layers. These cells consist almost entirely of keratin. It is the protector of the skin, preventing excessive dehydration of the skin tissues. As the cells near the surface they "desquamate" (shed) or are rubbed off during normal wear and tear of the skin.

The amount of water here is influenced by internal factors such as medication and health, as well as by external factors, humidity and climate. If the atmosphere is humid the horny layer will absorb moisture, If the atmosphere is dry, we lose water faster than it is replaced. The cells in this layer become brittle and curl-up causing cracks in the skin.

Dermis
The dermis is composed of dense fibrous tissue allowing for strength, and movement. The dermis is the underlying or inner layer of skin. Highly vascular and sensitive, containing blood vessels, lymph, nerves and oil glands, hair follicles, erector pili muscles and papillae.

Collagen and elastin fibres are abundant in the dermis. Collagen makes up about 70% of the dermis. It gives structure and support for cells and blood vessels, allow for stretching and contraction of the skin, provides strength and aids in healing of wounds. The space between the collagen fibres contain a protein called elastin, which gives the skin its elasticity.

Moisture is important in keeping this network supple. It is the skins collagen condition and not the facial muscles that cause the lines and wrinkles. Cells within the dermis called fibroblasts are responsible for producing the collagen and elastin fibres. As we age, the fibroblasts decrease their production ability. These fibres are supported in a structureless gel-like material called "ground substance".

It is mainly composed of mucopolysaccharide, particularly hyaluronic acid which helps retain water and hold cells together. This ground substance resists compression and acts as a shock absorber to help the skin resist pressure.

Subcutaneous tissue
This is a fatty layer found below the dermis, also referred to as adipose tissue. It attaches the skin to the underlying tissue and organs. It serves as a heat insulator and stores fats for use as energy, and acting as a cushion. It varies in thickness according to age, sex, and health, it gives smoothness and contour to the body.

Penetration routes of the skin
The skin, up until the 1960's, was believed to be a barrier and able to resist any form of substance from penetrating into the body. We know today, however, that it is an effective way to deliver medication and essential oils etc. into the skin to the body. This route is known as transdermal penetration. The substances will be carried through the skin directly into the blood stream. It must be realized that the size of the molecule is the deciding factor. Some molecules are too large to penetrate into the skin.

Essential oils are extremely small and are able to penetrate the skin with ease, through the lipids (saturated fats) and, as essential oils are soluble in fats, they can enter the dermis to reach the blood capillaries and lymph. Urine tested shortly after applying essential oils is found to contain that oil.

The four different way to penetrate the skin:
1. The hair follicle
2. Sebaceous/sudoriferous glands
3. Transcellular route, this route is through the skin cells, eventually into the dermal layer and on into the blood and lymph vessels.
4. Intercellular rout, this rout is the best for penetration of the epidermis. The lipids found in the intercellular cement (in between the cells) and will accept substances in that are similar in composition. In other words solubility in lipids allows for permeability.

Other factors that influence penetration
An excessively thick stratum corneum will hinder product penetration. This is obvious due to the large build up of dead skin cells.

People who suffer from an oily skin, will not have as in-depth penetration as well. The excess sebum will slow down any absorbency. Temperature of the skin will also influence penetration. A warm skin is generally more accepting due to the fact that heat causes activity within the molecules thereby increasing cellular activity. Also remember that hot or warm temperatures (steam, compresses etc.) will dilate the follicles while cool or cold temperatures will constrict the follicle.

Aging of the skin

The natural process of wear and tear will naturally affects the skin. At puberty, adjustment to increased hormonal activity usually manifests itself on the skin of the adolescent. By the age of twenty, the system of the body should be fully grown and developed. If the body is healthy, the skin should be at its optimum, glowing, firm and without lines and wrinkles.

Aging of the skin begins at age 25, and becomes more noticeable in the mid-forties. It is from the mid-thirties that facial skin starts to lose its firmness and fine lines and wrinkles arrear, and if there is any loss of muscle tone there will also be sagging of the skin.

In the forties and fifties, the lines of expression and furrows deepen and loss of muscle tone will accentuate this. This is largely due to subcutaneous fat and connective tissue losing its elasticity. The papillary (upper) layer of the dermis flattens out so that the skin is finer and thinner. During menopause the activity of the sebaceous glands is reduced and the skin becomes dryer.

As we grow older the cell's capacity to reproduce, grow and renew themselves decreases, and in older people cell regeneration slows down due to lack of nourishment as the arterioles thicken and venous circulation is impaired. Over the years the sebaceous glands and hair follicles atrophy and there is general loss of colour and thinning of the hair. More keratin is produced and the skin becomes dry and looks dull. Skin tags may appear and age spots occur, especially on the back of the hands.

This process is effected by environmental conditions (sunlight, weather, chemical irritants) as well as by intrinsic (hereditary) conditions.

To Summarize the Changes Within the Skin Due to Aging:

1)   breakdown of collagen and elastin fibres, resulting in wrinkles and sagging

2)   loss of subcutaneous tissue, resulting in sensitivity to temperature changes

3)   atrophy (wasting away) of the sebaceous glands, causing dry skin

4)   decrease in melanin production *(this is a pigment that is found in the hair, skin and eyes that serves as a means of protection by screening out any harmful ultraviolet rays)* that results in grey hair, and pigmentation *(age)* spots.

The Effect of Water on the Skin

The skin is 50 to 75% water. This is maintained by the secretion of sebum which creates a protective coating on the surface of the skin. This layer of oil that is produced slows down the evaporation of water in the skin and prevents any excess moisture from penetrating into it. If the natural oils are removed, or lost, the protection is lost. This is why when you are dealing with a dry skin type, you are generally finding dehydration present as well.

Effects of Ultraviolet Radiation on the Skin

Ultraviolet radiation, whether its from the sun or a sunbed, produces damaging changes within the skin. This damage is cumulative, over a period of many years, although one days overexposure can result in short term changes such as a severe sunburn. Long-term damage caused by excessive ultraviolet radiation results in increased wrinkling, loss of elasticity, liver spots, a *"leather type"* skin appearance, and skin cancer.

Unfortunately these effects do not appear for years, hence, uninformed teenagers and young adults accelerate the skins aging and open the door to skin cancers that may arise later in life. Tanning beds can increase these potential problems.

Skin cancers are the most common form of cancer. Most are curable through surgery. These are called Basil Cell Carcinoma and Squamous Cell Carcinoma. However, Melanoma Cancer of the Melanocytes spreads rapidly and if it is not detected in the early stages, it will result in death in 45% of the cases.

You can reduce the risks of overexposure to ultraviolet radiation by limiting the time in the sunlight between the hours of 11 am to 3 PM and by using a sunscreen with a minimum SPF 15. Remember that sunscreens are not cumulative. If you have applied an SPF 8 and then applied a SPF4 on top, you still only have a maximum SPF8 coverage. Also remember that sunscreens should be applied daily to any exposed area of the body irregardless of the season.

The Glands Of the Skin

There are two types of duct glands found within the skin:

1)   the sudoriferous or sweat glands
2)   the sebaceous or oil glands

1)   There are approximately two million sudoriferous glands in the body. They consist of a coiled base and a tube-like duct which ends at the skins surface to form the sweat pore. Almost all parts of the body are supplied with these glands. These glands are under the control of the sympathetic nervous system regulate the body temperature and help to eliminate waste products from the body. They are richly supplied with blood vessels.

There are two types of sweat glands:

i) apocrine glands - these have a duct that empties the secretion into the hair follicle. They occur primarily in the axillary *(underarm)* and the pubic regions. They produce a more fatty type of secretion than the eccrine glands. Breakdown of the secretion by bacteria leads to body odour under the arms and in the groin. Their activity is increased by heat, exercise, emotions and drugs of a certain type.

ii) eccrine glands - most of the glands are of this type. These are found all over the body and they secrete their secretions onto the surface of the skin. Practically all parts of the body are supplied with sweat glands, but they are more numerous on the palms of the hands, soles of the feet, forehead and the underarms.

The sudoriferous glands secrete perspiration or sweat. This is a mixture of water, salt, urea, uric acid, ammonia, amino acids, simple sugars and vitamins. It also has anti-bacterial substances which help the body's defence against infection.

2) The oil glands are small saccular, glandular organs. They secrete sebum out of their glands, through the hair follicle and then onto the surface of the skin. This sebum lubricates the skin and helps to prevent the evaporation of moisture. Sebum is a mixture of fats and lipids.

Some of the substances found within this mixture are triglycerides, sphingolipids, glycolipids, phospholipids, cholesterol, ceramides, fatty acids and waxes.
Sebaceous glands are found over the entire skin surface, excluding the palms of the hands and the soles of the feet. They are most abundant in the scalp and face and are very numerous around the apertures of the nose and mouth.

Sebum secretion varies greatly with age, state of health, etc. It is subject to the activities of certain endocrine glands and the nervous system. The secretion of sebum is more active during the warm months. It is very slight until puberty, when it greatly increases, then decreasing in the aged.

Excessive sebum is termed seborrhoea. Seborrhoea is often accompanied by an enlargement of the gland and a number of skin disorders.

Other skin conditions found
Acne - acne is a chronic inflammatory disorder of the skin. Common acne is known as acne vulgaris. It is the commonest of all skin disorders. The outbreaks are generally worse in males than females because the main cause is an increase in the production of male hormones. Normally, the sebaceous glands produces the sebum, but with acne, there is an overproduction that often plugs up the follicle. Acne appears in a variety of different types ranging from presence of comedones *(blackheads)* to deep-seated skin conditions.

STRESS AND ACNE
Acne is only one of the disorders that can arise from stress. Generally an acne skin can be brought under control *(not necessarily cleared up*!) in a relatively short period of time, but an acne condition resulting from stress could become a long-term ongoing problem. *(Whether or not an individual suffers from acne will be determined within their genetic makeup or in the DNA)*. But acne caused by stress can make acne appear for as little as a few days, or as long as years.

Stress does not cause acne in everyone. However, when stress does arise, whether or not it is positive (*i.e.; marriage*) or negative, there will be hormonal changes within the body. The sympathetic nervous system (*under the autonomic system*) begins to take charge in stressful situations and by doing so begins to increase the body's metabolic rate, the heart rate and constricts the intestinal blood vessels (*which can result in poor digestion*) as well as other internal changes. In response to these changes, the body's adrenal glands secrete hormones that causes the sebaceous glands to produce more oils, resulting in acne. The same is true with premenstrual acne. There is no quick fix under these situations, but realizing the cause and alleviating some of the stress may greatly improve the condition.

Understanding Sight and Hearing

<u>SIGHT</u>

The eyes

The eye is a globular structure filled with a jelly-like fluid under slight pressure to give it firmness. Our sense of sight is the response of the brain to light stimuli and these are received through the eye. The eyeball itself is a hollow, spherical structure, its walls consisting of three principal layers:

1.   The sclera or tough fibrous, opaque coat, the sclera being modified in front to form the clear, transparent cornea. In other words, the white outer surface, the "sclera" surrounds the eyeball except for the transparent cornea in the front.

2.   The choroid or middle coat which consists of an interlacement of blood vessels and pigment granules supported by loose connective tissue; the iris being a pigmented, muscular curtain suspended behind the cornea. In the centre of this iris is an aperture known as the pupil through which light reaches the interior of the eye.

3.   The retina forms the delicate inner layer of the eyeball. In this layer are found the receptor and sensory optic nerve endings sometimes referred to as rods and cones.

DIAGRAM OF THE EYEBALL

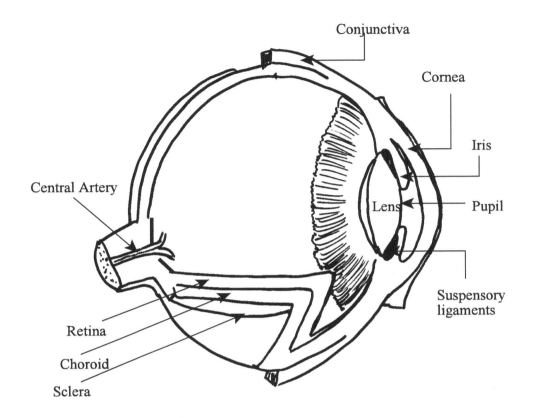

The eyeball has a number of appendages, primarily the various muscles which directionally rotate it and the lachrymal or tear glands which moisten and clean the outer surface of the eye. Excess secretion of the lachrymal glands overflow onto the cheeks as tears. From the inner corners of the eyes the tears drain into a channel which opens into the nose, which is why weeping is sometimes accompanied by sniffling.

The pupil controls the light image by contracting in bright light and dilating in dim light. These light images strike the retina as an upside down image which is then conveyed to the brain through the optic nerve. The brain then re-inverts the impulse so that it becomes a right side up image.

The pupil is a circular opening in front of the lens, varies in size very rapidly depending on the amount of light falling on the retina. The circular and radial muscle fibres in the iris are under the control of the autonomic nervous system. This prevents over-stimulation of the retina by brilliant light. The pupil can vary in size from 1-8 millimetres.

Iris
The iris is the continuation of the choroid in front of the lens. Its colour, genetically determined, depends on the way in which the pigments are distributed.

The lens
The lens is a soft, bi-convex, transparent structure in a thin, tough capsule. It divides the anterior third of the eye from the posterior two-thirds, being held by the suspensory ligaments to the ciliary muscle fibres.

The ciliary body contains the ciliary muscles, which alter the shape of the lens. It is close to the ducts that change the aqueous humour and together with the iris and the choroid coat, forms the uveal tract.

The conjunctiva
The conjunctiva covers the outer surface of the cornea as it bulges forward. Much of the focusing of the eye is made by the convex shape of the cornea, finer adjustments are made by the contraction of the ciliary muscle altering the lens shape.

The aqueous humour
The "aqueous humour" is produced by the ciliary body and circulates through the posterior, behind the iris, and anterior chambers of the eye to bathe the inner surface of the cornea and lens.

Vitreous humour
The vitreous humour fills the posterior two-thirds of the eyeball. Through the centre there is a thin, vessel structure that is the empty remnant of the foetal blood vessel that used to supply the lens in the foetus, known as the hyaloid canal.

Choroid coat
The choroid coat lines the inner surface of the sclera and has brown pigmented cells to absorb light.

Optic nerve
The optic nerve, containing one million nerve fibres, penetrates the sclera and choroid coats and the nerves spread round the inner surface of the eyeball to form the retina. The point at which the optic nerve enters is known as the "blind spot", as there are no light-sensitive nerve cells at this point. The optic nerve is accompanied by an artery and vein that spread over the retina.

Retina
The retina consists of light-sensitive cells or cones for red, green and blue, and the rods for shades from grey to white.

****Please note, you will not find a reference in the following pages in the treatment of eye disorders or diseases. Aromatherapy is not an indicated treatment for eye problems. Essential oils should never be used around or in the eyes. Caution should always be noted when preparations that contain essential oils are used in the facial area. If you happen to accidentally place any in the eye, immediately flush with water for 5-10 minutes. Seek medical attention if required.

HEARING

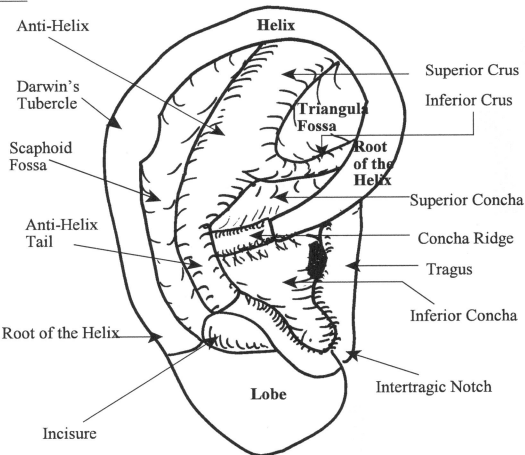

The ears

The ear is normally divided into three structures:

1. The external ear which consists of the auricle and the external acoustic sometimes called the auditory meatus. It also contains ceruminous glands which secrete cerumen or wax. In between the external ear and the middle ear is the drum or tympanic membrane which is a parchment-like membrane which lies obliquely across the external and middle ear.

2. The middle ear or tympanum is a small cavity about five eighths of an inch long by half an inch high by half an inch wide, two principal structures communicate with the middle ear.

    ▸ The auditory (eustachian tube) about one and half inches long, which passes from the nasal pharynx to the middle ear allowing passage of air from the throat to the ear, enabling air pressure on both sides of the drum to be equalised.
    ▸ The mastoid antrum which is an air-filled cavity above and behind the tympanum with which it communicates.

3. The internal ear. This consists of three parts:

    ▸ The osseous labyrinth.
    ▸ The membraneous labyrinth.
    ▸ The peril lymph which lies between the two.

    It is the osseous labyrinth which contains the three semicircular canals which are concerned with the control of balance.

The external ear collects and funnels sound waves or air vibrations to the tympanic membrane. When the sound waves strike the tympanic membrane it beings to vibrate.

These vibrations cause three tiny bones in the middle ear (the auditory ossicles) to vibrate as well. The auditory ossicles are popularly called the hammer, anvil and stirrup (malleus, incus & stapes).

The vibrations continue to the inner ear, to the cochlea which is filled with fluid and tiny nerve endings. These terminate in the auditory nerve which leads to the brain.

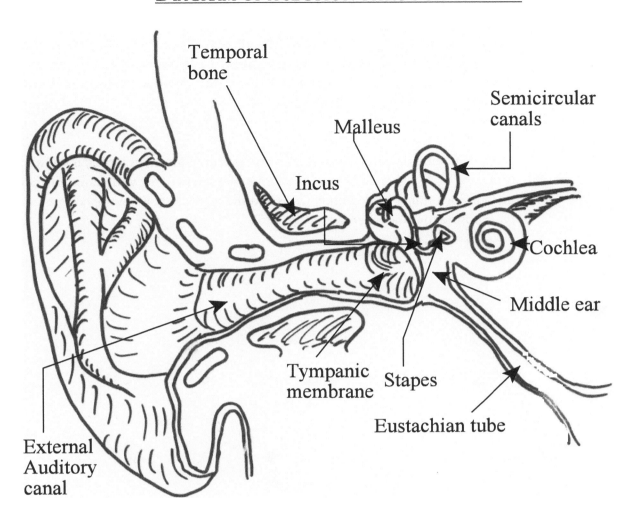

Temporal bone

Semicircular canals

Malleus

Incus

External Auditory canal

Tympanic membrane

Stapes

Cochlea

Middle ear

Eustachian tube

Conditions and Diseases of the Accessory Organs

Cataract

The lens of the eye is situated directly behind the pupil and in health is clear. With age and in some diseases such as diabetes it loses its transparency and becomes more and more opaque, gradually shutting out vision, this condition is known as cataract. It is not a growth but a biochemical change in the lens.

Conjunctivitis

This is inflammation of the conjunctiva. In its acute contagious form it is known as 'pink eye'. It is caused by various forms of bacterial and virus infections and includes swimming pool conjunctivitis and the type which is developed as a result of exposure to ultra-violet rays.

Disease or Disorder	ACNE VULGARIS
Description	Acne is a common inflammatory disorder of the pilosebaceous (hair follicle and sebaceous gland) gland with the appearance of blackheads, whiteheads, pimples (with or without pus) and/or cysts. The peak acne years in females are 14 - 17 years in females an 16-19 years in males. Clearing of this condition generally occurs in the twenties. Acne is caused by four different factors. These include an increase production of sebum (oil), an abnormality in the bacteria of the skin, an inflammatory process and hardening of the pilosebaceous area.
Possible Allopathic Treatment	Allopathic treatment includes drug therapy in the form of topical drying agents such as clindamycin, benzoyl peroxide, and other drugs with various sulfur-resorcinol combinations. Internal drugs such as antibiotics are prescribed. The most commonly used are tetracyclines (variants include minocycline and doxycycline). They do not know how antibiotics work in the treatment of acne. It is thought that it is due to the antimicrobial and/or antiinflammatory abilities. Isotretinoin also known as Accutane is a derivative of the Vitamin A that is taken orally. It is a powerful drug with severe side effects and should never be used in cases of pregnancy or for those attempting to conceive.
Possible Holistic Aromatherapy Treatment	Anti-inflammatory essential oils; *Caraway, Teatree, Camphor, Chamomile, Fennel, Geranium, Jasmine, Peppermint, Benzoin, Frankincense, Myrrh and Patchouli.* Analgesic (Pain-killing) oils; *Bergamot, Cajeput, Coriander, Eucalyptus, Lemon grass, Niaouli, Black-pepper, Chamomile, Jasmine, Lavender, Marjoram, Peppermint, Rosemary and Ginger.* Anti-depressant essential oil; *Basil, Bergamot, Lemon grass, Clary Sage, Geranium, Jasmine, Lavender, Melissa, Orange Blossom, Patchouli, Rose, Sandalwood and Ylang Ylang.* Astringent essential oils; *Cypress, Frankincense, Geranium, Immortelle, Juniper, Lemon, Lime, Myrrh, Peppermint, Rosemary, Sandalwood, Yarrow* Antimicrobial essential oils; *Myrrh, Thyme*

Disease or Disorder	CONTACT DERMATITIS
Description	An acute or chronic skin inflammation that often has distinctive boundaries with a similar appearance of a rash (erythema with pain or pruritis). Can be caused by an inflammatory reaction initiated by the immune system in response to a certain allergic substance. Its a hypersensitive reaction.
Possible Allopathic Treatment	Avoidance of irritating substance is of first importance. Topical corticosteroid creams may be prescribed and/or topical drying agents. In more serious cases, oral corticosteroids such as prednisone may be given.
Possible Holistic Aromatherapy Treatment	Anti-inflammatory essential oils; *Caraway, Teatree, Camphor, Chamomile, Fennel, Geranium, Jasmine, Peppermint, Benzoin, Frankincense, Myrrh and Patchouli.* Analgesic (Pain-killing) oils; *Bergamot, Cajeput, Coriander, Eucalyptus, Lemon grass, Niaouli, Black-pepper, Chamomile, Jasmine, Lavender, Marjoram, Peppermint, Rosemary and Ginger.* Auto-immune enhancers; *Cinnamon leaf, Clove bud, Frankincense.* Cytophylactic; *Carrot seed, Frankincense, Geranium, Immortelle, Lavender, Mandarin, Palmerosa, Neroli, Rose* Anti-allergenic; *Chamomile, Melissa*

Disease or Disorder	ECZEMA
Description	The word eczema comes from the Greek word of ekzein which means "to boil out". It is a inflammatory disorder that results from both internal and external factors. It is considered a superficial skin inflammation (dermatitis). The appearance of this disorder includes small vesicles (blisters), redness, oozing, crusting and scaling with itching present. Different forms include allergic contact eczematous dermatitis caused by chemicals from plants, fabrics, cosmetics, and medications. Photoallergic contact eczematous dermatitis caused by a combination of ultraviolet light and a causitive chemical. Another common type is infectious eczematous dermatitis which is seen with open draining wounds. This type clears when the wound, the primary cause is treated. **Do not attempt to diagnose the type of eczema and remember do not touch this problem as there are infectious types present.
Possible Allopathic Treatment	Avoidance of irritating substance is of first importance. Topical corticosteroid creams may be prescribed and/or topical drying agents. In more serious cases, oral corticosteroids such as prednisone may be given.
Possible Holistic Aromatherapy Treatment	Anti-inflammatory essential oils; *Caraway, Teatree, Camphor, Chamomile, Fennel, Geranium, Jasmine, Peppermint, Benzoin, Frankincense, Myrrh and Patchouli.* Analgesic (Pain-killing) oils; *Bergamot, Cajeput, Coriander, Eucalyptus, Lemon grass, Niaouli, Black-pepper, Chamomile, Jasmine, Lavender, Marjoram, Peppermint, Rosemary and Ginger.* Auto-immune enhancers; *Cinnamon leaf, Clove bud, Frankincense.* Cytophylactic; *Carrot seed, Frankincense, Geranium, Immortelle, Lavender, Mandarin, Palmerosa, Neroli, Rose* Anti-allergenic; *Chamomile, Melissa*

Disease or Disorder	TINEA PEDIS (ATHLETE'S FOOT)
Description	A fungal infection of the foot normally found between the 4th or 5th toes and on the soles of the foot. The cause is T. mentogrophytes, T. rubrum and E. floccosum. They generally have a fissures (cracks) in the skin, vesicular-like (small blister) appearance and there may be some peeling of the skin involved. Itching is sometimes present. Infection is most common during the summer months and is spread in moist damp areas like public showers, swimming pools, locker rooms, etc. **Whether allopathic or holistic treatment is chosen, it must be stressed that the foot and in between the toes should always be dried thoroughly. Cotton socks and permeable footwear should be used.
Possible Allopathic Treatment	Topical antifungal preparations such as miconazole, clotrimazole, ciclopirox olamine cream and naftifine hydrochloride cream are used for treatment. For more extensive or serious cases, oral medications such as griseofulvin are given for systemic treatment. Allopathic treatment generally takes a minimum period of 90 days in order to see any results. It is traditionally up to 6 - 9 months to see a benefit.
Possible Holistic Aromatherapy Treatment	Anti-fungal; *Cedarwood, Immortelle, Lavender, Lemon grass, Myrrh, Patchouli, Tea Tree* Antipruritic (reduces itching); *Chamomile, Lemon, Spearmint, Tea tree*

Disease or Disorder	PSORIASIS
Description	A chronic skin disorder that is characterized by red patches covered with thick, dry, silvery scales of varying sizes. The scaling is from an increase build up of epithelial cells. The cause is thought to be genetic in origin (though the pattern of inheritance is unknown) with the disease becoming apparent in childhood or early adulthood. The buld up is caused by an increased cell turn over and/or a decreased shedding from the top layer of skin (stratum corneum) Areas commonly affected include elbows, knees, trunk and scalp. Although the scaling is very thick in appearance, they are loosely packed and flake off fairly readily. There may be some nail involvement as well.
Possible Allopathic Treatment	Topical lubricating creams (hydrogenated vegetable oils or white petroleum products) are recommended. Corticosteroid creams, salicylic acid, crude coal tar or anthralin are prescribed sometimes on their own, or in combination with each other. Ultra-violet light therapy may be used.
Possible Holistic Aromatherapy Treatment	Antiseptic essential oils; *Basil, Bergamot, Black Pepper, Cajuput, Camphor, Cedarwood, Chamomile, Cinnamon, Clary Sage, Clove, Cypress, Eucalyptus, Fennel, Frankincense, Geranium, Ginger, Hyssop, Jasmine, Juniper, Lavender, Lemon, Lemongrass, Lime, Marjoram, Myrrh, Neroli, Niaouli, Peppermint, Pine, Rose, Rosemary, Sage, Sandalwood, Tea tree, Thyme, Vetiver, Yarrow* Anti-pruritic oils; *Chamomile, Lemon, Spearmint, Tea tree* Cytophylactic; *Carrot seed, Frankincense, Geranium, Immortelle, Lavender, Mandarin, Palmerosa, Neroli, Rose* Cicatrisant; *Bergamot, Cajuput, Chamomile, Clove, Cypress, Eucalyptus, Frankincense, Geranium, Hyssop, Juniper, Lavender, Lemon, Niaouli, Patchouli, Rosemary, Sage, Tea tree*

Disease or Disorder	EAR INFECTIONS
Description	There are many different types of ear infections including: Otitis Externa (swimmer's ear) The cause is trapped water in the canal, irritating the lining. The moist, dark environment is a perfect breeding ground of bacteria. Serous Otitis media An accumulation of fluid in the middle ear space that is not draining properly through the eustachian tube. It is generally caused by colds, allergies, etc. If the fluid remains in the ear fr an extended period of time, the condition will become chronic and the fluid becomes thick. Bacteria can develop and they may experience hearing loss. Otitis Media A term for middle ear infections. They are caused by either bactera or a virus. A common way for bacteria to
Possible Allopathic Treatment	Antibiotics are commonly prescribed. However, 1/3 of all ear infections are caused by a virus and will not be helped with this treatment as antibiotics are useul in the cases of bacterial infections.
Possible Holistic Aromatherapy Treatment	Anti-inflammatory essential oils; *Caraway, Teatree, Camphor, Chamomile, Fennel, Geranium, Jasmine, Peppermint, Benzoin, Frankincense, Myrrh and Patchouli.* Analgesic (Pain-killing) oils; *Bergamot, Cajeput, Coriander, Eucalyptus, Lemon grass, Niaouli, Black-pepper, Chamomile, Jasmine, Lavender, Marjoram, Peppermint, Rosemary and Ginger.* Auto-immune enhancers; *Cinnamon leaf, Clove bud, Frankincense.* Cytophylactic; *Carrot seed, Frankincense, Geranium, Immortelle, Lavender, Mandarin, Palmerosa, Neroli, Rose* Anti-allergenic; *Chamomile, Melissa*

Essential Oils

CAJEPUT OR CAJUPUT

The three main areas where this oil can help are:

1. Respiratory infections (common cold).
2. Head aches.
3. Tooth ache.

Properties	Uses
Analgesic	Toothache, headache
Antidontalgic	Colds, catarrh, sinusitis
Antirheumatic	Reduces inflammation
Antineuralgic	sore throats, headaches, toothache
Antiseptic	Sore throats, mouth infections
Antispasmodic	Reduce muscle tension
Decongestant, Expectorant, Febrifuge	Clear throat, chest and sinuses
Stimulant	To stimulate and tonify
Vermifuge	To expel parasite

Place of Origin
Cajuput essential oil is obtained from the leaves and buds of the tree "melaleuca leucodendron", originally found in Malaya, Australia and the Philippines. Trees of the melaleuca group are a sub-species of the family myrtaceae which includes all eucalyptuses, clove and myrtle.

The predominant property which is shared by all members of this family is the ability to combat or prevent infection. The tree has a whitish bark, which has given the oil its name, derived from the Malaysian "caju-puti" meaning "white tree". The odour is decidedly medicinal, camphorous and very penetrating.

Method of Extraction

Cajuput is extracted by steam distillation, and it is a greenish-yellow colour which distinguishes it from several other oils from closely related varieties of melaleuca. The greenish tinge is due to traces of copper found in this tree. The active principles of this oil include, cineol, terpineol, pinene, and various aldehydes.

Cajuput is best known for its use as an inhalation for the common cold and other respiratory infections. Used in a steam inhalation it will effectively clear the nasal passages while inhibiting the bacteria that proliferate in the mucus formed during colds and flu, and which can lead to catarrh and sinusitis.

It also has pain killing properties which are useful in reducing the discomfort of sore throats and headaches that accompany colds.

Cajuput can irritate the skin, so it needs to be used with caution, well diluted and must never be allowed to come into contact with mucous membranes.

For most situations where cajuput might be used on the skin, such as in a massage oil for the chest and throat infections, and pain-killing friction for arthritis, gout and rheumatism, it would be recommended to use an alternative oil that is non-irritant.

Cajuput can be used to dull a painful tooth. A single drop is put in or on the tooth (not gum) as a first-aid remedy until the sufferer is able to get to see a dentist. The only other oil that has this property is clove.

CAUTION: *Cajuput is a powerful stimulant, and is not recommended to use it just before going to bed, unless it is mixed with a sedative oil to counteract this effect.*

CEDARWOOD

The three main areas where this oil can help are:

1. Skin and hair, inflammation, acne, blemished skin, eczema, dandruff, oily hair.
2. Helps with depression or anxiety.
3. Assists the removal of mucus from the respiratory tract.

Properties   Uses

Antiseptic	Astringent	Acne, Bronchitis
Diuretic	Expectorant	Catarrh, Cancer
sedative	Antidepressant	Cystitis, Dysuria
Insect repellent		Pyelitis, Respiratory
		Skin diseases, Urinary tract

Place of Origin
The oil from Cedarwood *"Cedrus Atlantica"*, which is known as Atlas Cedarwood oil is produced in Morocco. Obtained from the twigs and the wood of the tree, with an harmonious sweet-sour, woody scent.

Unfortunately the Lebanon Cedar *(cedrus libani)* which was the one used by the ancients, no longer grows as abundantly as it once did. There used to be great forests of these enormous trees, but over the centuries they have been considerably reduced by the great demand for Cedarwood furniture. The wood was used in building temples and palaces in the middle east, and vast quantities were used to build Solomon's great temple in Jerusalem. Today only a few hundred trees survive.

"Cedrus Deodorata" is distilled in the Himalayas.
"Juniperus Virginiana" is distilled in Virginia, USA. A close relative of Cedarwood, but is in fact a Juniper.

Method of Extraction
The essential oil is extracted by means of steam distillation. Cedarwood oil was possibly the first essential oil to be extracted from a plant, and was used by the Egyptians in embalming and the mummification process. It was also one of the ingredients of *"mithridat"*, a famous poison antidote that was used for centuries. They also valued it highly as an ingredient for cosmetics, and impregnated papyrus leaves with it to protect them from insects.

Cedarwood oil has a pronounced effect on mucous membranes, and is good in all catarrhal conditions, especially coughs and bronchitis. It may be used with other oils for inhalations for all types of respiratory complaints. Having a sedative effect it could be used in conditions associated with anxiety and nervous tension. Generally it is more useful for chronic complaints than acute ones.

Cedarwood has a pronounced effect on the skin, and is of value in all types of skin eruptions. Its action is sedative, astringent, antiseptic and it relieves itching. This makes it good for acne, oily skin and seborrhoea of the scalp *(oily hair, dandruff)* and has been recommended for traumatic alopecia. It may also be of value in more serious conditions such as eczema, dermatitis, and psoriasis. In high concentrations it will irritate the skin.

It is a very good insect repellent, and is effective against a variety of fauna including mosquitoes, moths, woodworms, leeches and rats.   Since it has been shown to inhibit the mitosis *(cell division)* of tumour cells, it may be of value in cancer therapy.   This action is due to its oily consistency, and is shared by turpentine and various fatty acids.

CONTRAINDICATED: *During pregnancy.*
Toxic doses of cedarwood consist of more than 5-10 drops in any one treatment

NIAOULI

The three main areas where this oil can help are:

1. Cuts and Bruises
2. Respiratory disorders.
3. Cancer skin care treatments.

Properties   Uses

Antiseptic	Analgesic	Cuts and wounds, Infections
Bactericidal	Antirheumatic	Bacterial disease, Burns
Expectorant	Stimulant	Sore throats, Acne
		Respiratory problems

Place of Origin
Niaouli (melaleuca viridiflora) is from a flexible tree with spongy bark that flakes off. It is found growing in Australia, Tasmania and the East Indies. The healthy air in these regions and the absence of malaria is attributed to this tree. It appears that the falling leaves cover the ground and act like a strong disinfectant.

Method of Extraction
The oil is obtained from the leaves and young twigs, of the tree. The essential oil of Niaouli varies in colour, from pale to dark yellow. It has a strong camphorous smell and contains: cineol, eucalyptol, terpineol, pinene, limonene and various esters. Caution, this oil is often adulterated, and so care must be exercised when buying this oil.

Niaouli is very similar to cajeput (melaleuca leucodrendron) so that the two are sometimes confused. However, there are sufficient differences in the composition, odour and constituent properties of the two oils to make such confusion inexcusable, and no good supplier will substitute one for the other. You may occasionally find this oil sold under its old name of "gomenol" which originated from the fact that it used to be distilled near, and shipped from, the port of Gomen in the French East Indies, hence "gomen-oil". Now most supplies come from Australia.

The reason why it is so important to distinguish clearly between this oil and its cousin, is that unlike cajeput, which is a skin irritant, niaouli is well tolerated by the skin and mucous membranes when used in suitable dilutions. It can, therefore be safely used for massage, as a gargle and even as a vaginal douche. It has been used in hospitals in France as an antiseptic in obstetrics and gynaecology.

It is suited for cleaning minor wounds and burns, cuts and grazes, especially if any dirt has got into them. (Mix 5-6 drops of niaouli in ½ pint of boiled and cooled water and wash out the wound repeatedly.)

For burns, the oil can be sprinkled neat on a sterile gauze and fastened over the burn. It is a powerful tissue-stimulant and will therefore help healing.

Because it is non-irritant and powerfully antiseptic, this is a good oil for the treatment of acne and similar skin conditions such as boils.

Niaouli is good for all respiratory tract infections, whether they affect the nose, throat or chest, and is used in chest rubs as well as inhalations. It is quite a powerful stimulant, so it is better not to use it late in the evening, unless mixed with a more sedative oil.

A little-known but very valuable use of niaouli is in conjunction with radiation therapy for cancer. A thin layer of niaouli applied to the skin before each session of cobalt therapy gives some protection against burning of the skin and has been shown to reduce the severity of such burns. In line with this, it is also very beneficial for sun burns especially when combined with other oils such as lavender.

NEROLI (ORANGE BLOSSOM)

The three main areas where this oil can help are:

1. Sedative-antidepressant.
2. Skin care problems.
3. Diminishes cardiac contraction.

Properties   Uses

Antidepressant Aphrodisiac		Depression, Diarrhoea
Antiseptic	Antispasmodic	Hysteria, Insomnia
Cordial	Deodorant	Nervous tension, Shock
Digestive	Sedative	Palpitations, Skin care
Tonic		

Place of Origin

Neroli *(citrus aurantium)*, the origin of the name Neroli is uncertain, it is thought to come from the name of the Emperor Nero, but the most popular belief is that it associated with a certain Anne-Marie, Princess of Nerola, who first used it to perfume her gloves and bath water.   She was the wife of a famous Italian prince who lived in the 16th century.   Her glove perfume became very popular, and gloves scented with it were known as *"guanti neroli"*.

The orange tree is native of china. It is now cultivated in France, Italy, Tunisia, and the USA.

Method of Extraction

There are two types of orange tree;

1. The sweet orange *(citrus sinenis)* and
2. The bitter orange *(citrus aurantium)*.

The two types of Orange tree strongly resemble each other, except that the leaf stalk of the Bitter Orange, bears a small *"second leaf"* which when flattened out, forms a perfectly shaped heart.

Essential oil of Neroli is usually produced by the "Enfleurage method", though sometimes it is also extracted by steam distillation from the white blossoms of the bitter orange. Oil from the Sweet Orange flowers yield oil of an inferior quality.

It has a pale yellow colour with a bitter taste.

The principal known constituents are: linalol, geraniol, nerol, benzoic, anthranylic and phenylacetic esters, traces of indole and jasmone, enzoic esters.

One of the most important uses is for helping with problems of emotional origin, it is especially valuable for states of anxiety or shock and hysteria.

Neroli is particularly valuable in skin care for it has the special property of stimulating the growth of healthy new cells, and has therefore certain rejuvenating effects. It can be used for all skin types, but is perhaps most useful for dry or sensitive skins.

One of the physical actions of neroli is to relieve spasm in the smooth muscle, especially that of the intestines. This action makes it really helpful for chronic diarrhoea, especially where this arises from nervous tension.

The reputed aphrodisiac quality of neroli stems not from a directly hormonal or stimulant effect, as with some oils, but rather from its ability to calm any nervous apprehension that may be felt before a sexual encounter, and as many sexual difficulties arise from a state of tension and anxiety, and in turn give rise to further anxiety and depression, neroli can be one of the means of overcoming them.

MYRRH

The three main areas where this oil can help are:

1. Cuts and wounds.
2. Eczema type skin disorders.
3. Mouth infections.

Properties	Uses
Antiseptic	Amenorrhoea, Pyorrhoea
Antiphlogistic	Aphthae, Stomatitis
Astringent	Catarrh, Tuberculosis
Carminative	Chlorosis, Ulcers-skin & mouth
Emmenagogue	Cough, Wounds
Expectorant	Diarrhoea
Sedative	Dyspepsia
Stimulant(especially pulmonary)	Flatulence
Stomachic	Gingivitis
Tonic	Haemorrhoids
Uterine	Leucorrhoea
Vulnerary	Loss of appetite

Place of Origin
Myrrh is a resin produced by a small tough spiny tree which grows in semi-arid regions of Libya, Iran, along the Red Sea, and various Places in North East Africa. it is also found in The *"Garden of Eden"* which was part of Babylonia in the time of Moses. The tree or shrub, grows only to a height of nine feet, with small white flowers and trifoliate leaves which are also aromatic.

Method of Extraction
The liquid resin is exuded from natural cracks or cuts in the trunk of the tree, and sets into irregularly shaped brownish-red lumps. As with Frankincense, modern harvesting consists of making systematic cuts in wild trees, and to an extent, cultivated trees.

The essential oil is extracted from the resin by steam distillation, and is a deep reddish-brown and may need warming before it is possible to pour it from the bottle. It has a smoky aromatic smell.

The active principles include: pinene, dipentene, limonene, cadinene, formic acid, acetic acid, myrrholic acid, eugenol, several aldehydes and alcohols, and a number of resins.

In common with Frankincense, Myrrh was used in all the ancient civilisations as a perfume, incense and in medicine. It was highly valued as a healing ointment for wounds and it is said that no soldier of Ancient Greece went into battle without a paste of Myrrh in his pouch. This use is well justified by what we know of Myrrh's antiseptic, healing and anti-inflammatory properties. Myrrh is especially valuable for wounds that are slow to heal or for weepy skin conditions.

Eczema and athlete's foot respond to Myrrh, the fungicidal constituent sees to that. It will also heal cracked and chapped skin.

Myrrh is very good for gums, and quickly heals mouth ulcers and most gum disorders. The most convenient method is to use myrrh in the mouth as a tincture. It will sting and taste bitter *(awful),* but the healing effects are well worth the initial discomfort or inconvenience. It is used in many brands of tooth paste with essential oil of peppermint to mask its bitterness and to make it palatable.

Chest infections like, catarrh, chronic bronchitis, colds and sore throats, respond well to inhalations of myrrh. It is a good pulmonary antiseptic, expectorant and astringent. Best used in a massage oil or inhalations as it is very difficult to dissolve, even in alcohol.

Some care should be considered when using myrrh, as it is emmenagogic and should not be used during pregnancy.

Myrrh has a tonic and stimulating action on the stomach and in fact the whole digestive tract, and is a remedy for diarrhoea.

Because of the antifungal action of myrrh, it can be used in a vaginal douche against thrush. It will eliminate the itch and discharge effectively, but thought should also be given to the underlying candida infection which leads to these symptoms, and ti-tree oil, with perhaps a special diet used.

PATCHOULI

The three main areas where this oil can help are:

1. An aphrodisiac.
2. Promotes scar tissue and helps with skin care problems.
3. Uplifter for depression.

Properties   Uses

Antidepressant Antiphlogistic		Anxiety, Depression
Antiseptic	Aphrodisiac	Skin care, Wounds
Astringent	Cicatrisant	
Deodorant	Sedative	

Place of Origin
Patchouli *(pogostemon patchouli)*, comes from India, where it is known as *"puchaput"*. The plant of the labiate family, but the oil is unlike other labiate oils. The leaves of Patchouli are ovate, about four inches long and five inches broad. The stems grow up to three feet in height, and the flowers are whitish, tinged with purple. Patchouli first became known in Europe about 1820 when it was used to impregnate Indian shawls. In the east the oil is also used to scent linen.

Method of Extraction
Patchouli oil is steam distilled from the leaves of the plant and is a deep reddish-brown colour and somewhat thick in consistency. The active principles include: patchouline, patchoulol *(or patchouli camphor)*, norpatchoulol and traces of eugenol, cadinene, carvone, caryophylene, seychellene, humulene, benzoic and cinnamic aldehydes. Of these, it is interesting to note that patchoulene is very similar in structure to azulene *(found in camomile)* and has the same anti-inflammatory properties.

Patchouli oil has the unusual property of improving in odour with age. Not a great deal is known about the therapeutic properties of Patchouli oil. It has a fairly general but mild bactericidal action. It is a notable aphrodisiac, providing of course both partners found the odour pleasing. This is particularly relevant with regards to Patchouli, as the odour is very strong and distinctive.

It also promotes the formation of scar tissue and helps with skin care problems, such as inflamed or cracked skin, acne, skin allergies and certain types of eczema. It is reputedly said to be beneficial for aging skin and wrinkles, making it particularly suitable for mature skin types.

Patchouli has a pronounced effect on the nervous system, and is indeed a strong nerve stimulant. Taken to excess it will keep you awake at night. However, used correctly, it can have a definite uplifting effect on someone who is suffering from depression, anxiety or tension. It is also said to bring together the thoughts and assist in clarifying problems, allowing the person to see things more objectively.

Additionally, Patchouli is said to help in decreasing the appetite, and reduces fluid retention.

Question and Answer Sheets

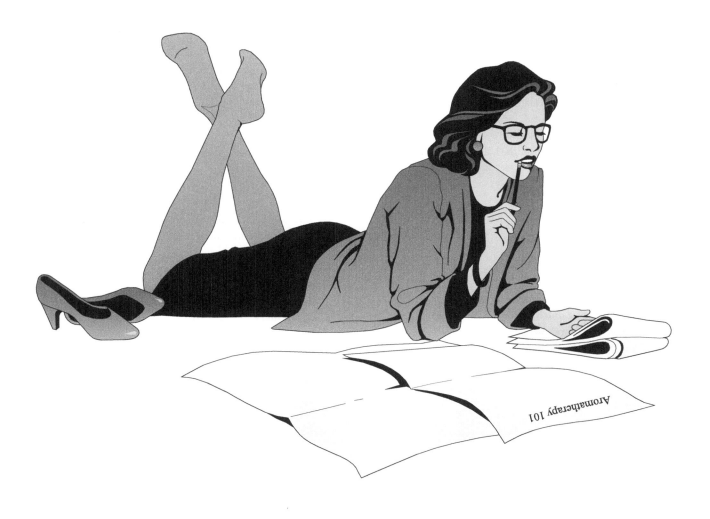

Please keep the questions for review.
Circle the correct answer/s on the Answer Sheets at the back of the book and
<u>return these sheets only</u> to your instructor.

Questions - Lesson #10

1. Three primary functions of the skin are:
a. protection
b. Skin covering
c. temperature regulation
d. sun screen
e. a sensory covering of the entire body

2. Skin has two principal divisions:
a. epidermis
b. subcutaneous
c. dermis
d. dead cells

3. The erector pili muscles:
a. contract in response to cold and fear
b. contract in response to exercise
c. help hair follicles maintain the hair root in good condition

4. The sebaceous glands secrete:
a. sweat
b. sebum
c. salts and urea
d. pheromone

5. The sensory nerve endings:
a. cause the hair follicles to become erect
b. give sensations of touch, pain and temperature
c. give sensations of well being
d. send signals to the brain to move muscles

6. Adipose tissue is made up of:
a. nerve endings and no blood vessels
b. connective tissue with supporting blood vessels
c. fat
d. cellulite

7. Apocrine sweat glands differ from the eccrine sweat glands in that they:
a. are located all over the body
b. are located in the axillary and genital areas of the body
c. act as heat regulators
d. are present from birth
e. develop with puberty

8. Label the diagram of the skin.
(SEE ANSWER SHEET FOR DIAGRAM)

9. The layers of the eyeball are:
a. the duroid
b. the choroid
c. the sclera
d. the lens
e. the retina

10. The sclera is:
a. clear, transparent and tough
b. fibrous, opaque and tough
c. the middle coat
d. the white outer coat

11. The following gland moistens and cleans the surface of the eyeball:
a. the apocrine gland
b. the thymus gland
c. the lachrymal gland
d. optic gland

12. The contraction of the pupil is controlled by:
a. the autonomic nervous system
b. the cerebrum
c. the amount of light in the area
d. blinking

13. The ciliary muscles are in:
a. the face and control eye movement
b. the ciliary body and control eye movement
c. the ciliary body and control the shape of the lens
d. eye lid

14. The vitreous humour differs from the aqueous humour in that:
a. it circulates through the posterior and anterior chambers of the eye to bathe the inner surface
b. fills the posterior two-thirds of the eyeball
c. it covers the outer surface of the eye not the inner
d. this is a trick question

15. The retina contains light sensitive cells. They are:
a. cones for red, green and blue
b. rods for shades of grey to white
c. cones for shades of grey to white
d. rods for red, green and blue

16. Label the diagram of the eyeball.
(SEE ANSWER SHEET FOR DIAGRAM)

17. The three structures that make up the ear are:
a. the external ear
b. the membraneous labyrinth
c. the middle ear
d. the osseous labyrinth
e. the inner ear

18.   The gland which secretes wax is called:
a. the tympanum gland
b. the ceruminous gland
c. the lachrymal gland
d. eustachian gland

19.   The purpose of the eustachian tube is:
a. allow passage of air from the nasal pharynx to the middle ear equalising air pressure
b. to act as a connection from the ear to the brain via the auditory nerves
c. allow passage of air from the external ear to the inner ear equalising air pressure
d. to allow mucus to enter and lubricate the inner ear

20. Three parts of the internal ear are:
a. the osseous labyrinth
b. the mastoid antum
c. the membraneous labyrinth
d. the tympanic membrane
e. the peril lymph

21. The osseous labyrinth contains the following which control balance:
a. the hammer, anvil and stirrup
b. the ear drum or tympanic membrane
c. three semicircular canals
d. Auditory meatus

22.   Label the diagram of the ear.
(SEE ANSWER SHEET FOR DIAGRAM)

23. The four kinds of papillae found on the tongue are:
a. sweet, sour, bitter, and salty
b. filiform, folioform, vallate and fungiform
c. parotid, sublingual, mandibular and ptyalin
d. large, small, long and short

24. Palatability is assessed by what part of the brain?
a. the parietal lobe of the brain in conjunction with the thalamic taste centre
b. the parietal lobe of the brain in conjunction with the limbic taste centre
c. the frontal lobe of the brain in conjunction with the thalamic taste centre

25. Smell is perceived through:
a. odiferous molecules striking the cranial nerve and entering the limbic system
b. odiferous molecules striking the olfactory nerve and passing into the olfactory bulb before entering the limbic system
c. odiferous molecules striking the olfactory nerves passing through the pons varolii on its way to the limbic area of the brain

26. Acne is caused by:
a. over-secretion of sexual hormones
b. chocolate
c. over-secretion of sebaceous glands

27 Alopecia is:
a. patchy baldness
b. an highly contagious skin condition
c. a skin condition characterised by dry scaliness
d. a skin condition similar

28. A cataract is:
a. an inflammation of the conjunctiva
b. the lens of the eye becomes opaque and shuts out vision
c. inflammation of the eye ball
d. Nasal congestion

29. Pink eye is also known as:
a. conjunctivitis
b. Tineacapitis
c. hirsutism
d. Downs syndrome

30. Psoriasis is characterised by:
a. dry, peeling patches
b. elevated reddish, scaly patches
c. weeping, itchy patches
d. discolouration of the skin

31. Verrucas are caused by:
a. viruses
b. bacteria
c. incorrect cleansing
d. infestation

32. What is a blister?
a. a point of pressure between the epidermis and dermis
b. an elevated area under the skin
c. a collection of fluid between the epidermis and dermis
d. another name for a boil

33 What is athletes foot?

a. an highly infectious bacterial infection

b. an highly contagious viral infection

c. an highly contagious fungal infection

34. Vertigo is caused by:

a. imbalance of hormones

b. sensation of loss of balance

c. a disease of the eyes

35. Colour blindness is as a result of:

a. improper care of the eye during bright light

b. eye infection common to males

c. an inherited condition passed down via female carriers

36. The mammary gland in the breast is called:

a. alveolar tissue

b. connective or fatty tissue

c. lactiferous tissue

d. chest

37. The lactiferous sinuses expand:

a. in response to pregnancy

b. as a woman's weight increases

c. to create a reservoir for milk

d. during sex

38. Which gland affects the development of the breasts?

a. the thyroid

b. the pituitary

c. the axillary

d. mammary glands

39. Prolactin starts what?

a. breast development

b. lactation at the end of pregnancy

c. onset of menstruation at the end of pregnancy

d. childbirth

40. Prolactin is secreted by what gland?

a. the thyroid

b. the pituitary

c. the axillary

d. the adrenal

41. Can essential oils be used during pregnancy?

a. Yes, during the entire pregnancy

b. Yes, but you must avoid certain oils

c. No, they will cause miscarriage

d. No, all essential oils are dangerous

42. Aromatherapy can help what conditions in pregnancy?

a. nausea

b. low back pain

c. miscarriage

d. stretch marks

e. bleeding

43. Which three categories of oils must be avoided during pregnancy?

a. those described as emmenagogue

b. those recommended to strengthen labour

c. those described as stimulants

d. those considered toxic

e. those considered anti-inflammatory

44. Which oils should be avoided during the initial stages of pregnancy?

a. aniseed	b. arnica
c. angelica	d. basil
e. black pepper	f. clary sage
g. chamomile	h. cypress
i. fennel	j. geranium
k. hyssop	l. jasmine
m. juniper	n. marjoram
o. myrrh	p. neroli
q. origanum	r. pennyroyal
s. peppermint	t. rose
u. rosemary	v. mugwort (Armoise)
w. sage	x. thyme
y. wintergreen	z. ylang ylang

45. When recording client information, why is it important to state the client's occupation?

a. this states what takes up the client's time

b. this assists in assessing possible environmental problems

c. this assists in assessing other occupations

46. Why is taking medical history from a client valuable?

a. this will give you an overall picture of client health

b. this will give an indication of a hypochondriac

c. this is necessary to have

47. What information can be obtained from recording any medication your client is taking?

a. you need to check possible side effects before treating

b. you need this to have an overall clear picture of health

c. you need to determine spending habits on health needs

48. With regards to body analysis - why is posture important?
a. this is to ascertain discomfort in relation to posture
b. this is to determine where stress is held
c. this is to analyze body language

49. Test lines are done how and where?
a. these are on a sheet of paper after initial questions
b. these are done on the clients back, using thumbs to draw a line down either side of the spine
c. these are done on the clients back, using a pen to draw lightly a line down either side of the spine

50. What is revealed by these test lines?
a. these determine potential eye problems
b. these determine whether the spine is straight
c. these determine whether there are congested areas on the back

51. When examining a client's legs, what as a therapist, are you looking for?
a. bruises, thread-veins, mobility in knee & ankle joints
b. bruises, tan lines, muscle tone
c. bruises, hairiness, muscle tone, lymph glands

52. How would you know if a client had deep circulation or poor circulation?
a. the hands and feet would be cold with poor circulation
b. the hands and feet would be cold with deep circulation
c. hand and feet would be cool but nails pink with deep circulation
d. nails would be bluish with poor circulation

53. What are the two main things to look for when examining the eyes?
a. stress and anemia
b. the depth of colour around the eyes
c. tiredness and bags under the eyes

54. What would a marked roughness on the outer, upper arm indicate?
a. poor state of cleanliness
b. poor circulation
c. respiratory problems

55. If your client wakes up tired after sleeping, what will this tell you?
a. their sleep pattern is interrupted and not restful
b. they should take something to help them sleep
c. stress level is too high

56. List the seven ductless glands which secrete hormones into the blood stream.
a. the axillary
b. the pituitary
c. the thyroid
d. the parathyroid
e. the gonadotropic
f. the thymus
g. the eccrine
h. the supra-renal or adrenals
i. part of the pancreas
j. parts of the ovaries and testes

57. Which gland is described as "the leader of the endocrine orchestra"?
a. the thyroid
b. the pituitary
c. the thymus

58. How many lobes does the pituitary gland have?
a. two
b. three
c. four

59. What is the name of the growth promoting hormone which controls the bones & muscles?
a. adrenocorticotropic
b. somatropic
c. thyrotropic
d. metabolic

60. If this hormone is over secreted in childhood, what condition occurs?
a. dwarfism
b. cretinism
c. gigantism

61. If this hormone is under secreted in childhood, what condition occurs?
a. dwarfism
b. cretinism
c. gigantism

62. Which lobe within the pituitary gland produces gonadotropic hormone?
a. the posterior lobe
b. the anterior lobe
c. the middle lobe

63. Which hormone regulates the thyroid?
a. adrenocorticotropic
b. somatropic
c. thyrotropic
d. gonadotropic

64. What two things does adrenocorticotropic hormone regulate?
a. the adrenal cortex and the metabolic hormones
b. the adrenal cortex and the kidneys
c. the metabolic hormones and the circulatory system

65. The posterior lobe of the pituitary gland produces two hormones, name them.
a. thyroxin and oxytocin
b. oxytocin and insulin
c. oxytocin and vasopressin

66. What is the function of the hormone oxytocin?
a. causes contraction of the diaphragm
b. causes contraction of the uterine muscle and mammary glands
c. causes contraction of the blood vessels in the heart and lungs

67. What are the functions of the hormone vasopressin?
a. increases the amount of fluid the kidneys absorb
b. contracts the diaphragm in the breathingprocess
c. contracts the blood vessels in the heart and lungs increasing the blood pressure
d. contracts the uterine muscles and mammary glands

68. Where in the body is the thyroid gland situated?
a. in the frontal lobe of the brain
b. on either side of the trachea
c. on top of both kidneys

69. What two hormones does the thyroid gland secrete?
a. thyroxine and tri-iodothyronine
b. thyroxine and cortico-steroids
c. cortico-steroids and tri-iodothyronine

70. What is the function of the hormone thyroxine?
a. it controls the sodium/potassium balance
b. it controls the general metabolism
c. it controls the fluid level in the cells

71. If this hormone is under secreted in childhood, what condition occurs?
a. dwarfism
b. cretinism
c. gigantism

72. If thyroxine is under secreted in adulthood, what condition occurs?
a. high metabolic rate
b. diabetes
c. low metabolic rate

73. How many parathyroid glands are there, and where are they positioned in the body?
a. four, two on each side of the thyroid
b. two, one on each side of the kidney
c. two, one on each side of the pituitary

74. Name the hormone that the parathyroid gland secretes.
a. tri-iodothyrnonine
b. parathormone
c. paratetany

75. Under secretion of this hormone causes something called tetany, what is that?
a. muscles go into spasm
b. calcium to be lost to the blood from the bones
c. softened bones and depression

76. Where in the body is the thymus gland positioned?
a. in the lower abdomen
b. in the frontal lobe of the brain
c. in the lower part of the neck

77. What is the function of the thymus gland?
a. to control the metabolic rate
b. control the development of the sex organs
c. to control growth

78. How many adrenal glands are there, and where are they positioned in the body?
a. there are two, one on top of each kidney
b. there are four, two on each side of the thyroid
c. there are two, one on each side of the pituitary

79. The adrenal glands are divided into two parts, they are?
a. the cortex and the medulla oblongata
b. the medulla and the cerebrum
c. the cortex and the medulla

80. What is the name of the hormones produced by the cortex part of the adrenal gland?
a. cortico-steroids
b. adrenalin
c. noradrenaline

81. What is the function of cortico-steroids?
a. control sodium/potassium balance and stimulate the storage of glucose
b. control the blood pressure by constricting the smaller blood vessels
c. controls the output of sugar from the liver

82. What part of the adrenal gland produces adrenalin?
a. the medulla oblongata
b. the cortex
c. the medulla

83. Describe the two functions of the hormone adrenalin.
a. control sodium/potassium balance and stimulate the storage of glucose
b. controls the output of sugar from the liver
c. controls the blood pressure by constricting smaller blood vessels
d. supplements the production of sex hormones

84. How is the amount of adrenaline secreted, affected?
a. in response to excitement, fear or anger
b. in response to exercise
c. in response to a large meal

85. The female gonads and hormones are called?
a. ovaries with oestrogen and progesterone
b. ovaries with oestrogen and testosterone
c. testes with testosterone and oestrogen

86. The male gonads and hormones are called?
a. ovaries with oestrogen and testosterone
b. testes with testosterone
c. testes with testosterone and progesterone

87. Where are the "Islets of Langerhans" found?
a. the pituitary gland
b. the thyroid gland
c. the adrenal gland
d. the pancreas

88. What hormone is produced by the "Islets of Langerhans?"
a. insulin
b. thyroxine
c. vasopressin

89. What is the function of this hormone?
a. controls blood pressure
b. controls the blood sugar level
c. controls growth

90. If too little of this hormone is produced, what disease occurs?
a. high blood pressure
b. diabetes mellitus
c. cretinism

91. What is addison's syndrome?
a. adrenal-cortical insufficiency characterised by hypotension, wasting, vomiting and muscular weakness
b. adrenal-cortical insufficiency characterised by hypertension, bloating and dizziness
c. adrenal-cortical excess characterised by moon face hypertension and muscular weakness

92. What is meant by the term Amenorrhoea?
a. absence of menstruation
b. absence of appetite
c. absence of muscle tone

93. What is Cushing's syndrome?
a. adrenal-cortical insufficiency characterised by hypotension, wasting, vomiting and muscular weakness
b. adrenal-cortical excess characterised byhypertension, bloating and dizziness
c. adrenal-cortical excess characterised by moon face, hypertension and muscular weakness

94. What is hyperthyroidism?
a. increased metabolic rate
b. decreased metabolic rate
c. alteration of function of thyroid

95. What is meant by the term menopause?
a. cessation of menses at the end of reproduction cycle
b. absence of menses
c. absence of male influence and hormones

96. What is a steroid?
a. a generic name given to various compounds of internal secretions
b. a hormone used to increase muscle size
c. a hormone used to counter inflammation of muscles and joints

Answer Sheet - Lesson #10

(Keep the questions for review. Circle the correct answer/s and return these sheets only to your instructor.)

1.   A.   B.   C.   D.   E.

2.   A.   B.   C.   D.

3.   A.   B.   C.

4.   A.   B.   C.   D.

5.   A.   B.   C.   D.

6.   A.   B.   C.   D.   E.

7.   A.   B.   C.   D.   E.

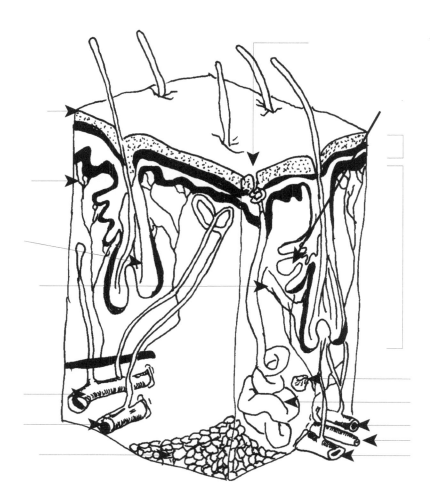

8.   Label the following diagram of the skin:

---

9.   A.   B.   C.   D.   E.

10. A.   B.   C.   D.

11. A.   B.   C.   D.   E.

12. A.   B.   C.   D.   E.

13. A.   B.   C.   D.   E.

14. A.   B.   C.   D.   E.

15. A.   B.   C.   D.

16. Label the following diagram of the eyeball:

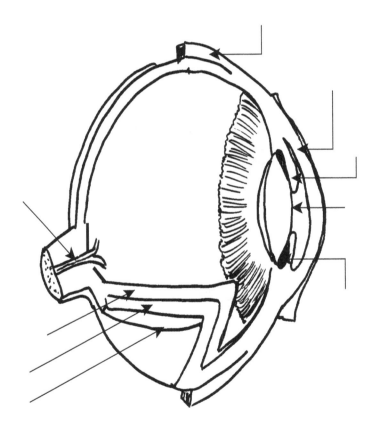

17. A.   B.   C.   D.   E.

18. A.   B.   C.   D.   E.

19. A.   B.   C.   D.   E.

20. A.   B.   C.   D.   E.

21. A.   B.   C.   D.   E.

22.   Label the following diagram of the ear:

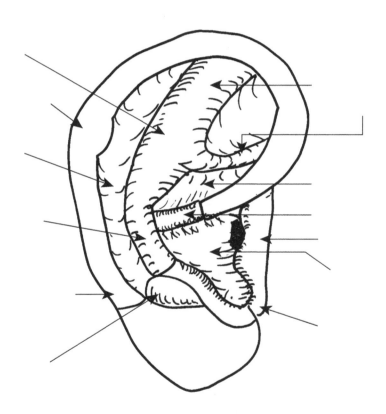

23. A.   B.   C.   D.

24. A.   B.   C.

25. A.   B.   C.

26. A.   B.   C.

27 A.   B.   C.   D.   E.

28. A.   B.   C.   D.   E.

29. A.   B.   C.   D.   E.

30. A.   B.   C.   D.   E.

31. A.   B.   C.   D.   E.

32. A.   B.   C.   D.   E.

33 A.   B.   C.

34. A.   B.   C.

35. A.   B.   C.

36. A.   B.   C.   D.

37. A.   B.   C.   D.   E.

38. A.   B.   C.   D.   E.

39. A.   B.   C.   D.   E.

40. A.   B.   C.   D.   E.

41. A.   B.   C.   D.   E.

42. A.   B.   C.   D.   E.

43. A.   B.   C.   D.   E.

44. A.   B.   C.   D.   E.   F.   G.   H.   I.   J.   K.   L.

     M.   N.   O.   P.   Q.   R.   S.   T.   U.   V.   W.   X.

     Y.   Z.

45. A.   B.   C.

46. A.   B.   C.

47. A.   B.   C.

48. A.   B.   C.

49. A.   B.   C.

50. A.   B.   C.

51. A.   B.   C.

52. A.   B.   C.   D.

53. A.   B.   C.

54. A.   B.   C.

55. A.   B.   C.

56. A.   B.   C.   D.   E.   F.   G.   H.   I.   J.

57. A.   B.   C.

58. A.   B.   C.

59. A.   B.   C.   D.

60. A.   B.   C.

61. A.   B.   C.

62. A.   B.   C.

63. A.   B.   C.   D.

64. A.   B.   C.

65. A.   B.   C.

66. A.   B.   C.

67. A.   B.   C.   D.

68. A.   B.   C.

69. A.   B.   C.

70. A.   B.   C.

71. A.   B.   C.

72. A.   B.   C.

73. A.   B.   C.

74. A.   B.   C.

75. A.   B.   C.

76. A.   B.   C.

77. A.   B.   C.

78. A.   B.   C.

79. A.   B.   C.

80. A.   B.   C.

81. A.   B.   C.

82. A.   B.   C.

83. A.   B.   C.   D.

84. A.   B.   C.

85. A.   B.   C.

86. A.   B.   C.

87. A.   B.   C.   D.

88. A.   B.   C.

89. A.   B.   C.

90. A.   B.   C.

91. A.   B.   C.

92. A.   B.   C.

93. A.   B.   C.

94. A.   B.   C.

95. A.   B.   C.

96. A.   B.   C.

Index

Lightning Source UK Ltd.
Milton Keynes UK
UKOW07f2335091015

260237UK00002B/3/P

9 780982 031803